Gabriele Zerbi, *Gerontocomia:* On the Care of the Aged

and

Maximianus, Elegies on Old Age and Love

Fig. 10

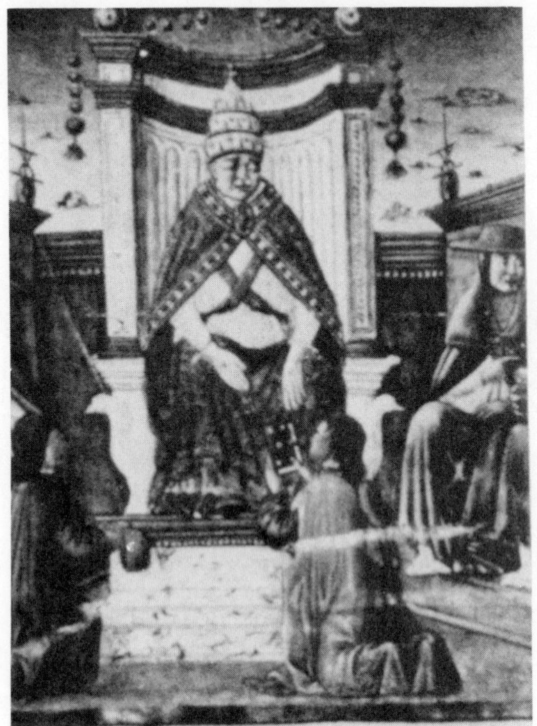

Gabriele Zerbi (? 1455–1505): This Italian physician had an important career in philosophy, medicine, and medical history that began precociously at the age of 21 and ended with his assassination before he reached the age of 40. His work on aging, *Gerontocomica Scilicet de Senium Atque Victu* contained: "a very clear picture of the medical features of old age." The book was dedicated to Sixtus IV. The kneeling figure on the right is said to be that of the author.

Gabriele Zerbi, *Gerontocomia:* On the Care of the Aged

and

Maximianus, Elegies on Old Age and Love

Translated from the Latin

by

L. R. Lind

American Philosophical Society
Independence Square Philadelphia
1988

Memoirs
of the
American Philosophical Society
Held at Philadelphia
For Promoting Useful Knowledge
Volume 182

Cover illustrations from *Hortus sanitatis* (1517) and *Historia Mundi Naturalis* (1582) in the Library of the American Philosophical Society

Library of Congress Catalog Card No: 87-72873
International Standard Book No.: 0-87169-182-5
US ISSN: 0065-9738

For Elena, Through All the Years

Contents

Part One

Zerbi's Gerontocomia: *On the Care of the Aged*

1.

Introduction to Zerbi and His Works

GERONTOLOGY

When the history of gerontology is written it will look back to the Renaissance and the late Middle Ages for its chief source and inspiration as well as its starting point. The article on aging in the latest edition of the *Encyclopedia Britannica* is based upon the following admirable definition but it is one without a precise historical perspective: "Gerontology, the study of the aging process, developed from man's awareness of the inevitability of decline and death, an awareness that has long been a major influence in religious and philosophic systems and continues to shape man's intuitive conceptions about the nature and origin of aging. See the articles Life-Span and Death for related information." The article begins with the statement: "Gerontology is devoted to the understanding and control of all factors contributing to the finitude of individual life."

The study of gerontology and its related science, geriatrics, which treats the physiological and pathological aspects of the aging process primarily from the medical point of view, is, strictly speaking, a recent one especially in the growth of wide popular interest beyond its base in scientific scholarship. The *Rivista di Gerontologia e Geriatria* was founded at Rome in 1951. American journals in the field were founded somewhat later, except for the *Journal of Gerontology,* 1946. Geriatrics as a branch of medicine in its own right seems to have been created by I. L. Nascher in his book, *Geriatrics: the Diseases of Old Age and Their Treatment,* etc., in 1914. It contains an introduction by Abraham Jacobi, who in 1860 had begun to practice pediatrics as a separate branch of medicine. Much work had been done, of course, in the fields of gerontology and geriatrics by nineteenth-century writers (e.g., Seidel, *Diseases of Old Age,*

1890) and others, including those who had written Latin dissertations in the seventeenth and eighteenth centuries (see the bibliography in Thewlis's *Geriatrics,* 1919, 237–42).

In the introduction to my verse translation of the *Elegies* of Maximianus (sixth cent. A. D.) in the latter part of this book I have referred briefly to the treatment of aging among the classical writers of antiquity from Homer to Aristotle among the Greeks and from Horace to Juvenal among the Romans. Bessie Ellen Richardson has written an exhaustive account in her work, *Old Age Among the Ancient Greeks;* I know of no similar book for the Romans. The Middle Ages with its generally melancholy view of life here and hereafter made something of a topos of old age in its literature and thought, not adequately treated by E. R. Curtius in his *European Literature and the Latin Middle Ages,* which deals with topoi of all kinds. The topos, or common place, reached its greatest height in the personal, almost clinical, analysis of both old age and love in the *Elegies* of Maximianus, unknown to or at least neglected by all writers on old age since his time except by Zerbi and Max Neuburger. Zerbi quotes him liberally and recognized his unique value as a witness to the decline of strength and its ravages in old age.

It was in the early Renaissance that the subject of human longevity and ways to achieve it became of general interest. Various regimina and consilia dealing with health and its preservation were written especially in the period between A. D. 1300 and 1350 by medical men for those who were going on the Crusades. Among these was the *Liber conservacionis sanitatis senis* by Guido da Vigevano (really of Pavia) in 1335, intended for use by older men going to the Holy Land on pilgrimage. It forms part of a manuscript (11015 fonds latin in the Bibliothèque nationale, Paris, still unedited; see Sarton, *Introduction to the History of Science* 3. 1, 1947, pp. 285, 846). Even earlier Roger Bacon had written his *Libellus de retardandis senectutis accidentibus,* composed probably before 1236 but listed by Sarton among his dated writings in 1243 and printed as late as 1590 by J. Barnes at Oxford. Of this book Sarton writes (op. cit., 2. 2, 1931, p. 959; see also p. 894): ". . . the longest and best known of these writings [on medicine] . . . was also the poorest. It was relatively early (it was probably his first publication) when his mind was still undeveloped. In spite of its mediocrity it was plagiarized c. 1309–1311 by Arnold of Villanova under the title *De conservanda juventute et retardanda senectute* and Villanova's edition was translated into Italian and into English [by Jonas Drummond in 1544]. Bacon's own work was Englished by Richard Browne (London, 1683).''

Bacon's *Libellus* consists of thirty-one pages divided into sixteen chapters with about two pages to each. In summary fashion he covers the causes of old age, its remedies, chief phenomena, wrinkles and other signs, debility of the senses, the food and drink appropriate for the aged, the preservation of individual natural humidity, the means for retarding old age and preserving its strength, the care of the skin, and finally some medicines and a regimen for reviving the imagination, reason, and memory.

In order to complete this review of early works on aging it is necessary to speak at least briefly about two other books from a time later than Zerbi's *Gerontocomia* (1489). Francis Bacon wrote as the third part of his *Instauratio Magna* a long work, *Historia Vitae et Mortis* in 454 pages, published in 1623. Quoting very few authors he covers somewhat the same ground as Roger Bacon and Zerbi, recognizing as Zerbi does the two-fold objectives: (1) to halt as much as possible the inroads of old age, and (2) to comfort and maintain the current condition of tolerable health. He discusses the value of bathing, exercise, food and drink, care of the emotions, medicines, and especially of diet, where (at p. 242) he refers to Luigi Cornaro's self-discipline in this respect, who observed his regimen so carefully for so many years that he lived to be one hundred, sound in strength of body and senses. An English translation of Bacon's work appeared in 1638: *The Historie of Life and Death. With Observations Natural and Experimental.*

Bacon's reference to Cornaro brings us to the last of the books worth mentioning here as forming the historical setting in which Zerbi's book may be placed. Luigi Cornaro (Alvise Cornèr: 1467; actually 1475–1566) of Padua falsified the date of his birth in order to claim an age of one hundred years. He was more interested in architecture and hydrostatics than in gerontology but he is known today for his treatise *Della vita sobria,* a charming how-to book on living a long life. His friend Ruzzante in one of his dialogues portrayed Cornaro as something of a charlatan. Yet his book is an extremely readable and convincing discussion of longevity from an intensely personal point of view. In the anonymous translation which eventually became a Haldeman-Julius Little Blue Book (No. 93), the title ran thus: "How to Live One Hundred Years, wherein is demonstrated by the author's own example the method of preserving health to extreme old age." The first edition came out in Padua in quarto in 1558 and at Venice in 1612, followed by translations in London, 1779, Philadelphia, 1810, with a new version in Milwaukee, 1905, with essays by Joseph Addison, Lord Bacon, and Sir William Temple.

Cornaro was a wise and genial soul who described his reform from a life of gluttony and intemperance. At doctor's orders he reduced his intake of food and drink and then adopted a regimen which effectively combatted his fevers, aches, and pains as follows: "I have carefully avoided heat, cold, and extraordinary fatigue, interruption of my usual hours of rest, excessive venery, making any stay in bad air, and exposing myself to wind and sun; for these, too, are great disorders." He attributes ill health to a mismanagement of the humors; his own were well united, harmonized, and disposed. His principal recipe for good health is a moderate intake of food and drink and regular, sane habits of life: "O holy and truly happy regularity!" he apostrophizes. His recreations consisted of horseback riding, climbing stairs and hills, reading good books, and playing with his eleven grandchildren when they were from three to five years old. He vacationed in the Euganean hills near Padua and spent much time at his villa on the plain nearby. In a brief Compendium at the end of his book he discussed the pros and cons of sobriety with good-natured logic and demolished the arguments of critics. He once said: "I never knew the world was beautiful until I reached old age."

THE GERONTOCOMIA

The *Gerontocomia* (the title is misspelled throughout as *Gerentocomia*) is a unique title. The word occurs in the Justinian Code as gerontokomeion, an alms house or hospital for the aged (1. 3. 45. 1); gerontokomos, a warden of such a hospital, appears at Justinian, *Novellae* 7.1; the Suda has gērokomeion. It was published on 27 November 1489, at Rome by Eucharius Silber alias Franck, 134 folios in quarto and in semi-Gothic type (Klebs 1057. 1; Goff

No. Z–26), with the subtitle: *scilicet de senium cura atque victu.* The book exists in very few copies today. Beyond the copy (lacking a frontispiece) in the National Library of Medicine, Bethesda, Maryland, which I have used in making my translation I know of one in the library of the University of Pavia, one in the Biblioteca Malatestiana at Cesena, and three copies at Rome in the Alessandrina, Angelica, and Casanatense libraries, as well as one in the Göttingen University Library. There is also a copy in the Vittorio Putti library of the Istituto Ortopedico Rizzoli at Bologna; Putti is well known for his Italian translation of Berengario da Carpi's *De fractura calvae sive cranei* (1937). Gaetano Marini, *Degli archiatri pontifici,* I (Rome, 1784): 311, says there was a copy in the Biblioteca Barberina at Rome and one in the monastery of San Martino in Palermo. I have made no effort to list other copies than those I have seen in Italy.

This book, in the words of my late friend, Signor Ladislao Münster, practicing physician at Bologna during my stay there in 1962 and lecturer in the history of medicine at Ferrara, is the "first practical manual on the problems of old age." Its primacy can be clearly ascertained by comparison with both the earlier and later books on the subject which I have briefly described above. Münster has, to date, written the chief articles on Zerbi and his place in the history of medicine as anatomist, physician, writer on medical ethics and old age, and philosopher. In general, the topics handled in these other books are also handled by Zerbi but in much greater detail and with a stronger emphasis on the personal care of the aged in a rest home especially selected for the purpose as to climate, exposure, equipment, a caretaker (gerontocomos) with assistants, and in all other important respects appropriate for achieving the desired results. Münster in his article "Il primo trattato, etc." (see the bibliography at the end of this book) has set down an admirable summary which was helpful to me when I wrote my chapter on Zerbi in *Pre-Vesalian Anatomy,* etc. (1975), pp. 148–51.

The structure Zerbi follows in his book is clearly set down in his prologue directed to Pope Innocent VIII and in his table of contents. Chapters 1–10 deal with the various periods and causes of old age and with the prognostication of longevity. At chapter 11 his procedure is described as two-fold: (a) conservative, that is, the preservation of old age and its physical and mental resources, and (b) the resumptive method or the renewal of declining energies, reducing the unequal mixture *(intemperantia, dyscrasia)* of the humors and re-establishing their former equilibrium. Since (b) is the more important approach of the two, the word resumptive appears very frequently. Zerbi employs the ancient system of humors, complexions, powers, qualities, operations, and spirits then in general use by all who dealt with the human body and based upon the writings of Aristotle and Galen. These terms are well described in an older medical book, R. Dunglison, *A Dictionary of Medical Science* (1860); modern medical dictionaries have abandoned the entire terminology of an earlier era. Since old age is dry and cold these conditions must be restored by a constant and assiduous supply of their opposites, heat and humidity, as these are depleted in old age. There follow the physiological and pathological phenomena of aging according to the six non-naturals. These are defined by Dunglison as follows:

> Under this term the ancient physicians comprehended air, meat and drink, sleep and watching or waking, motion and rest, the retentions and excretions, and the affections of the mind. They were so called because they affect man without entering into his composition, or constituting his *nature;* but yet are so necessary that he cannot live without them.

Zerbi then describes with eloquent detail the choice of a caretaker or gerontocomos in chapter XIV. He should be liberally educated, frugal, experienced, with some medical training, sympathetic toward his charges, clean, zealous, vigilant, efficient, a good manager of both his establishment and his assistants, whom he must be careful in choosing. Their habits both private and at their task should be constantly monitored by the gerontocomos. The nationality of the assistants is also of great importance; Zerbi discusses this subject frankly and fully.

The atmosphere, climate, region, and exposure of the home *(mansio)* are then discussed. The proper exercise, baths, massage, rest, food and drink, water and wine, bread and meat, both domestic and wild game, with respect to the especially beneficial parts of animals, milk, cheese, oil, salt, plants and vegetables, spices and herbs, fruits in season and out are examined closely for their usefulness in the resumptive diet.

Sleep, bodily elimination, the emotions, sex, retardation of gray hair and baldness, means of purifying the blood and those for reviving the spirits (vital, animal, and natural) through the use of snake flesh, water of flesh, human blood, and potable gold are then discussed. The book ends with the description of gems, syrups, and electuaries prescribed for the elderly by various authors.

The text is replete with references (at least 645 of them) to writers from Aristotle and Galen to Celsus, Pliny, and Isidore of Seville (for etymologies), with heavy dependence upon their statements. This method of corroboration was, of course, standard practice during the Renaissance; Galen, for example, maintained his position for centuries to follow as an incontrovertible authority. This habit reflects the unwillingness of writers on natural science and medicine to depart from earlier knowledge and pseudoknowledge and accounts for much absurdity conveyed solemnly and uncritically from age to age. In the discussion of antidotes and medicines for all purposes writers were content to heap up a multitude of ingredients prescribed by Avicenna in his *Canon Medicinae,* any one of which might be well omitted without apparently disturbing the net result of the compound to be administered.

It is unfortunate that Zerbi rarely mentions women and regards them as inferior (except at raising chickens), following in this respect Aristotle and Pliny. Yet all of the *Gerontocomia* may be taken to apply to women as well as to the old men he has in mind. While much of his book may sound strange to modern readers, they must realize that he represents the current attitudes and conventions of his time in his scholarship and could scarcely be expected to deviate widely from prevailing views. Yet in what amounts to a highly sensitive and sympathetic understanding of the problems, maladies, and sufferings of the aged, he represents a unique approach to his purpose: to relieve the aged physically, mentally (his words on amusements and recreations for the old people are particularly perceptive and timely in view of the modern psychological approach), and spiritually, as he shows in chapter XLII devoted to this subject. His work is indeed the first enlightened manual for the use of those who manage rest homes and as such well worth reading by all who are interested in this aspect of their eventual experience.

ZERBI'S LIFE

Gabriele Zerbi (1445–1505) was one of the most remarkable medical men and anatomists of his time, a man of great energy who was active in his profession as a practicing physician, a professor of anatomy, and author for many years at Padua, Bologna, and Rome. He was born at Verona of an old and aristocratic family; his father held various offices in civil government there and was prominent in the guild of the wool merchants.

We have no record of a university degree for Zerbi. He probably studied at Padua, where he began to teach medicine in 1467, having obtained the doctorate at the age of twenty-two. From 1475 to 1483 he taught medicine and logic at the University of Bologna, although he was not a Bolognese citizen. Among his distinguished colleagues were Baverio Bonetti, Gerolamo Manfredi, Alessandro Achillini, Giovanni Garzoni, and Aristotile Fioravanti. In 1480 he was promoted to ordinary professor, replacing Nestore Morandi, and in 1482 he published his first book, *Quaestiones Metaphysicae,* a commentary on Aristotle's *Metaphysics,* dedicated to Pope Sixtus IV.

The next period of his life was spent in Rome, where he lived and worked accompanied by two sons for ten years, from 1483 to 1494. Pope Innocent VIII, to whom he dedicated the *Gerontocomia,* showed him special favor in a letter dated 11 March 1490. At the end of this year Zerbi was offered a two-year contract in the chair of the theory of medicine at Padua. He returned there to teach for eleven years, from 1494 to his death in 1505. His working career may be summed up thus: I. First period at Padua, 1467–75; II. Stay at Bologna, 1475–83; III. Stay at Rome, 1483–94; IV. Second and last period at Padua, 1494–1505. From this period date five letters from Benedetto Rizzoni to Zerbi, so far the only correspondence known to me and containing some interesting facts concerning the friendship between the two men. In letter 1, for instance, we hear of Zerbi's fame as a physician at the court of Pope Innocent VIII (1484–92) and that Zerbi owned property at Rome.

The details of Zerbi's biography are few and scattered among the archives of Verona, Venice, Padua, Bologna, and Rome. The famous diary of Marino Sanuto, published at Venice in 1879, contains a few items of information. In 1499 Zerbi practiced medicine at Venice during the vacation from the university in Padua. He also helped to hire Antonio Fracanzano, then teaching at Ferrara, to lecture on philosophy at Padua in 1502. The entry for August, 1500, in Sanuto's diary (III, 654) gives Zerbi's teaching record. In May, 1503, he went to Florence to attend Lorenzino dei Medici, who lay ill. In July, 1503, he traveled to Corfu to aid the captain-general, who was suffering from a flux.

On 15 October 1504, there arrived a messenger from Skander Pasha to the Signoria of Venice, asking for a physician to attend him in his illness. Zerbi, accompanied by his son Marco, set out for the Turkish court in Bosnia at the request of the Venetian consul at Constantinople with a leave of absence from his duties in Venice. On 5 November it was learned that the Pasha had died. Zerbi, attracted no doubt by the high fee which had been offered (300 ducats a month), had accomplished a cure of the affliction (dysentery) and Skander, chief minister to the Sultan, had loaded him with precious gifts and given him safe conduct through infidel territory back to Venice. Then as Valerianus tells the grisly story in his remarkable book on the unhappy lives of well-known literary men (*De Litteratorum Infelicitate Libri Duo;* Venice: Jacob Sarzina, 1620; new ed., Geneva, 1821, pp. 38–40) the Pasha resumed his lustful habits and quickly died of their excesses. His sons, eager to regain the gold and gems which Zerbi carried on his pack mules, caught him near the border of Dalmatia, brought him back, and murdered both him and his son by sawing them through between two planks of wood.

Zerbi's will, which he had made before he left for the East and which I have published in my account of him in *Studies in Pre-Vesalian Anatomy,* etc., pp. 323–24, is dated 13 October 1514, the very month in which he left Italy for Bosnia (Sanuto, *Diarii,* VII, 77). He was to be buried in the church of St. Francis at Padua. After his death his property was to go to his four sons. He left the usufruct of his estate to his wife, Elena dei Metaselimi, of Bologna. He also had a daughter, Taddea, to whom he bequeathed an income determined by his executors, one of them his wife, the other Pietro of Mantova. His mother, who was at least eighty-eight at the time Zerbi's will was drawn up, was to receive part of the income as well. Another daughter, Hermodoria, and his sister, both nuns, received specific sums of money as did his sister Angela and his brothers Giovanni and Benedetto.

ZERBI'S PUBLISHED WORKS

Zerbi's published works are as follows:

1. *Quaestiones Metaphysicae,* 1482
2. *Gerontocomia,* 1489
3. *De Cautelis Medicorum,* 1495
4. *Liber Anathomie Corporis Humani,* etc., 1502
5. *Anathomia Matricis Pregnantis,* etc., 1502, published at the end of no. 4.

Quaestiones Metaphysicae is an original study of Aristotle's *Metaphysics,* replete with the quotation of many authorities, however. Both theology and philosophy are drawn upon in the usual scholastic manner. This book, for all its value, is completely ignored by modern students of medieval and Renaissance philosophy.

Gerontocomia: this is discussed above.

De Cautelis Medicorum is, like the *Gerontocomia,* one of the first practical treatises on its subject: the study of duty or moral obligation. It is certainly the chief Renaissance contribution to this important branch of medicine. Zerbi begins with a prologue in which he quotes Aristotle, Haly Abbas, Mesue, Damascenus, Avicenna, the New Testament, Galen, and Haly Rodoan on the relationship of the physician both to God and to his patients. He emphasizes the great moral responsibility of the physician's calling, a career full of perils, temptations, fraud, and error which he must avoid. *Cautela* means both caution and precaution and, in legal language, security. Zerbi defines it thus: "the avoidance, with diligent attention, of deception, fraud, and delusion, infamy, ignominy, and shame which can occur to the physician in his operative activity upon the human body while his practical reason directs him to preserve the honor and usefulness of his profession." He thus expresses in Aristotelian terms the material, formal, efficient, and final causes of *cautela*.

The work is divided into six topics according to the means of attitudes by which the physician must seek to preserve himself from danger. The first is drawn from the nature or character of the physician himself, his physical appearance, and his training. The second is his attitude toward God, the third his attitude toward himself, the fourth his behavior toward his patient, the fifth his relation to other people present in the sick-room, women, disciples, ordinary folk, and druggists. The sixth describes the image he presents to the world outside the sick-room. It will be seen at once that Zerbi's preoccupation is with a series of problems in public relations well known to all modern physicians. In fact, he presents a compendium on the subject well worth reading today. I have given a fuller account of this book in my *Studies in Pre-Vesalian Anatomy*.

The *Liber Anathomie* is a vast work covering in great detail and according to the scholastic organization of material the structure of the body and its organs, systematized for inspection on the basis of Aristotle, *De Incessu Animalium* 705 b, where the six positions of living creatures are listed: superior, inferior, before, behind, right, left. The three books into which Zerbi divided his study fall into I. Anterior Parts; II. Posterior Parts; III. Lateral Parts. As a detailed anatomy it can be compared only with the *Commentary on Mundinus* by Berengario da Carpi (1521). Zerbi cites all the authorities, Arabic, Greek, and Latin, abundantly but with some emphasis on independent conclusions based on personal observation.

As an appendix to the *Liber Anathomie* Zerbi printed his short essay on the embryo, *De Generationis Embrionis,* also printed by Johannes Dryander in 1537 as part of his own brief *Anatomia.* This is one of the few specialized treatises produced by the pre-Vesalian anatomists and bears the variant title, *Anathomia Matricis Praegnantis*.

An unpublished work which I have recently edited is Zerbi's *Libellus de Preservatione Corporum a Passione Calculosa* in the Biblioteca Comunale of Verona, No. 775, Cl. Medic., 91, 1, Busta A. It consists of 130 folios and is a treatise on the causes and cure of kidney and bladder stone. He does not mention it anywhere, not even in the appropriate section of the *Liber Anathomie* on the illnesses of the kidneys, ff. 36, r, v, although he quotes the same authors as he does in the *Libellus.* He does, however, make use of the latter in the portion on diet in the *Gerontocomia,* where the sequence of the foods and drinks discussed is identical; he even repeats some phrases from the *Libellus.* From the biographical facts concerning the Cardinal Gabriele Rangone, of Verona, to whom Zerbi dedicates the *Libellus,* I conclude that it probably preceded the *Gerontocomia* and is therefore his second book after the *Quaestiones Metaphysicae.* Whether or not it was intended for publication and why it was not printed during Zerbi's lifetime as were his other writings are questions difficult to answer. Zerbi probably met the cardinal during his stay at Rome in 1483–94 but before 1486 when the cardinal died. The *Libellus* may then have been written between 1483 and 1489, when the *Gerontocomia* appeared.

José Riesco has recently emphasized the fact that Zerbi was patronized by two popes during his stay at Rome (1483–94), Sixtus IV, who died 8 December 1484, and Innocent VIII, who died 7 July 1492. Zerbi dedicated his *Quaestiones Metaphysicae* (1482) to Sixtus IV; its frontispiece shows Zerbi at the right kneeling before the pope and offering his book to the pontiff. On the left kneels a person whom Münster (*Nuovi Contributi Biografici,* p. 79) believes might be the creator of the miniature. Since the people shown in such portraits were usually represented with great fidelity we cannot doubt that we have here the unique existing portrait of Gabriele Zerbi, if only in profile. A letter of Innocent VIII to Zerbi (*Ex Reg. Brev. Innoc.* VIII, t. IV, p. 465) speaks of the latter's high qualities and learning as well as of the special favors the pope has awarded him. Marino Brocardo in the laudatory letter he published in the front matter of Zerbi's *Anathomia* (Venice, 1502) deals with the high regard in which both popes held Zerbi. On 11 March 1490, Innocent VIII raised Zerbi's salary from 150 to 250 florins, an undeniable indication of his esteem (*Ex Reg. Brev. Innoc. VIII,* ibid.)

Verification of the numerous references made by Zerbi, especially to Arabic authors in their Latin translations, has been sometimes difficult in consideration of their rarity and general lack of adequate indices. In the case of Theodorus Priscianus as well the Teubner text of the *Euporista,* edited by Valentin Rose in 1894, has been of no help at all except for one citation from the preface. All other references to Theodorus are to be found in the section entitled *De diaeta* (Rose, p. xxi) but not included by this editor in his text. It is to be found in MS Città del Vaticano F. IV. 57, f. 184v–96r printed in *Experimentarius medicinae, Theodori dieta,* etc.; Argentorati Apud Joannem Schottum, 1544, pp. 232–45, referred to by short chapters called *capitula.* This book is no. 1411 in Richard J. Durling, *A Catalogue of Sixteenth Century Printed Books in the National Library of Medicine* (Bethesda, Md., 1967).

Isaac Israeli, also known as Judeus, has been cited from the *Opera Omnia* (Lyon: Bartholomew Trot, 1515), f. 11r–156r, *De diaetis universalibus et particularibus* and by the folio numbers. Other texts used are as follows:

Averroes, *Colliget;* Venice: Scotus, 1542.
Rabi Moysi Aphorismi; Venice: Jacobus Penchius de Leucho, 1508, which also contains *Aphorismi Jo. Damasceni = Mesue = Yuhanna ibn Serapion.*
Pietro D'Abano, *Conciliator;* Venice: Boneto Locatello, 1496.
Rhazes, *Opera;* Basle: Henricpetrus, 1544 (Book IV, *De diaetis medicinis et cibariis*).

Abulkasim (Abū'l Qāsim Khalaf ibn Abbas al-Zahrāwī) was born in or after 936 and died probably between A. D. 1010 and 1013 according to Sami Khalaf Hamarneh and Glenn Sonnedecker, *A Pharmaceutical View of Abulcasis al-Zahrāwī in Moorish Spain with special reference to the "Adhān"* (Leiden: E. J. Brill, 1963), pp. 20, 22. He wrote a large medical compendium, *Kitāb al-taṣrīf liman 'Ajiza an al-Ta'lif,* usually shortened to *Al-taṣrīf,* in thirty treatises. Several parts of this work were translated into Latin in the fifteenth century and published as *Liber Servitoris, Liber Theoricae nec non practicae,* and *Methodus Medendi,* the latter covering surgery. This became quite influential upon later European medicine.

The section on hygiene and diet to which Zerbi makes frequent reference embraces treatises 26 and 27. It is not available in Latin or in any other language since *Al-taṣrīf* has not been published in its entirety. Hence I have not been able to verify his references in a printed text. Hamarneh and Sonnedecker, pp. 60–61, give a brief account of these sections. Here Abulkasim discussed diet in general, useful and harmful foods, special diets for certain diseases and their preparation, the faculties of regimen and the properties of drugs, clothes for use in hot and cold weather, and other matters. The authors of *A Pharmaceutical View,* etc., give an excellent and very thorough presentation of Moorish culture in the time of Abulkasim, the transmission of the manuscripts with printings of his writings, the content and structure of his work, and a special study of the *Adhan,* "the fatty or oily essence that could be extracted from certain substances by pharmaceutical processes." (p. 78). To their ample bibliography may now be added the article on Abulkasim by Sami Hamarneh in *Dictionary of Scientific Biography* 14 (1976):584–85.

It seems that Zerbi must have had access to an Arabic manuscript of *Al-taṣrīf* and either read it himself or had the assistance of some one who knew Arabic in making his copious references to the book. The other Arabic authors he used were generally available in Latin translations.

The Gerentocomia [Gerontocomia] by Gabriele Zerbi of Verona Dedicated to Pope Innocent VIII Happily Begins

PROLOGUE

According to the ancient and ancestral agreement induced by nature and reason among almost all people it is acknowledged that all things are fashioned by some immense power without whose will nothing first of all can be preserved. This power, whether it be called God or some other name, bestows as is fitting the complete abundance of its perfection upon individual beings and has done so quite bountifully even though because of the inadequacy of the individual subject to this power the latter has not been able to attain perfection. Although the individual being exists with the desire of a long life and health as well as of the other perfections which proceed from God as constituent parts of nature it has retained none of the essential goodness which corresponds to those perfections and which is inherent in the first beginnings of things. For nature our parent gave to man alone of all animals along with a better or a sadder fate (I do not know which) such a great desire and joy of life as companions of his existence that although life is brief and full of trouble both young and old long for it, and those who are suffering do not wish to die even when they perceive that they are miserable. Thus it is that most men wish to grow old in spite of the fact that they curse old age when they have reached it.[1] Moreover, the breath of life itself is so sweet for each man that no one is so old but that the hope of another year of life at least survives in him while death itself is at his door and his passing away brings its dread. That life which humans so greatly desire is fulfilled in the same period of time for few or none until its final and

[1]Cicero, *De Senectute* 4; 24.

natural end, indeed, certainly not for those who reach the brink of old age, since not only sloth but loose living destroy their good habits (as they say), those vices by which human bodies are accustomed to be afflicted, to say nothing of many accidents and adversities which intervene in their lives before the arrival of those who, insofar as it is possible, seek to oppose these ills. I speak here of those people whose business it is to handle skillfully the care of the aged, whom the Greeks call gerontocomos, that is, those in charge of the health of old people. In order to retard old age and to extend life they employ only those means by which the old are guided and preserved and which should lead them to the natural end of life in accordance with the beginnings of their generation. Nevertheless, the health-care of the aged is still a difficult and most laborious task with its conservative method alone, for the nature of old age is cold and dry[2] and the collection of phlegmatic humor at that age is abundant and moist. The strength of old people likewise ebbs away and their bodies grow heavy with cold. "Diseases, forming ranks, leap all around them."[3] As they say, there are more than three hundred perils and uncertain diseases of all kinds which attack the old so that one may declare that there are as many of them as there are nations in the world. According to the very ancient Hippocrates, a man outstanding in the medical art and in that of writing, Galen, and Cornelius Celsus, a few of these diseases out of many are dyspnoea, catarrh, dysentery, cough, strangury, dysuria, pains in the joints, the erosion of the nerves which the Greeks call paralysis, kidney disease, the formation of stones, dizziness, apoplexy, the bad condition called cachexia by the Greeks, itching of the entire body, melancholy, insomnia, fluids in the stomach, dripping of the eyes and nostrils, dimness of vision, cataract, illnesses of ears and nostrils of rather long duration, stomach trouble and the contortions of the intestines which accompany it, and other ills of the abdomen. In addition to these there are progressive emaciation, loss of appetite, pains in the sides and in the viscera, ills of the throat, coryza, and gibbosity on the front, back, and sides. Finally, many old people who are obese die suddenly from weakness of breath and strangulation. Since this variety of

[2]E.g., Aristotle, *Probl.* 875 a.
[3]Juvenal 10. 218–19.

diseases is more powerful through long illnesses in old age and because of a general sluggishness which afflicts old people and all kinds of accidents which befall them one must labor to protect the old from the torture of their bodies, to ward off death by proper care of their health as far as is possible, to extend the services of the gerontocomos and to stand guard against those forces which bring on premature death so that with their health intact the old people may live out the rest of their lives as peacefully as possible. That medical process for the advantage of old age which is called resumptive or reductive by the ancients is helpful for this purpose. It is especially adapted as something divine to the desire and joy of living and is suitable to be embraced vigorously and to be imitated for it conduces greatly to the extension of life. A rather long span of life is by no means the least among those good things which nature has given us. Therefore I cannot wonder sufficiently at that man of a deservedly great name, Pliny of Novum Comum,[4] who held the belief that nature had given men nothing better than brevity of life but even proclaimed it as a basic principle no less to be admired. This great man added that of all the good things nature had given to men there was nothing better than a timely death and the best thing about it was that each man could provide it for himself. For to man alone among living creatures a more fragile life had been given; hence many men[5] thought it best not to be born or, having been born, to perish as quickly as possible. This view is of course at variance with the beginnings of nature; it is in the interest of human life to refute it. For since man just as also every kind of animal is wise in this regard by a sort of natural instinct he not only wishes to preserve his health and to avoid destruction, as Boethius says,[6] but through his great desire as I have said he as one among all living things longs for life, nor is this desire fruitless, since nature does nothing in vain.[7] It is reasonable beyond doubt that as long a life as possible is desirable and the wish for brevity of life by no means to be reckoned as an attribute

[4]Pliny, *N. H.* 28. 2. 9.

[5]Cf. W. C. Greene, *Moira, Fate, Good, and Evil in Greek Thought,* 42, n. 189 for this topos, beginning with Theognis 425–28.

[6]Boethius, *Cons. of Phil.* 3, Prosa 11. 49.

[7]A frequent quotation from Aristotle by 15th- and 16th-century anatomists. I have collected a number of passages in my *Studies in Pre-Vesalian Anatomy,* etc., p. 220. See also H. Bonitz, *Index Aristotelicus,* 836.

of human nature. Otherwise we should be forced to admit that the best gift among all those given to man by nature is to be deprived of that which men by instinct labor so hard to attain, expend their energies upon, and strive after eagerly. This naturally immense desire for human life is hampered by the view that brevity of life is a good thing given us by nature although the natural inclination of man is in favor of reaching its intended culmination. All this speculation is highly absurd for the end is loved and desired as perfection moves toward it, designed as being perfectible. Neither by law or nature is it proper to believe these frivolous arguments. Not brevity but longevity of life is to be considered the more desirable goal, which each individual is able to attain if he observes what is suitable by way of the resumptive or restorative method of health-care and is advised in the use of those means by which hastening age and its causes are halted and life is extended. Nor is human frailty to be borne with pain because the human condition and each man's fate determine the place of birth for him, but his continuous memory is to be weighed equally with his life in the scales, and he must live in such a way that no one will consider that he has been born in vain.

Therefore in this *Gerontocomia,* divided into fifty-seven chapters, I shall set forth insofar as my feeble intellect may foresee the theory I have referred to as ideal for the useful purpose mentioned in the recovery or resumption of old age nor shall I hesitate to make use of earlier authorities in summary form. I shall follow most especially as far as I can the opinions of the famous medical men through whose work this discipline which is so salutary for old people has been developed. It is proper to follow them carefully so that it may be realized by what method these authors have studied the retardation of old age and whose beliefs are worthy of mention in this book. For it is as Pliny says[8] the part of a kindly and sincere person to admit the benefits one has received from others. I have assumed this undertaking especially for this reason because few of our recent physicians have attempted the task not through contempt for it or because it is widely accessible but because they have touched rather lightly upon the subject within

[8]Pliny, *N. H., pref.* 21.

narrow limits and with excerpts merely. I now begin this little work under the auspices of your name, Innocent the Pope, in order that having observed the resumptive regimen you may survive through a longer life and reach the height of your blessed pontificate to which by your merits the greatest God will have brought you after having led a most happy life.

Contents of This Book

Chapter I

The Various Periods and Peculiar Qualities of Old Age

Old age, which Galen[1] calls the pathway to death, as correctly defined, is a certain disposition attached to the general aggregate of physical characteristics of a living individual of a warm natural innate humidity and caused by the influence of the heavenly bodies extending through a period in which the living creature decreases and clearly declines, the first part of which is called old age. In man this period begins from the thirtieth or thirty-fifth or fortieth year more or less and is held to extend to the fiftieth or sixtieth year. Its inception is not perceptible nor does the deficiency it brings appear at all clearly in the substance of the faculty of the members in quality or in quantity. Hence Judeus[2] calls this the unrecognized period of old age in which

> We decline imperceptibly and grow old in silent years.[3]

In this period there does not yet occur a contraction of the nerves (or sinews), there are no wrinkles in the skin, nor are the vertebrae of the back curved, and in the members which have like parts or similarity of composition[4] no diminution can be discerned because they retain more heat than in the other periods of aging, if the heat-loss is well restored since the heat is not yet entirely lost. There is nevertheless after some passage of time beyond doubt in this first period of old age a diminution in the like parts for not only does the natural consistency of heat begin to diminish but also whatever tendency in the way of corruption there is in old men begins to set in, and for this reason they say the old man is corrupt because he is on the way to corruption, for corruption,

[1]Galen, 7. 680; 1. 582.
[2]Isaac Judeus or Israeli, *Opera Omnia,* f. iii r.
[3]Ovid, *Fasti* 6. 771.
[4]Galen, 4. 741; 10. 48.

especially that of nature, is part of the process of great age, as Aristotle says.[5] There are, however, as they say certain differences as in every mean between extremes, for the first part of this period coincides in certain qualities with the period immediately preceding which they call the age of consistency, beauty, and flowering and which they describe as hot and dry. The latter part of age shows to some extent the qualities of final old age which is cold and essentially dry but accidentally humid. It has, however, something like a middle equidistant between these two periods, where the natural humidity by evaporation becomes cold and dry. Therefore in this period they attribute to those who are of this age constancy, strong understanding, and wisdom.[6] When men become old, in the first part of old age they understand more perfectly and fully because the intellect in us when we become old is more efficient. Constancy indeed is more adapted to the same people because this age retains cold and dryness well. Similarly, because of the lack of heat it retains and mingles understanding among the operations of reason and wisdom because of much experience and the memory of many things associated with cold and dryness. In old men in addition the loss of youthful playfulness and sexuality is increased because of the immobility of cold which is continual in that period and of the dryness which is not easily removed. The astrologers say that Jupiter dominates the first period of old age, providing the person with guidance for about twelve years, the planet of the future lifetime, of peace and tranquillity, under whose sign the person born is engaged in good works of religion. To this part of old age another one succeeds which is the latest or the last or the decrepit period of old age, which they call the old age of the old men or the end of life, differing from the first period of old age in its humid superfluity in the manifest decline of the entire body. For then almost all the elderly feel that their old age is rendered weaker; in this period old age is full of many great and continuous ills; many difficulties surround the aged, as Flaccus says.[7] The lack of strength appears clearly in

[5]Aristotle, *Probl.* 909b.

[6]Cael. Aur., *Acut.* 1. 8; 2. 28; *Tard.* 5. 4.

[7]Horace, *Ep.* 2. 3. 169. On the theory of localization of cerebral ventricular function see Edwin Clarke and Kenneth Dewhurst, *An Illustrated History of Brain Function;* Berkeley and Los Angeles: University of California Press, 1974, and the classic article by W. Sudhoff, "Die Lehre von den Hirnventrikeln in textlicher und graphischer Tradition des Altertums und Mittelalter"; *Arch. Gesch. Med.* 7 (1913):149–205.

almost all old people as the actions and sufferings of the members reveal. First, the active workings of the limbs in continuous succession are imperfect so that they finally begin to find pleasure in and to do childish things. All this happens, as the experts have taught, because the thickness and sluggishness of the animal spirits in the limbs do not penetrate to the ventricles of the brain, the seat of the cogitative and discretionary forces, nay rather, they remain in the inner part of the head with their deficiency and because of this reason the power of fancy is not checked since then according to the act of reason they discourse imperfectly and out of their wits. They say this is because the harmony of the animal powers is discordant like a dissonant lyre. Therefore they also say old men are called thus *(senes)* because they know not *(nesciant),* or from a diminution of the senses, for finally in old people the power to understand and to reflect maturely dwindles away with a sort of inner corruption of the organ of fancy. Older people are forgetful just as children are because memory shifts in both of them, increasing in the latter and decreasing in the former. Their memory is bad as to reception because cold and dryness are dominant in them. Among so many difficulties of old age with all the loss in their members the greater loss in old people is dementia, so that, as the poet[8] says:

> But worse than any loss of limb is loss
> Of memory, which cannot name his slaves,
> Cannot recognize the friendly face
> With whom he dined the night before, nor those
> Children whom he created and brought up.
> For with a savage testament he cuts
> Off all his heirs.

More fully and generally, the senses become less acute in old people; we see their limbs distorted, their sight grow more feeble, their hearing, gait, even their teeth and the instruments by which they eat their food likewise, feeling becomes more dull to such an extent because of their frigidity that they are not adequately sensitive to pain, as Galen says.[9] The vision grows dull as it grows less, or "They lose both eyes or envy the one-eyed,"[10] their hearing is

[8]Juvenal 10. 232–37.
[9]Galen, 17 B.5.
[10]Juvenal 10. 228.

dulled so that they scarcely hear "The blare of horns and trumpets blown all together."[11] Their movement becomes difficult and they are properly called decrepit because on account of old age as they say they can neither move nor make any creaking *(crepitum)*. Their taste becomes dull. "Their voices tremble like their legs, their torpid taste finds no more joy in wine or food."[12] Furthermore, the sex-urge in older people is lulled to sleep, for

love fades into a long oblivion
and if they try, their little tool lies still
[with a hernia] and helpless even though they work all night.[13]

There is furthermore a trembling in the limbs of the aged because of excessive frigidity, as Aristotle says.[14] The stature of a particularly tall body is distorted, curved, and humped; those who are tall are stooped over, as Galen says.[15] Thus the tall stature which is an ornament in youth is ruined in advanced old age. By excessive lack of innate heat and humidity their members are wrinkled and contracted. Thus so many are the difficulties of old age that one may repeat that saying of Pliny:[16] The years of old age as penalty for the time of a vigorous life are not to be counted for so often is death invoked in old age that no prayer is more frequent.

Yet now since age is useless, heavy, long,
Since live I cannot, give me power to die.
Death's sweet to the old but, hoped-for, it recedes.
Yet when it's bitter it comes at break-neck pace.[17]

For to many old men old age is so odious, according to Cicero,[18] that they say they are sustaining a burden heavier than Mount Aetna. But it happens that when they are already worn down with years old age enervates and afflicts them. There are certain differentiae in this period of life, for that part of old age nearest to its beginning does not have so much coldness and humidity as that part which is immediately close to death which they call the period

[11]Ibid. 214–15.
[12]Ibid. 203–204.
[13]Ibid. 204–206.
[14]Aristotle, *Probl.* 875a15.
[15]Galen, 18 A. 552.
[16]Pliny, *N. H.* 7. 167.
[17]Maximianus, *Elegies*. 1. 111–16.
[18]Cicero, *De Sen.* 4.

of termination. This period although almost devoid of natural warmth and humidity still has a phlegmatic humidity adhering to the outer members and softening them. This humidity is accidental, inducing the coldness of death and the suffocation of natural warmth. For this reason also old people in the last stage of old age are afflicted with a heavy cough so that their voices become more feeble; almost all old people breathe with a certain musical wheezing sound. They say the cause for this is that their lungs become filled with a superfluous viscous matter. The midmost part of this period of life has median dispositions. Finally, this age measures its years with the end of life. The astrologers say this final period is dominated by the planet Saturn, which is cold and dry, treacherous, brooding, gloomy, full of suffering and difficulty, the planet which governs the person born under this sign according to the number of his earlier years around thirty; he suffers many infirmities and much sadness so that finally the querulous old man says

> What I was once, I am not; the best has perished;
> Illness and fear possess what's left of me.[19] . . .
> Bowed age comes forward burdened with its evils.[20]

Compelled by these misfortunes the poet[21] has imagined wretched old age at the gates of Hell saying:

> There on the very threshold and in the jaws
> Of Hell crouch Sorrow and avenging Cares.
> There dwell pale Illnesses, and sad Old Age.

[19]Maximianus, *Elegies* 1. 5–6.
[20]Ibid. 261.
[21]Vergil, *Aeneid* 6. 273–75.

Chapter II

The Causes of Old Age in Man

Among authorities it is agreed that there are two kinds of causes of old age, extrinsic and intrinsic. The extrinsic indeed and especially in a universal manner touch upon that which the astrologers who examine the causes of old age have not scorned, namely, the influence of the planets, that is, of Jupiter in the first period of old age upon the animate body and of Saturn in the last period, bringing the individual finally to about the age of ninety-eight of the years in which the person is governed by the planets as computed from the beginning of his exit from the mother's womb down to the end of his life. For very few men are *gymnestes,* or long-lived, that is, living beyond one hundred years except with the loss of almost all their faculties. Those who do live that long are said to pass from the leadership of Saturn to that of the moon, which governs those who are older than twenty-five years. Crates of Pergamum calls those who exceed one hundred years by the name of *gymnestes,* but not a few others call them *macrobii* (long-lived).[22]

The intrinsic causes of old age are more truly to be sought out by more experienced physicians; they say that the human body has the beginnings of its generation from the sperm of both man and woman. Hence, since the beginnings of human substance are from blood and sperm the substance of each of these is humid and fluid which does not attain a great coagulation because the substance thus formed by the two liquids is made quite soluble and fluent by exposure to many kinds of harmful influences, some of which are casual and extraneous such as a congealing frigidity, poisons, a pernicious destruction of continuity, and everything fatal which occurs by chance to the human body, as Galen says.[23]

[22]Schol. to Juvenal 10. 150.
[23]Galen, 1. 582.

Physicians cannot prevent these unfortunate effects of chance since they are of a random sort and beyond human control, but after these influences or events have exerted their force the physician will be able to check their injurious effect. Yet the astrologer as they say since such things are not for him accidental but necessary or for the most part contingent therefore is able to prevent the greatest share of them. The best astrologer will be able to prevent most adverse events which are to occur according to the stars for when he knows the figure of the region of the city and of the horoscope constructed suitable to the individual he will be able to foretell expertly the events which happen to the person. These two masters, the physician and the astrologer, must in particular consult and provide for human nature. There are also two other types of ill to which the human body is exposed that must be especially examined by the physician. The first of these is the resolution or decline of the innate heat which comes in some kind of order. The other is the putrefaction, corruption, and alteration of the restorative humor by which heat is fostered, which is not suitable for the fomentation of life. Each of these ills has an intrinsic and an extrinsic cause. Both forms of ill lead men to a double species of death and cause a sickly as well as a natural old age.[24] For animate creatures are destroyed either by illness or nature; old age necessarily precedes a natural death. Thus the beginnings of old age in the order of events, as the physicians touch upon them, are the decay of the natural humidity caused by the innate heat and containing that which they say is earthy. It is the cause of natural death which is the cause of the old age that precedes death which is itself the way of death, as has been said.[25] For since life is the act of living by means of a natural heat as an instrument life is thus a persistence of the spirit in natural heat. A particular characteristic of this heat is an innate humidity because of which the act of living is a process combining warmth and moisture. This happens to the natural consumption of the innate humidity which is created in it with the wasting away of nature while that humidity is not entirely consumed because the natural heat is diminished and hence old age follows. When the innate heat is extinguished old age ends and

[24]Aristotle, *G. A.*, V. 784b30.
[25]See note 1.

that death which they call natural follows. It happens by reason of an intrinsic origin since a natural and continuous action occurs between heat and humidity. Hence it happens that death occurs quickly in old age with the advent of even small illnesses since there is slight heat with great evaporation in the aged; if any discomfort is created in the first particle which is the heart the body is quickly destroyed. Hence it happens that death occurs in old age without sadness for old people die without the occurrence of any violent suffering and the taking away of their spirit is accomplished quite gradually, as Aristotle says.[26] They call this death into which old people finally pass *tabes* or *marasmus (tabes senum, gerontatrophia).* Beyond doubt it is a corruption of the living body by reason of a dryness which is not saddening since it is not caused by great violence due to the great inclination old men have toward corruption. Such a death takes place when a man who has completed his span of life has reached the ultimate period of old age, for then his natural heat by consuming the humidity proper to his body becomes the cause (accidentally, however) of his extinction when the humidity has wasted away since this is the cause of the consumption of the material body like the flame of a lamp which is extinguished because it consumes the material which feeds the flame. In reference to this situation Seneca[27] says: "He who arises with me dies with me, and he who revives me kills me." And this death which is a corruption is caused through a wasting away which comes in old age. If therefore such a death is nothing other than an extinction of natural heat then old age is like some drying-up and almost disappearance of that heat since they properly call dry that which has lost its natural humor or moisture. Because it has destroyed the humidity subject to the innate heat it has destroyed as it were the spirit of the old people. The heat which nature has given us is first humid in the young, as Galen says,[28] and then increases up to the age of those who survive and shines and increases to the greatest magnitude. From this point on due to the lack of aliment it gradually dwindles away and thus later old age is extinguished because death is on all sides of it. Rightly therefore

[26]Aristotle, *De Resp.* 479a20.
[27]The word *vivificat* proves that this quotation is ecclesiastical Latin and not by Seneca.
[28]Galen, 15. 154, 156, 262.

Galen commends Aristotle's[29] statement, saying, O how good it was because Aristotle likened old age to the dryness of plants which when new and fresh are soft and humid. When they are older their dryness persists and increases until they are entirely dried out and this is death and the end in them. For old men die, as Cicero says, as if by their own will without any application of force as a fire is extinguished and as ripe fruit falls from trees.[30] Thus ripeness carries away the life of old men until they arrive at the end of their days as a natural terminus, which is nothing other than a natural arrival at the ultimate frigidity and dryness because of which the spirit in the human body cannot persist. This end few or none can reach as was said because of many accidents and illnesses which intervene. These debilities can be resisted by the conservative or resumptive art of medicine and by the avoidance of ignorance and impotence in the matter. A regimen has been discovered which prevents the domination of the causes which accelerate dryness and as a defence against immoderate dryness in order that the natural humidity of the body should not be swiftly consumed. Hence thus much has been said about the causes of old age. Its ills are not of the entire body but a disposition in member by member. Quality and disposition are normal, for age and complexion are of the same kind and are connected with age. Since the approach of age cannot surely be far from the end of old age as a complement of all the living organs and especially of the heart such a natural extinction of the natural heat is also identical with death.

[29]Aristotle, *De Resp.* 479b; Galen, 19. 341.
[30]Cicero, *De Sen.* 5.

Chapter III

The Extrinsic Causes of the Swiftness and Slowness of Old Age in Man With the Exception of Causes Arising from Food

Old age is prolonged by those factors which extend the span of life, just as it is accelerated by the causes which make men old, the reasons for which have been stated. Some of these are universal and to be examined more truthfully by the astrologer just as are the celestial aspects and influences of the heavens, especially, according to the assertions of the astrologers, when the planet called Alcochodem which gives the years of life to the individual, just as beauty or the father or marriage, with benevolent aspect has gazed upon the house of life. This planet is called Ylech in Persian and it is proportioned to the mother of the bride or to the wife. Whatever years are taken away or added to the individual horoscope itself are done so according to the will of fortunes or misfortunes by Alcochodem. Nevertheless, according to the natures and properties of the planets which bring fortune or misfortune integrity or wholeness is brought about or the perversion of the inner human nature. They say that the leadership of Jupiter and the sun with Venus in particular invigorates and extends old age and the life of man. This is accomplished more in one part of the universe than in the other because the leadership of the planets is more vigorous in one part than in the other just as it is at one time more than the other. For at the time when the heads of the equinoctial and tropical signs of the movable zodiac occur directly in the eighth sphere under the heads of the aforesaid signs of the immovable zodiac in the ninth sphere then the causes and virtues are ordered in a more perfect manner so as to impinge upon this lower sphere and thus vigor and a longer span of life are offered for the individual person. It is no wonder therefore if in the more temperate regions in early times men possessed a larger body, more robust powers, were very handsome and were giants, with a longer span of life which it is not only right to believe on principle but which can also be proven by reason. When the aforesaid zodiacs are separated from each other by a great distinction men's days become short. Avicenna[31] agrees with this statement when he says: In no species of living creature are placed the ends of life because of nature alone but the cause of the reception of longevity is the influence from the stars as long as life is in harmony with the resolution of some one or of many stars.

Among the particular and especially extrinsic causes of age the air which contains us and the period of the sun and moon are assigned. The cause of a long life for any living creature, according to Aristotle,[32] will vary according to the air containing it and particularly to the periods of the sun and moon, for it is reasonable that the students of the subject should wish the times of all lives to be measured in reference to the nature of the given period. The simile of a mean which contains is to be compared to these causes since the cause of a long life is a lesser disposition to corruption. The fatherland is the beginning of each generation just as the father is, according to Porphyrius,[33] because it has been discovered through experience that men live longer in their own fatherland as being more similar to them than a foreign land. The fatherland has given the individual as a mode of generation brief or long days with strength or weakness of his powers. Those born of youthful parents have strong and healthy principal members proper to each, as Damascenus writes,[34] wherefore it is set down in Book 7 of Aristotle's *Politics* that men of thirty-five [thirty-seven] should copulate with a wife of eighteen so that the combination of their seed may be more excellent because of feminine vigor at the time of conception and gestation of offspring.[35] If coition is unseason-

[31]No such statement appears in the *Canon.* The index to the Giuntine edition of 1562 by Julius Palamedes, printed separately as *Index in Avicennae libros nuper Venetiis editos Julio Palamede Adriensi medico;* Venice: Giunta, 1584, has been used. The effects of a temperate climate on man are drawn from Hippocrates, *On Airs Waters Places* 12. 30–40.

[32]*Probl.* 909b.

[33]*Aristotelis Opera cum Averrois commentariis* I, pt. 1, 2v (*Porphyrii* Introductio); Venice: Giunta, 1562 (repr. 1962).

[34]Johannes Damascenus, *Aphorismi,* f. 24.

[35]*Pol.* 7. 16.

able rather frequently with the body indisposed and especially when full of food and drink the offspring is sickly, weak, and prone to an early old age or at any rate it will not be a male. In similar fashion one must regard as most salutary to the length or brevity of life the proper use of the six non-naturals necessarily appropriate for the human body and especially of the surrounding air. For some men have a long life and some have a short one according to their distance apart in other regions, as Aristotle says,[36] because although life is longer in the warm individuals and shorter in the cold ones the discussion will be more lengthy when it deals with the habitation which produces old age. Warmth which resolves and liquefies the humidities makes the innate heat weaker and there follow the cold and dryness of old age. The unsuitable use furthermore of the other non-naturals we must regard as the cause of an early old age and the brevity of life just as the suitable use of them makes for a tardy old age and a long one. Labor which exceeds a mean is also a cause of old age for whatever male animals are laborious grow older because of their labor since toil dries up the body, and old age is also dry. Immoderate exercise is also harmful especially if it is followed by the drinking of cold water; this immediately cools the viscera and frequent use of what is cool causes coolness to dominate; this leads to weakness of the body and old age. Such cold things prohibit the nutritive powers from their complete function. They also affirm that no less than these causes just mentioned unnecessary rest is the cause of a swifter old age; to remain at ease and to be completely quiet is harmful to old age. The accidental complexion of old age is rendered greater by these causes, humid, watery abundance of crude humor, and by the lack of innate warmth with lessened digestion. Furthermore, there follows upon immoderate quiet among old people a certain sluggishness which they call impotence toward the initiation of movement, relaxing the animal powers and complexion of the body, inclining it toward the nature of phlegm, as Avicenna[37] says, and this is the cause of a swifter old age. Sluggishness also brings about from stronger causes the nature in old people of one who suffers from something like melancholy. Excessive venery

[36]*De Longitudine et Brevitate Vitae* 465a5.
[37]Avicenna, *Canon,* I, 33.

also happens to precipitate a man more swiftly into old age, for on account of rather frequent coition men grow old more rapidly, as Haly Rodoan says.[38] Excessive inanition of the body or that which causes hunger such as fasting or lack of food or thirst or blood-letting or the evacuation of any other humor hastens old age, for evacuations chill and dry out while they are proceeding. The same thing happens also in over-abundant repletion for both lack and super-abundance lead to the same results. Because of this fact it is possible to see from the repletion of the evacuated members and the evacuation of superfluities that the organs which undergo these states or conditions are not stopped-up nor made weak. It follows necessarily that man does not grow old swiftly, as Galen says.[39] The inordinate use of food leads to the creation of bad juice or a thin and soluble composition of slight and delicate liquids, humors in flux and slender weak powers of generation and to old age. Wakefulness which exceeds a modest norm brings on an untimely old age, just as intemperance of lust, over-work, and excessive use of the eyes causes old age, as Johannes Nazarenus says.[40] These excesses dispose a man toward aging and corruption since they weaken the natural heat and take away the spirit. Nocturnal vigils diminish the strength of the body; too much sleep makes life shorter following long hunger and inanition of the body because the radical humidity is consumed more than in a body properly fed. Immoderate accidents of the soul are the causes of a swifter old age especially for those whose bodies dry out excessively; thus it happens generally when the frequency of all the animal movements of the body dry it out. The same thing happens with anything that dries up the body such as excessive sadness; this stupefies a person and corrupts the person's nature for sadness is an evil beyond doubt and to be avoided, as Aristotle says.[41] It is nothing other than a certain pain on account of the loss of some good whose recovery is hoped for. When this does not happen although one's suffering is acute sorrow is created by the hopelessness of

[38]Ali ibn Ridwan, *Commentum Galenum;* Pavia: Michele and Bernardino de Garaldi, 1501; also Venice, 1496. He is also known as Haly Eben Rodan or Rodohan Aegyptius (circa A.D. 908).
[39]Galen, 7. 669.
[40]Johannes Nazarenus: I have not been able to identify this author.
[41]Aristotle, *N. E.* 14. 1153b1.

that recovery, and this is a great sadness. The same thing happens they say with inordinately frequent cogitation which accelerates the arrival of old age. Of this type also is the suffering called hereos [eros] in Greek, that is, a deep love, hilichi in Arabic, or excessive love, which arises when one thinks continually of a beloved object, through which there grows an immoderate desire under the power of a mistaken estimation for whose sake all other activities are rendered secondary to the attainment of that object. With all these maladies there is created a vehement and laborious motion of the vital spirit just as in distress or of the animal spirits beyond those which are to be avoided as in sadness or by the union and fixation of the same in the inner regions as in strong cogitation and excessive love. For it happens due to the immoderate frequency of these troubles that they persist a long time since the heart is heated by external dryness which finally hastens old age. Distressful thought diminishes the bodily strength. The same thing is accomplished they say by the frequency of anger which becomes like madness or fury, for fury is a strong and impetuous anger mingled with agitation. Nor is old age rendered less swift by constant great fear, for these emotions are like the others, labored, inordinate, and sudden movements of the spirits followed by dryness of the body. In anger there is first created a more subtle motion of the spirits and the blood from the extremities to the inner parts because they are inflamed near the heart with the evaporation of the gall which contributes to the process. Because of this motion the angry grow pale at the beginning of their wrath. There follows a similar movement of spirits in return from the heart to the exterior parts; this is the reason why the faces of the angry which had turned pale before now turn red.[42] Thus the inner and outer parts grow warm in anger. In fear, however, a violent, inordinate, and sudden movement toward the inner parts constrains the warmth because of this flight of spirits. The result is that sometimes in fear both the stomach and urine are emptied, as Aristotle says.[43] When fear is great not only does it bring on the illness called melancholy and frigidity but it sometimes increases so much that it kills the patient, as Averroes says.[44] The cause of this is the regression of the natural

[42]Aristotle, *Probl.* 947b3.
[43]Ibid., 948b8.
[44]Averroes, *Colliget* I, 10r.

heat to the heart brought on by fear, but the experts say anger does not kill as does fear in this situation because anger increases the heat in the center and circumference of the body. Jealousy is classified with fear as also bringing on old age; along with it fear becomes a certain continual loss of a good which is much beloved and which is accompanied by suffering and worry.

The Extrinsic Causes of the Swiftness and Slowness of Old Age in Man Arising in Part from Food

Many men grow old more swiftly through weakness not only of the natural heat brought about by its decrease due to time or through the inordinate regimen of the non-naturals of which I have spoken but also by reason of those things by which we are nourished, whether food or drink, which are created to be swallowed down, as they say. First of these is the use of those substances which thin and dry the forces of the body and which are called stimulant in medical terms and nourishing, such as aromatic foods and *acrumina* [pungent] foods. Through the use of these foods insofar as they heat the body they can be prescribed as of medicinal benefit to the stomach and the digestion for old people. Those foods which dry out the body are to be avoided; those which humidify it are of value because of their humidifying nutrients. In similar fashion fresh humid vegetables and fruits are of great value since the alteration or putrefaction or corruption of the restorative humor often makes old age swifter. The heat of natural putrefaction is mixed with that humor, injuring it and impeding its natural action, thus accelerating an untimely old age and creating that crude phlegm they call watery and undigested. A humor of this kind enters the passages of nutriment, preventing the natural heat from passing through and invigorating the members. Many foods are of this disposition, especially fresh juicy humid fruits which are ready for putrefaction. Men are checked from eating foods which make one thin, such as herbs and the inner part of fruits of trees which have a hard bark; men grow old more swiftly by their frequent use, as Judeus says.[45] These are the fruits from which the blood receives aqueosity, such as peaches, cherries, and similar food. Their humidity is not easily separated by the first or second digestion because their complexion is said to be strong so that parts of their substance are not easily separated in relation to human heat although absolutely speaking in relation to fire or to its heat as heat they have a weak complexion. The same thing is true of oil whose parts are so tightly joined and strongly binding in nature that art and nature are unable to separate them. For if oil should be boiled forever its parts would not separate except when they are impure since most of its parts are humid, airy, moderately fiery, thin, and penetrative. Other viscous terrestrial foods are to be discussed elsewhere. But watery fruits whose nature is weak, such as are figs and fresh grapes, are in large part separated by the first digestion from the chyle in the stomach. Thus they soothe the belly for they are not like the watery fruits which generate phlegm for the blood does not receive their aqueosity. They say the same thing about humid melons from which a large part is segregated by the second digestion, thus setting the urine in motion. Therefore the blood generated from the fruits mentioned above is the cause of gray hair, which I shall discuss in chapter V.

[45]f. cliv.

Chapter IV

The Intrinsic Causes of the Swiftness and Slowness of Old Age

Among the chief intrinsic causes of a swift old age are a continual sluggishness and especially a bad corruption of the concoction of the stomach which not only leads to an early old age but to many other malignant ills of the stomach. These include epilepsy, melancholy, ills of the mirach *[epigastrium]* and similar ones. In fact, Avicenna calls this sluggishness the mother of illnesses and the origin of chronic infirmities. The coldness which dominates with weakness of the body preventing the nutritive power from its full operation creates a disposition toward old age and the character of debility with dryness. They say it brings a swifter old age because heat and humidity which are the two principal and particular intrinsic causes of a long life in its perfection and vigor do not preserve a proper proportion. This state leads to a decline over a determined period of time which is prolonged. They either generate a humidity which fosters heat insufficiently or a superfluity of it which they do not dispose of or alter or temper. In fact, they hasten or impede it in some other way. Heat and humidity which are the principal conservative elements of life are said to be distinguished by certain conditions, that is, the humidity should be digested and airy so that heat may be properly fostered by it. It should not easily putrefy nor become smaller lest it dry out more swiftly nor should it become superabundant lest it fail to be controlled by a proper heat. Both have a suitable proportion when heat dominates over humidity; otherwise humidity would putrefy or congeal and the heat would be extinguished. The particular non-principal cause on which depend the tardiness and the deferment of old age is assigned as the domination of the active qualities over the passive, of heat over cold, and of moist over dry. The operation of all life of the soul is caused by heat as its proper and greatest instrument as no one will doubt, for they say that heat is sustained and fostered by humidity. The domination of passive over active qualities, however, leads to putrefaction, while the dominance of dryness over moisture is less hot. These are the causes which assist a long life and conserve it from among the six non-naturals whose moderate use is of benefit to the body. There is required in addition to these a suitable measure of active and passive qualities related to a third, which is the heart. For it seems that a longer space of life follows upon as much as possible a hidden complexional preparation of the heart. It happens that a man of a well-mixed complexion who uses a proper regimen will end with a swifter death, although this rarely happens, while another man may live longer although he follows an ill-mixed or evil regimen. In fact, it is not impossible, as Averroes says,[46] that there may be two men of similar complexion directed equally by the same regimen; one, however, will reach the optimum length of life according to nature while the other will incur death on account of the evil humors which are generated in him. Averroes says that the cause of this situation is the bad preparation fixed in his complexion which creates his ill even if we do not know just what this preparation is. The reason for this ignorance is that in natures there are so many fixed preparations that we are unable to recognize them by their signs. They call these preparations certain individual dispositions following assigned material from the astrological sources named Ylech and Alcochodem according to which they are associated with these variables. They are perhaps properly such as one composed from the four elements, according to greater and lesser proportion of these elements in composition determined by chance according to the influences of the fixed stars in regard to an inferior form of components and they influence these according to the suitability of the material for forms which are given in accordance with the merits of the material. That which has given material of form under the diversity of dispositions just as under the diversity of merits is the mingling of the heavens as can be observed more fully because nothing is brought to birth by the nature of things without some hidden cause. But with all these

[46] 6. 94v.

causes which induce old age more quickly and death through violence a death thus brought about is called properly an extinction because it is caused by the putrefaction of the humid nutriment from an improper regimen of things happening by necessity to the human body. This condition must be resisted by a regimen prohibitive of the generation of putrefaction for the protection of the body from the power of extraneous intrinsic and extrinsic heat.

Chapter V

The Causes of Certain Accidental Accompaniments of Old Age, Especially of Gray Hairs, Wrinkles, and Baldness

Gray hair and wrinkles of the skin are special accidents consequent upon old age, accompanied sometimes also by baldness, more rarely however than the other two. Those who examine the causes of these accidents and first of gray hair say that what they call true grayness and Plautus[47] calls *canitudo* is a feebleness of hair caused by aging of the body declining in this manner to frigidity and nothing other than a bad cold and dry disposition. This occurs since the proper innate heat is the power of digestion of food, putrefying and corrupting external matter through the lapse of the body to coldness and dryness with cold dominating the aliment coming to the members, diminished by the heat of digestion for the most part putrefied and corrupted by that action to a watery frigid humor which is phlegmatic and putrescent. Thus the vapor which is the material of hair arising from such aliment with its viscosity by weakness of its propelling heat does not easily pass through. Therefore throughout its length like a pore it putrefies through the heat of its contents and when it putrefies it grows gray because it has very much air closed up in it through its viscosity, wherefore the hair grows gray. Hence gray hair is so called as a shining *(canities)* is called from *candor.* This happens in every digestion for this indigestion which is caused in flesh creates gray hairs, as Aristotle tell us.[48] They say it is an indication that this happens by a certain putrefaction of vapor because we see that hairs covered with hats and coverings of other kinds grow gray more quickly because the covering prevents the wind from blowing the hair and thus preventing putrefaction. Also more gray hairs are

[47]Apud Paul. ex Fest. p. 62 Müller; Lindsay 54.
[48]Aristotle, *G. A.* 784b30; 785a1–25.

first created on the temples[49] because the phlegmatic humidity in the muscles of the temples which irrigates them is intercepted. Hence they call such men *temporicani* (of gray temples), as is handed down in the old lore, for example, by Alexander on Problems.[50] According to the explanation of the generation of gray hairs just given they declare that fruit and watery vegetables produce gray hairs, for while the blood remains thick, heavy, warm, and viscous the hairs are black but when it tends toward wateriness the hairs incline toward grayness. Hence Avicenna[51] bids us to avoid fruit in order to ward off gray hairs; we should also avoid humid vegetables, milk, rye boiled in water, gruel, and drinking much water. He also tells us that excessive sexual indulgence creates gray hairs for it sends the superfluous humors to the extremities of the body and dries out the warm putrid vapor coming to the upper part of the skin where it putrefies. Since the cause of the whiteness of hairs is similar to that of wrinkles in the skin which they call "goatified" skin from its similarity to the horns of goats therefore they have said that the subcutaneous vapor which is manifest in the body is earthy and has very much the nature of heavy air. This touches and congeals it and then it is like a flat piece of ice, or it is not congealed, as it happens, and when putrefied it makes wrinkles in the thinner, more exposed parts of the skin. The thicker parts are contracted because that vapor does not congeal them but covers them against the cold. Corrugation is an adverse condition of the body caused by some kind of icy congealing. Wrinkles and ice are similar in consistency as to their cause, for they arise from a vapor existing in a non-similar form although both are somehow a putrefaction of vapor;[52] hence Homer[53] rightly called old age wrinkling and ice. Wrinkles are caused by a too great drying-out of the skin with coldness, for when dryness is increased men become wrinkled, as Galen says.[54] Dryness causes

[49]Ibid.

[50]Alexandri Problemata, ed. A. Poliziano, 203, in *Problemata Aristotelis ac philosophorum medicorumque complurium,* etc.; London: George Bishop, 1583. Homer, *Iliad* 8. 518; Bacchylides, fr. 21, 2, use the word *poliocrotaphos,* gray at the temples.

[51]Avicenna, II, 569.

[52]Aristotle, *G. A.* V. 784b5–10.

[53]Not found in Homer, but see *Com. Adesp.* 650 a, cf. 381, ed. T. Kock, CAF; 3 vols., 1880–88: mould and frost of old age.

[54]Galen, 17 B. 650.

laxity and coldness causes corrugation because coldness by stretching a fold of the skin over another folds them together and thus creates wrinkles. White hairs and wrinkles are caused by the malfunction or error of the third digestive power which is abundant in the members. The salutary remedies for all these conditions in the body will be set forth in their places, especially in chapter XLIV. In addition baldness, which is nothing other than a certain natural lack of hair, sometimes occurs and more in old age than in any other period, for at that time due to the superabundant dryness in the entire extent of the aged body the material to be converted to hair is taken away. A greater rarefaction of the pores occurs by which the retention of hair is prevented with the cooperation of excessive dryness of the anterior part of the head which is called the skull. A great dryness of the sinciput results in a paucity of the brain and its shrinkage from the cranium by which the latter is dried so that the glutinous humidity of the hair roots does not remain glued to the skin. This happens more in the anterior part[55] of the head than in the more sensitive and thinner part for which it is rendered more suitable because of dryness with the result that the hair grows less in dimension. In the anterior part the skin is closer to the skull and more free from flesh by which it must be humidified. Thus when the brain is diminished and along that part of the skull the skin dries out and withers the hairs fall. For this reason their regeneration does not occur further. Those men who undergo this change are called *recalvastri* [bald in front]. Among the three accidents which especially accompany old age are wrinkles and gray hairs; these afflict the elderly of whatever nature and more or less inseparably. Thus it is as appropriate in old age for a man to grow gray as it is to have wrinkles. Thus there is no one through all the periods of age running to the end of life who is not hampered and marked by such disgraceful disfigurement. Although in all people who become progressively weaker the innate heat decreases in some, however, the process is swifter than in others. They point this out because when an idea in the cold dry brain of man is put in motion swiftly around the head all men become old and thus grow gray more quickly, which does not happen with the ideas of other bad tem-

[55]Aristotle, *G. A.* V, 784a.

peraments of the brain. For it is said[56] also that white hairs are attributed to man alone of the animals in old age because man alone among all the animals properly grows bald and gray for the brain in the heads of other animals in proportion to the size of their bodies is small but not very humid.[57] Therefore the heat which digests or consumes it completely overcomes the humidity. Among other animals white hairs sometimes appear, however, as in horses because the bones of the horse's head are softer and thinner than the bones of other brutes.[58] They say that a proof of this fact is that a slight blow delivered on a horse's head, especially on the temples, will kill it at once. Often gray hairs appear before old age sets in. This is due to continual illnesses, fear of a terrible death, a long period of grief, or the lapse of the natural brain toward cold and dryness. Isigonus Nicaeensis[59] writes that some men in Albania are gray from childhood. No one says that the same thing occurs with wrinkles, however, except by chance through a wasting illness and atrophy, which is a substantial consumption of the radical humidity that happens in the case of hectic fever of the third kind. According to the old proverb gray hairs are an undependable sign of old age but wrinkles are a sure sign of it. Baldness does not necessarily accompany old age nor is inseparable from it, for one can find old men to whom baldness does not come even before they die. Baldness occurs in man alone just as does gray hair but not always and not to every man, which is easily perceived as Galen tells us.[60] Those whose brain inclines by nature toward warmth and is temperate and dryer beyond equality do not grow bald easily or swiftly. Those of a moister brain do not grow bald at all or do so at least somewhat more slowly. For this reason Galen[61] says that a person whose skin with advancing age is more inclined toward dryness and hardness will find that all his members grow cold, dry out, and wither. The skin becomes earthy in consistency and unsuitable for the growing of hair for it remains like solid ice which compresses the pores and prevents the en-

[56]Ibid., *Probl.* 891b; 898a30; *G. A.* V, 780b5.
[57]Ibid., *G. A.* V, 784a; *De Long. et Brev. Vitae* 466a25.
[58]Aristotle, *G. A.*, V. 785a10.
[59]Pliny, *N. H.* 7. 27.
[60]Galen, 1. 621.
[61]Ibid., 1. 620.

trance of anything. Therefore they also say that baldness shines like a mirror. Such a condition does not occur in those whose brain is warm and humid by nature; in fact, these people do not easily grow bald. This does not occur in like fashion with those whose brain is cold and dry, for coldness is more dominant than dryness, nor with those whose brain is cold and humid.

Chapter VI

The Signs Indicating Old Age Both Prognostic and Demonstrative

There arise with old age certain revealing indications which are accidents proper to and associated with it. The accidents proper to old age lead to a knowledge of the subject. These indications are wrinkles in the skin of the body and especially of the face and white hairs due to a progressive loss of innate heat. Not only do these appear as the stigmata of old age but they are what they call the banner of approaching death. If anyone grows bald with age so that his head is rendered naked old age is very close to him, for the natural loss of hair they say takes place closer to old age because at that time the causes of baldness are more vigorous. If the hairs of the eyebrows grow abundant and the eyes become hollow spontaneously these are indications of old age, as the poet who has grown old says:

> And where neat eyebrows brought together lashes
> Now a rough forest overhangs and covers
> As though the eyes were stowed in some dark cavern:
> What fierce and frightful thing they see I know not.[62]

In some old people the eyebrows[63] become so long that they brush the parts that lie below in the conjunction of the bones, and while they grow old a greater humidity penetrates because the bones are apart from each other. The more the consumption of the humidity proceeds which is conjoined and which drills through more sections which are in the bones of the eyebrows the more the vapor emitted extends the hairs and the construction of the senile body is rendered almost like a ruined and broken building, as Aristotle

[62]Maximianus, *Elegies* 1. 139–42.
[63]Aristotle, *Probl.* 878b25; *P. A.*, II. 658b20.

says.[64] Such people especially experience being subject to continuous meditations because the heat and spirit in them move more to the anterior part of the head. Hence they say they are in greater need of shearing, just as with the hair of the head. The witnesses of old age are the loss of some of their operations or of all the animal powers which serve voluntary motion and when the spontaneous power of love-making is no longer felt nor its accustomed delight experienced in it, according to the poet stricken with old age:

> The gifts of love and wine are now unpleasant,
> And now sweet banquets and delights grow harmful.
> We must abandon everything that pleases;
> That we may live, we are deprived of living.[65]

Those who for a long time suffer the continual and painful prostration of nature with eventual involuntary resolution of power grow old twice. This is what the poet also means when he says:

> Dejected nature abides, which hour by hour
> Dwindles and dribbles away with its own weakness.[66]

The next line declares that old age is not spontaneously pleased by what used to please. Hence:

> No medicines avail though I often take them,
> Nor anything which once could soothe my cares.[67]

If a change of form should happen against his will, a change of color, dryness of skin, stiffness of tendons, itching of the body, so that he who once was of fuller and more handsome coloring becomes emaciated, deformed, discolored, it is clear that old age is at hand, while the old poet says:

> The handsome looks I loved have now departed,
> And now I seem to be as dead as they.
> Instead of my healthy red and white complexion
> A pallor stains my face, bloodless as death.
> My parched skin dries, stiff tendons stand out on it,
> And claw-like hands now scratch my itching limbs.

[64]Aristotle, *P. A.*, II. 658b14–26.
[65]Maximianus, *Elegies* 1. 163, 154–56.
[66]Ibid., 165–66.
[67]Ibid., 167–68.

To gaze at an old man now brings fear, nor can you
Believe that he's a man, who lacks man's reason.[68]

I have told in the prologue with which sufferings the aged are afflicted. These are difficulty in breathing and in urination, catarrh, strangury, and so forth, especially insomnia, nightmares which press upon old men with the sadness old age brings them, as Galen says.[69] Of this kind are also doubtless unaccustomed troubled dreams. The old poet says:

Rest also, which for all is very pleasant,
Sleep flies away, scarce comes back late at night,
Or if it ever honors our tired limbs
Disturbs and horrifies with what strange dreams!
I'm forced to rise at midnight in distress
And suffer much lest I should suffer worse.
I'm conquered by an infirm body; whither
I do not wish I'm dragged unhappily.[70]

If an old person is distressed by his accustomed foods which without noticeable alteration have the power of restoring the forces of the body dreaded old age is thus stricken by both satiety and inanition, as the poet says:[71]

I whom no raw or adverse foods had troubled,
See how a regimented diet burdens!
I liked big meals; soon I'll regret I ate them.
It's better to abstain; abstention grieves me.
That which was good for me now is forbidden.
My pampered taste is gone that once delighted.

An old man, they say, exists in ills when he is troubled by spontaneous sadness, envying those things which used to delight his sight, which the poet also feels when he says:

Why do not public spectacles relieve me?[72]

If without apparent cause destruction or removal of the forces of external feeling occur to a person or diminution or corruption of

[68]Ibid., 131–36, 143–44.
[69]Galen, 5. 416; 8. 342; 11. 59; 16. 175.
[70]Maximianus 1.249–52, 255–58.
[71]Ibid., 157–62.
[72]Ibid., 175.

their operation he fears lest he fall into old age almost immediately. The poet says:

Now hearing is less, taste less, my very eyes
Grow dim; I barely know the things I touch,
No smell is sweet, no pleasure now is grateful:[73]

When anyone is unable to see small objects up close which however he can see at some distance,[74] if this happens to him without cause except through the limitation of age, this is old age. The vision of older people is weak because of their lack of humidity due to the sharp reduction of it by light, as the experts say. When therefore the color which exists in the act of vision has light joined with it it will greatly alter things too close so that they can see nothing else; that which is remote will be more within their sight, wherefore the visual impression will be weaker and more fleeting, as the poet says:

If I read books, the letters split in two,
The page I knew seems larger than it was.
I seem to see a bright light through the clouds;
The clouds themselves are brighter within my eyes.
Daylight is gone though I still live; who will
Deny that hell is fenced with opaque darkness?[75]

If constantly and without any other cause the eyes fill with tears it is clear that old age is near, as the poet says:

Once smiling eyes now weep with endless tears,
Both night and day deplore their punishment.[76]

They say that a three-fold damage of the mind's operation occurs: lessened activity, that is, alienation and corruption especially of the voluntary inward activity of the cognitive powers because of which old men are said to be delirious; this is a fault of old age. For the poet says:

Lethean oblivion comes upon my mind
Nor can it now, confused, remember itself;

[73]Ibid., 119–21.
[74]Aristotle, *Probl.* 960a, 960a20.
[75]Maximianus 1.145–50.
[76]Ibid., 137–38.

It rises to meet no demand, with the body weakens,
Is stupefied, concentrating on its ills.[77]

Change of accustomed habits without manifest cause is also a sign of impending death and especially with a certain maturity and gravity. His time is given to each of us, as Cicero[78] says, as weakness to children, great vigor to youth, and gravity to advancing age. Thus they attribute maturity or gravity to old age but frivolity to childhood, as the poet says:

The boy delights in games, old age in sternness.[79]

Stability of will is also appropriate to old age, as Avicenna[80] tells us. Everything concerning habits is understood as having its appropriate nature at each stage of life. For it can be regarded as almost monstrous or a perversion of the stages of life for a boy to have the habits of an old man or for an old man to have the habits of a boy. This is beyond doubt a sign of premature death, as Cato the Censor[81] was accustomed to say. To be stricken with continual long illnesses both of body and mind which are spontaneous testifies to an old age not only to be dreaded but to be feared, for just as from both such forms of illness sometimes gray hairs arise which are particular companions of old age, as has been said earlier, so also there comes with them a swift, nay precipitous, old age. They call[82] an old age that comes because of disease "acquired" old age and old age a "natural disease," whence the poet:

Thus itches trouble, thus wracking cough fatigues us.
Sick old age has nothing but complaints.
Thus cares concerned with everything torment me,
Thus no repose is given to my soul.
I who can't pile up wealth strive to retain it,
Yet feel that while I keep it I've kept none.[83]

Yet they assert that old age is to be expected, nay, we must stand ready for it; it is at hand, full of a willing although not customary

[77]Ibid., 123–26.
[78]Cicero, *De Sen.* 10, 33.
[79]Maximianus, *Elegies* 1. 105.
[80]Avicenna, I, 53.
[81]Cicero, *De Sen.* 33, 36.
[82]Aristotle, *G. A.* V. 784b30.
[83]Maximianus, *Elegies* 1. 245–46, 191–94.

expectancy, credulity, and madness toward all coming events, as the poet says:

Trembling, doubtful, the old man is expectant
Of ill, dreads foolishly his every act.
He praises the past, despises the present years,
Thinks only that is right wherein he's wise . . .
His listener's gone but he keeps right on talking:
Brave oldsters, brave in babbling alone!
He fills the air with clamoring in vain:
Nothing's enough; he shrinks from what once pleased him.
He laughs with those who mock him and, applauding
Himself, grows happier in his very shame.[84]

When without cause anyone is troubled by whatever change of the season whether natural or non-natural, that is old age as the complaining old men say:

The torture's being alive; we burn with sunshine, . . .
The gentle days of Spring and Fall afflict us.
The dewdrops injure, we melt in a little shower,
The clouds are harmful, cold and air annoy us.[85]

Well known to all old age are the spontaneous changes of habitual gait and color as if suddenly color and grace have faded and been lost, the curvature of limbs, the shrinking and bending over of the entire body, all of which happen to an old man; now his future welfare must become doubtful to him, if we believe the poet when he says:

First fruits of death, age flows down in his limbs,
Seeks his extremities by these degrees:
His carriage, color, walk as he goes by,
His shape are not the same as they once were.
His cloak falls down from shoulders hunching over
And what was short now seems to him quite long.
Though thin, the bed clothes press with heavy weight.
We shrink together, grow wonderfully smaller;
You'd think our very bones have been diminished.
We can't look upward; old age now looks downward
At earth from which it came, soon to return,

[84]Ibid., 195–98, 203–208.
[85]Ibid., 241, 244, 243, 242.

Becomes three-footed, four, like little babies,
And creeps in sorrow on the filthy ground.
Thus leaning on his cane old age decaying
Strikes sluggish earth with his repeated blows
In rhythmic steps that bring a sure applause.[86]

When all these ills appear in old age old men fall backward as though in a kind of ruin for then there occurs what was destined to happen, he becomes ready to fall, that is, frequently falling.

[86]Ibid., 209–14, 254, 215–20, 223–25.

Chapter VII

The Foreknowledge of the Brevity and Longevity of Life

This especially must be known to begin with that the fate of every creature in the world depends upon the signs of their planets, as iron clings to a lode stone, as Ptolemy says.[87] To arrive at a judgment as to the extent of a man's life one must carefully observe the powers of the aspects of his stars and their conjunction in both strength and weakness. Their duration for the extent of the life of a man as also of other generative factors is of great importance although (as is believed by law) not every kind of necessity is imposed by them. Men's actions can be impeded by these factors either through free will or by some disposition of matter. Thus you will know that the duration of all aspects and of all conjunctions and the powers of all the stars in the circle of the heavens which come forth in the first conception of a man concerning the brevity or longevity of life can be known in advance. Nonetheless, so that we may approach the subject insofar as it pertains to the physician we must say that the following factors are particularly conducive to the extension of life: a good celestial aspect; moderate use of the six non-naturals; more healthful foods; a more perfect complexion, especially the influence of the principal members upon the entire body by necessity, particularly of the heart itself. Thus for all members, and most of all the heart, their complexional proportion must be observed in order to predict the length or brevity of life. These factors which form the inherent material basis for reasoning must not be departed from, according to the experts, because the man in whose complexion the natural active powers dominate the passive powers with a proper proportion between them and furthermore of all these in respect to the heart has a longer life. As was said, the life of man universally follows his

[87]Ptolemy, *Tetrabiblos* 1. 3. 13.

complexional proportion, and they say a man is of a well-mixed complexion when this proportion prevails. Often to men whose viscera and powers are strong pernicious diseases befall by which they incur a premature death. Others of weaker power reach ultimate old age although their regimen is similar. Some men also troubled by severe illness live a long time while many of good consistency die young. They ascribe the difference in life-spans to their variation in this complexional proportion with an abundance of heat and humidity and the domination of active powers. For this reason they think that very many who have a complexion suitable for a long span of life have a complexion unknown to the science of medicine or that it is difficult to know since it is very hard to perceive through the senses; it is indeed rather more perceptible through the reason than through the senses. The proportion, as Averroes says,[88] is naturally unknown. What, however, it is has been explained in the previous chapter IV in its place. Haly Rodoan,[89] upon whose statement the preceding opinion is based, has said that the complexion of a warm and humid man is carefully preserved; in him the humors *[chimi]* are balanced, and he escapes from the illnesses brought on by putrefaction; as a consequence his nature is one of a longer life than that of a man with a different complexion, for, as Galen says,[90] those of a very humid and warm complexion are the longest lived, nor does this prevent, as the experts affirm, the complexion of a longer life from having less perfect operations. In fact, such a person is more prone to illness with an equable complexion because of the intemperance or lack of proper mixture of hot and humid; nevertheless, he is more likely to have a longer life because he has an intrinsic cause for longevity. Therefore, if the complexion is a little excessive in heat and humidity it will escape as they say from the putrefactions to which especially while he is young he will be prone. This will prove a cause for the extension of his life. The median complexion, however, is not prone to these putrefactions. Men of good consistency do not die young because they do not have that complexional proportion which Averroes touched upon but because they misuse it in one way or another and hence there arise pernicious diseases

[88]Averroes, *Colliget* II, 50r.
[89]See note 38.
[90]Galen, 6. 400.

nor does the physician in brief judge them to have long life because this does not depend alone upon an intrinsic cause which preserves it. Haly[91] in his *Theory* discusses the subject in this manner: that man is of a shorter life by nature whose complexion is from the beginning cold and dry. That man comes next in brevity of life whose complexion is cold only; the latter is followed by the man whose complexion is dry only; next comes the man whose complexion is warm and dry, then the one whose complexion is equable, finally, the man whose complexion is warm and humid. Hippocrates[92] says that fat men furthermore according to their nature die more quickly than more slender men. Galen[93] properly agrees that bodies not very fat nor very thin are best for extending life; if they remain thus constantly they will live to an ultimate old age. Averroes[94] says fleshy old men live longer since the cause of abundance of flesh is warmth and humidity. Further, they wish that the sixty-third year of life which Augustus called the ladder of life should be particularly observed, for it has been much tested by the memory of men, as Aulus Gellius[95] says, for often older men in that year of their lives experience peril and some misfortune through a rather severe illness, destruction of life, or sickness of mind. The word "ladder" *[scalarius]* just as *scandarius* comes from *scandendo,* climbing, that is, ascending, or *scalenon,* that is, graded by steps, for a *gradus* [step] is what all old men use when they climb. Thus far men whose parts from the umbilicus downward toward the pecten are larger than those which stretch from the umbilicus to the cavity of the chest, that is, at the pomegranate, which is a certain scutal cartilage made to protect the mouth of the stomach the physiognomists say are short-lived and with a bad quality of complexion. They are sickly, for their stomachs are cold because of their small size, their stricture, and their position in the body. Therefore, they cannot digest their food since digestion is completed with the aid of heat. When this happens an excessive amount of raw matter is generated in their bodies and gathers to-

[91]Haly Filius Abbas, *Liber Totius Medicinae, Liber Secundus, Theorice;* Lugduni: J. Myt, 1523, f. 142r.
[92]Hippocrates: see Galen, 17. B 547.
[93]Galen: see note 90.
[94]6. 94v.
[95]Aulus Gellius, 15. 7. 2; 3. 10. 9.

gether. This makes the person sickly since the excess of matter is the antecedent cause of illness, which easily passes to the adjoining parts. It is further to be observed that men of long life are curved in the shoulders. The rarity and weakness of the teeth also indicate the weakness of the entire body and a brevity of life. This must be understood as applying to many men, for the scarcity of teeth as the physicians say can result from the small amount of the material of generation. With the domination of the formative power which then prevails when it lacks sufficient material it elects rather to make few teeth by not sending forth material to them since from that power and that material the more principal parts are created. With the proper medical regimen, however, life can be extended even with a rarity of teeth and their weakness. Nor similarly do the heavenly bodies refuse to give any individual long years because of the scarcity of their teeth. There is reason in the statement of Rhazes[96] that from the rarity of teeth it is recognized that the bone of each jaw will be depressed and compacted and that every bone of the cranium is compacted and non-porous by which it is indicated that the humidity was not sufficiently obedient to the formative power in obtaining extension wheresoever and figuration of the bone according to that power. Hence it happens that the brain is rendered infirm because the superfluity brought to it cannot be removed from it. When it is thus retained the brain becomes naturally very humid and more moistened and then happens to be suffocated and quickly putrefied. On account of the respiration which is thus prevented the brain becomes associated with external heat; thus there are two perfective causes of putrefaction. That which putrefies is not of long duration. Those who have many teeth furthermore, especially more than thirty-two, as in many people, are said to be longer-lived. Those who have less teeth or are without them are shorter-lived. Averroes is authority for the statement that a scarcity of bile results in a good temperament and long life. These words are ridiculed by some who are surprised at them as erroneous, but the cause of the error, as Albertus says,[97] is that they have considered some animals with soles and hoofs such as

[96]Rhazes, *Liber Rasis ad Almansorem, Opera;* Basle: Henricpetrus, 1544, IV, 18.
[97]Albertus Magnus, *De Animalibus Libri XXVI,* ed. H. Stadler, 1920, II, 1373–74; Aristotle, *H. A.*, II, 506a20, 33; 506b4 is his source. On the chiromantic signs see Aristotle, *Probl.* 896a35; 964a30–35.

deer and such like creatures which lack bile and live a long time and have similarly considered those creatures without soles of this kind such as dolphins and camels which have hoofs and have not taken into consideration other animals which have bile and are long-lived. If they had considered these they would not have said that the lack of bile was the cause of long life because perhaps it will be the cause of a short life if the bile is not expunged from the food or if the bile does not sting the intestines. From the lack or diminution of the bile or from the obstruction of the bile-duct which leads to the intestines sometimes colic is caused. It is more correct to say that the nature of the liver is the cause of a long or a short life since the liver is a principal organ in all blooded animals. The liver is the organ which has such a superfluity of bile or requires it, and the other principal organs do not have such a superfluity since neither the heart nor the lung nor the brain has bile. It is impossible for the bilious humidity to approach the heart since it cannot suffer any such strong infirmities. But the liver is one of the organs which requires that such a superfluity takes place in it and therefore it happens that bile occurs in the liver only. The chiromantics say that very long fingers are a sign of a short life. The protraction of lines which appears extended within the entire palm of the hand indicates a shorter life. The experts assign this cause, for when these lines are symmetrically and ideally shaped by the formative power they are at an extreme distance from the heart. This is a sign that the power existing in the closer parts is very strong in the body as to influencing life. But when there are two short lines in the palm they signify that the material from the inordinate and endless formative power dominates and thus the period of life is rendered shorter because it putrefies before its time. The equilateral triangle which results in the palm from three large lines naturally protracted therein signifies a faithful long life and a man lovable and famous. This triangle results from the line which passes through the length of the palm diagonally caused by the curvature of the thumb to the interior of the palm and from the line which stretches toward the side caused by the curvature of the index finger with the other fingers to the inner part of the hand beginning from the upper side of the hand and from another line arising near the base of the palm with the resulting fold of the thumb toward the fingers and the fold of the hand toward the inner part along its length. This is agreed among authors. They report the cause as follows. The extension of these lines through the entire hand and their manifest dearticulation show the material by which the hand and the entire body have been animated to be sufficiently digested and tempered uniformly so that it receives the extension perfected by the dominant formative power, for if the formative power can thus form parts so distant from the heart and distinguish them separately this denotes its great power over the heart and other principal organs in influencing life and that the hands are suitably proportioned to the heart since also in the exterior substance of the heart there are to be found linear sections like sutures to such an extent that hearts more articulated and characterized by separations with manifest sections are present in more sensitive animals. Those animals with less sensitivity have hearts which are articulated, such as pigs, as Aristotle says.[98] For such a natural power which is thus manifested in the parts of the body causes life and its continuation for a long time. Those who are called *auriti* have long ears. They are said to be stupid and long-lived. Rhazes[99] also says that when a man appears to be like a boy and his entire face and eyes appear to be smiling he is happy and will have a long life. These are the words of the wise which have been collected from their statements. Thus there is no doubt that in bodies themselves something can be foreknown of the longevity or brevity of life nor is this foreknowledge to be regarded as empty and frivolous since its reasons are assigned by the experts. Whatever Pliny has marvelled at he attributes to Aristotle.[100] In fact, nothing has yet been said of the signs as to the leaden color and many incisions which are temporary in the hand and are the signs of a short life. On the other hand, the signs of a long life are curved shoulders and two incisions in one hand, according to the experts, since the judgment can be made by the aforesaid signs. There are certain properties of men without cognizance of which it is not easy to predict anything in the future; therefore they do not wish to depend on only one sign but insofar as is possible their aggregation must be considered to discover if there occurs any contrariety among the significations and to measure their powers and their

[98]Aristotle, *P. A.* 667a5.
[99]IV, 19.
[100]Pliny, *N. H.* 8. 16. 43–44.

testimony and then to incline toward the stronger indications and witnesses also when there are many of them upon which to base a judgment. For it is the basic confidence in the reliability of these signs which much oftener and to a greater extent reveals old men. One must listen to reason and to what is said as in many other matters. For they say that the universals of medicine and everything which concerns perceived matter should be verified in common and at length since that skill becomes conjectural with which often not only conjecture but experience does not correspond. Even when they correspond these factors quite often deceive us anyway, wherefore each man should persevere to persuade himself as to the truth of what appears evident to him the more he sees it because signs taken from the defect of the powers of the spirit and of the body spontaneously signify old age. However, they say that this defect does not occur in each and every old man. For Cyrus when he was dying as Xenophon describes him[101] gloried in the fact that he had never felt his old age to be weaker than his youth had been. Old age has not incapacitated or afflicted some who are even decrepit, by a miracle; they say that this is a solitary example. Xenophilus the musician lived one hundred and five years without any discomfort of body.[102] This defect of powers in old age is more often brought about by the vices of youth, as Cicero[103] says, than by old age, for a libidinous and intemperate youth brings an infected body to old age. This is the judgment concerning the actions of the spirits, for among old men the natural disposition abides as long as zeal and industry abide.

[101]Xenophon, *Cyropaedia* 8. 7. 6.
[102]Valerius Maximus 8. 13, ext. 2; Pliny, *N. H.* 7. 50. 51, 168.
[103]Cicero, *De Sen.* 29.

Chapter VIII

The Necessity or Inevitability of the Advent of Old Age; Of Man As He Passes Through the Stages of Life to Death in an Orderly Manner

They say that death by its nature cannot be avoided by any kind of benefit since the nature of man's condition provides a place for it, generally corrupting everything at some time or other, according to the poet:

> All things seek whence they rose, seek out their mother,
> Go back to nothing, which nothing was before.[104]

Because death is inevitable it is not possible to find any kind of medicine which will prevent it and to preserve life forever, as Haly Rodoan[105] says. Old age is also inevitable for all animals as they proceed through the stages of life to its very last day however much they are nourished and cared for with moderation. It is impossible therefore to prevent the wasting away of old age, but it is possible to combat it and to resist it considerably, as Galen[106] says, unless by chance this may be regarded among the miracles of nature. For they say that in those places where there are no shadows during the day men live one hundred and thirty years and do not grow old but die in middle age. Leaving aside such cases as being prodigies and passing on to matter beyond doubt we must more truthfully agree with Rabi Moyses[107] and other experts who tell us that the advent of old age although it can be slowed cannot be prevented. For this conclusion the experts, advised and informed by the principles of nature, adduce many effective reasons. First, the argu-

[104]Maximianus, *Elegies* 1. 221–22.
[105]Haly Rodoan, see notc 38.
[106]Galen, 7. 681.
[107]Rabi Moyses, *Aphorismi,* f. 24.

ment is taken from the extraneity and dissimilarity of the food of the animal body from its beginning. After it has incorporated in the members something of the extraneous it contains this for some time altering the powers of the members since every physical action has its reaction and everything that is acted upon acts in some manner. However, the alterations of the powers acting upon each other by confusing and dulling the organs of the limbs and the complexional qualities also render some of these powers weak. With all of these actions following each other often and for a long time it is necessary that the member itself should incur putrefaction through old age. Furthermore, that which is composed of particulars such as is every animal will sometime separate its mingled components to a distance, such as the light parts upward and the heavy parts downward before they disintegrate together with a little melting. Thus the powers, mixed and especially animated and more perfected, will begin to be slowed down as to qualities and for a space of time to be impeded and thus to incur what we call old age. They argue further that no generated animate creature even if it should be nourished with recently absorbed nutriment can avoid the end of old age which is coming to it for the nourishment cannot be assimilated, whatever it may be, except by a heat which opens the substance of the member and divides the substance of the nutriment through the pores of the member. For everything which is thus often divided by heat must be thickened and hardened after some substantial humidity is swallowed and the more it does this so much less susceptible it is to restoration.[108] Thus it is necessary for the member to contract and stiffen when a substantial humidity is drawn forth from it. Furthermore, the warmth of the surrounding air dissolves the body of the animal by drawing forth its humidity when that too is warm. Hence it results that the members remain dry inside and cold, but on the exterior they are humid with external moisture, and of such a disposition is old age, as has been said above. Furthermore, every animate creature is either quiet or in motion. If it is quiet its frigidity of complexion grows strong and is thickened and humidity and heat are extinguished; consequently, death and dissolution are induced. Of this condition old age is a prelude. If the creature is in motion its heat

[108]Aristotle, *G. A.* V. 783a35-b5-10; 84a35-b3.

by frequent movement is kindled; this draws out the humidity in cooperation with the heat, thus inducing old age. Furthermore, living creatures cannot refrain from motion which exercises the powers for all of them, such as imagination, feeling, thinking, and so forth, which by drawing out spirit and heat to the surrounding area destroys humidity and induces old age. They argue further as follows. Just as every animate creature whatsoever regulated in its species is for some time strengthened in power if it observes what is convenient for itself so also its power is rendered weaker by that very same regimen which has been mentioned, for just as by the accession of natural heat to the members it grows so by the recession of heat it grows less at which time there is less restoration in it because natural resolution is equal in time to the corruption of substantial generation and old age is correctly called corruption, since it is the path to corruption whose cause is a defect of nature from within because the human powers in time begin a withdrawal of heat from the members which is debilitating to all species. Thus it is necessary for every living thing whatsoever to undergo some old age even if unimpeded it observes its own convenience. Physicians use these and many other reasons to demonstrate the necessity of old age; nevertheless, it concerns the doctor to proceed in another way. The principles of particular sciences such as that of medicine should receive credit. The art of medicine does not pass over or dispense with the consideration of those things which concern sensible or perceptible matter because the entire basis of demonstration is sense-perception, as Galen says,[109] and in that which passes beyond the senses there is no consideration of medicine since the intellect of the physician examines almost everything by the senses. Therefore the inevitability of old age insofar as it pertains particularly to the physician nevertheless, with Galen, is proven by the following reason. The universal works of nature are inevitable since they possess a necessary order of generation. Old age, however, although it may not be according to nature just like those works of nature, is none the less nourished and increased beyond doubt following the necessity of nature. For old age and whatever accompanies it arrive naturally since nothing occurs so much according to nature as death for old

[109]Galen, 18 B. 648, 652.

men, as Cicero[110] says. For if old age did not occur naturally one could continue to live and to be preserved from death as one is preserved from an illness, which is false. Therefore old age by necessity follows according to the works of nature. Thus necessity orders the situation everywhere so that no living being proceeding through the stages of its existence will ever be found who does not grow old. Not undeservedly therefore Galen [111] reprimands that mad old physician who published a book showing how anyone can remain ageless and produced the book when he was already forty years old. That physician having reached the age of eighty was then admonished to collect his gear before he passed from life, to use the words of M. Varro.[112] His face began to become livid, thin, and dry, sallow, deformed, hideous and unlike its former self, with dry skin, hanging cheeks, and with such wrinkles

> like those an old baboon carves on her jowls[113]

so that the Hippocratic face would be justly compared with it, whose nose was sharp, eyes hollow, temples sunken, ears cold, limp, and contracted, their fleshy part [lobe] turned inward, the skin of the forehead dry and stretched. This old physician, being derided, had not dared to teach thereafter but, correcting himself, put out another edition of his book which he called one about "admirable non-aging." In it he said that not all men could remain without aging but those who were best suited for it from their birth and had taken care of themselves could wish to make their bodies immortal.

[110]Cicero, *De Sen.* 71.
[111]Galen, 6. 63.
[112]M. Varro, *De Re Rustica* 1. 1.
[113]Juvenal 10. 195. The Hippocratic face: Hippocrates, *Prognostic* II.

Chapter IX

The Uncertain Termination of Old Age

They say that of blooded animals capable of walking the longest-lived are men and elephants.[114] The course of life of the man concerning whom the previous description was made is certain, with one simple way. It is not possible to give precisely the day and year of the span of life nor of old age nor any other stage of life except according to a certain latitude. All is uncertain, not only the location, as will be told in the following chapter XV but also the lot of birth and life assigned to each person, as the experts tell us. The natural or innate heat is mixed thoroughly in various ways, varied by those factors physicians call natural, that is, the elements, the natural humors which they call complexions, members, powers, operations, spirits, and what are contained in them. That heat is diversified also by those things which the physicians call non-natural, that is, air, food and drink, motion and rest, sleep and waking, inanition and repletion, and the affections of the mind which accompany these. It is varied likewise by things beyond nature and extraneous which physicians call illness, the cause and accident of illness. Furthermore, as those more skilled experts among physicians agree, a period of life can be prolonged and death retarded by the benefit of the science of medicine operating upon the human body. It is not therefore possible simply to assign a terminus to old age or any other period of life, as Galen[115] first of all declared in these words: We grow old by a cold mixture of fluids or temperament, some more swiftly, others more slowly according to one's nativity from the beginning as the temperament results from that source or additions to it or diet or illness or worry or such as immoderate dryness. Some people shortly after

[114]Aristotle, *G. A.* IV, 777b1.
[115]Galen, 7. 679–80.

their thirtieth year experience the beginning of decline, some after thirty-five. Since the change is different in each man it is not possible to find in all of them one span of life according to truth which is common to them, for the youth of many men arrives on account of the first complexion and different dispositions to which the body is changed on account of accidents which occur to it or because of change of habit in the middle space between two termini. Old age thus has no certain terminus;[116] the experts agree upon the uncertain period or term of life, for those who say the days of man are numbered follow the way of ignorant physicians, as Averroes says, with whom Cicero[117] agrees in these words: "For it is certain that one must die, but it is uncertain as to the day itself." Nor does death lie under human power. This can be asserted with reason, for, as was said, death as well as old age can be retarded. Those who ignore a healthy diet, as Galen says,[118] it is fitting for them to die more quickly according to the reason of nature and for those who are of opposite mind to live longer, which situation could not exist if a certain terminus were fixed to life. For a healing or salutary diet or the restorative art for old men is established for the postponement of death and consequently for retarding old age by which we learn that the innate heat and radical humidity which are the more perfect and vigorous principles of life can be conserved by prolonging a proportion of them for a long time or by generating sufficient humidity by drawing out the superfluous fomentation of heat or altering and tempering it. Nor is the restorative method in vain, for we call fruitless the shoe of one who has no footwear, as Aristotle says.[119] This opinion is contradicted, however, by some authors who voice an opposite one, speaking figuratively. When Aristotle says that the time and life of each man has its number and that it is determined, that is, that the order and extent of time and life of each man are measured by a period, for they call a period the time of duration which is determined by the revolutions of the heavens[120] by which it is fixed, on account of this a period is so called as if it were a circular measure

[116]Cicero, *De Sen.* 74.
[117]Ibid., 74.
[118]Galen, 14. 693.
[119]Aristotle, *G. A.* I. 723b30 (?).
[120]Ibid., IV. 777b15–778a10, and Appendices A and B (LCL).

from *peri-*, which is "around" and *-ydus (-odos)*, which is "modulation or consonance." Furthermore they object when he says: It is reasonable to expect that the times of all gestations and lives should be measured by their periods. They adduce the words of Job when he says: And thou hast appointed his bounds that he cannot pass.[121] Further, there is the opinion of Avicenna:[122] Each individual has fixed bounds which are diversified because of the diversity of complexion, and all this issues forth from divine precept. One must know how to understand all this because the extension of life, the period and limit of each living creature are determined by the kind of complexion which is contained within him or is dependent upon the specific modes of that complexion in that individual. First of all it must be said simply that the limits and period of life which are assumed in this way cannot be prolonged nor can that specific complexion be changed while life lasts into a complexion which must be appropriate to another living species for just as a man cannot be changed into an elephant so his complexion cannot be changed to another nor his limits of life to other limits. For to all men (since they are of one nature and species) there is adapted one period which is due them as a human species and a complexion which they call specific. Because of this it is rightly said that, speaking in absolute terms, insofar as it is part of the heavenly circle there is one period not only for an individual man but for each species whichsoever proper to one and the other. You may consider the discussion concerning the terminations of life and the period thereof in a second manner. It is possible for the terminations of life and of its period to be prolonged for, as was said, the complexion that is worse, such as the choleric, can be changed to a more perfect complexion such as the sanguine or temperate. Hence nothing prevents the terminations of an individual to be changed to the terminations and period of another. For the human species is preserved in its material with different forms of complexion which are specific to it, of which some are more perfect than others; one is born with a longer life-span conserved in a specific form of matter. Taking the terminations in a third manner the terminations of life of any one individual, sub-

[121]Job 14. 5.
[122]Avicenna, I, 53.

stantial and capable of generation, and especially of a man, could not be changed just as an individual of the same species could not be changed into another. The transmutation is primarily impossible. Hence the permutation of the complexion of one individual which they call hidden cannot be effected for that of another and for his terminations and periods in exchange. These complexions are individual preparations which are hidden; they have been discussed in chapters IV and VII previously. These preparations differ from the celestial powers which dominate the nativity (or horoscope) since they are as was said the result of these powers. For it is reasonable to say that since the individuals of the human species originate with one or the other constellation so they should be measured by one or the other period. Therefore Asclepiades[123] said that the determined space of life was to be accepted from the stars. Hence two authorities, the first from Aristotle, may be heard concerning the terminations of life and period commonly set down and the specific complexion with its consequences. For Aristotle believed the period he called determinate was of any species, not indeed narrow nor precise nor particular, but rather vague and indeterminate. There is given a determinate time inclusively or exclusively which is due the human species beyond which man cannot naturally live by art or nature even if he observes whatever conservative or resumptive regimen and such is as rightly said the minimum time past which any man cannot continue to live, for the life of man as man is not extended from within his sixtieth year nor as they say can this time be extended to the two hundredth year. But within these two broad limits human life is found to be terminated at various points. They do not assign the limit of life absolutely but only on an individual basis. Hence another period of life follows his manifest complexion such as sanguine, choleric, temperate, and so on; it is variable in respect to length, long or short. Another period follows his hidden complexion, entirely prefixed, immovable, permanent, and based upon the beginnings of his generation, that is, the measure of heat and humidity acquired from the beginnings of his generation. This pe-

[123]Asclepiades Prusensis: none of his works is extant but he is frequently quoted by Galen; see the index vol. 20 to C. G. Kühn's edition of Galen. See Pliny, *N. H.*, 2. 23, 28; 7. 160, on the relation of the stars to human life and Galen, 19. 530, on their place in medicine.

riod measures the natural arrival of this man insofar as he is a man. To the ultimate bounds of cold and dryness this period and the limits of life correspond nor can they pass beyond them. Concerning them, induced by the last two authorities, we must accept them, and such beyond doubt is the maximum time through which this man insofar as he is this man with such a complexion as this can last in life.

Chapter X

Old Age Must Be Called a Certain Disposition Beyond Nature and Also Natural

When the body is deficient in the highest degree of health it declines, as Galen says,[124] or because the foetus is poorly constituted from the beginning, or because thereafter from some cause it reaches a disposition beyond nature, or by reason of age it reaches by ultimate means an old age as a disposition beyond nature. This is a disposition absolutely deficient in equality not related to youth or adolescence, which are attended at any rate with hope. But death follows old age nor can an old man return to those earlier ages by any means whatsoever although the rate of its approach can somehow be retarded. Old age is furthermore called a disposition beyond nature because the health of the old man does not provide perfect operations with the perfection which the health of the young man provides. The mark of this is the fact that a boy grows well more easily after he or the young man is wounded than the older man on account of the natural difference in ages. Therefore the health of boys gives no cause for complaint, as Galen says,[125] but that of old men certainly does, for in all his actions an old man has no strength. Hence it is rightly said by Aristotle[126] that old age and all powerlessness make one weak. Therefore some call this disposition of decline neutral, others call it natural languor, the ancients called it simply a bad age, just as they were accustomed to call youth a good age. In absolute terms however old age is a natural disposition insofar as it is effected by some intrinsic principle, for growing old is according to nature, as Aristotle says.[127] The aged body while it maintains itself according to nature is healthy with a health it owes simply to that age, or as the experts now say old age is a form of illness which proceeds from

[124]Galen, 6. 389.
[125]Ibid., 7. 256–57.
[126]Aristotle, *De Resp.* 479a, b.
[127]Ibid., 479b.

the necessity of nature, as was said previously, for it follows the action of intrinsic and natural principles of innate heat and basic humidity. Those who thus bring in the resumptive art of old age will speak as many do concerning old age and of the end of the first stage of old age which now almost strikes at the door of final old age as suggested by its nature more frequently in the aged male as being nobler and stronger. For the female is a deformed male.[128] In old age they say a disease of the anus occurs in women, that is, a disease of old women just as aging is a disease of old men. Males similarly in all animal species are stronger except in panthers and bears, as Pliny[129] writes, and the female is universally more imperfect than the male, as Aristotle says,[130] especially in the human species. In fact, she seems to participate in no virtue except loyalty and the life of the male human they say is more easily prolonged than in the female[131] because the male is better able to digest food and to expel that which is superfluous and thus to live longer. His humidity is less watery and his heat more commensurate, which is the cause of long life. For this reason the male almost always is longer lived than the female in whatever species except where coition takes place,[132] as Aristotle writes. For the species which copulates and has much sperm grows old more quickly. For this reason a mule created from a horse and an ass is of longer life and the male sparrow is shorter-lived than the females. The discussion will concern principally the old man who is in good health. Physicians have well treated commensurate complexion according to all treatises and more according to the sanitive regimen. Hence the bodies of old men will be restored by whatever regimen, for when they decline that which harms the healthy also harms the sick, as Galen says.[133] Whatsoever will be brought forward in this *Gerontocomia* will be for the sake of extending old age and will be an assistance to life, not as a punishment. For life is not to be so extended, according to Pliny,[134] that it should be protracted by any means whatever.

[128]Aristotle, *G. A.*, II. 737a25; IV, 775a15; V, 784a10. On anal disease see Paulus ex Fest. 29, Müller; Placid. 435, Mai.
[129]Pliny, *N. H.*, 11, 263.
[130]Aristotle: see note 128.
[131]Aristotle, *Probl.* 896a35.
[132]Ibid., 896a35.
[133]Galen, 6. 403–404; 10. 41; 14.727.
[134]Pliny, *N. H.* 28. 9.

Chapter XI

The Purpose of the Gerontocomos in Caring for the Aged

They tell us that old age should be retarded along the path of resumption but not of conservation. The conservative method consists in the administration of those factors which properly preserve old age to that limit of life which is due the old man according to his first complexion and by this way the life span cannot be extended beyond that which is due to the first complexion of the individual. Yet it endeavors to preserve the old man's life and to extend it to its ultimate natural limit if he observes what is helpful to him. For this reason the conservation of life because of its difficulty the experts have not approached in caring for the aged, as was said in the prologue. For since old age is cold and essentially dry its conservation might be accomplished by means of similar things which must be brought near to them [old people], things dry and cold for their conservation, both of which are, however, inconvenient for old age and as harmful as can be to it, first, because cold things are injurious since they generate phlegm quickly in the stomach and veins, as Galen says.[135] Dry things are also not assimilable for old people. An indication of this is the fact that if sometimes dry things are used in the care of their health old people actually at any rate desire humidity so that they will penetrate more readily through the passages of the body already contracted by cold and dryness. Every immoderate temperament is harmed by what is similar to it and is aided by the moderate use of its opposite. Old age is not only a bad complexion, frigid and dry, but has a dominance of dryness in the body, as Rhazes says.[136] Therefore they assist old age with the resumptive art which is considered more understandable than the conservative art of health

[135]Galen, 5. 676, 689, 701.
[136]4. 18.

insofar as it is so to speak the art of alleviation, that is, soothing old age to resist its increase and thus to prevent its acceleration and the approach of death beyond that which the art of conservation could prevent in the same endeavor. They resist their dryness with those things which moisten but are not very much elevated toward heat. For the aged body is better and more easily nourished by these things although the natures of old man are not homogeneous. Nor is the resumptive or restorative art curative of old age for he who is restored by another regimen does not need the curative one, as Galen[137] says, for he does not grow ill; but because he is among the healthy that does not mean he is perfectly sound of body. Among the old we cannot assume the same things we can assume among the healthy, for the resumptive art of old age is not that of its conservation, for conservation is accomplished through similar things, resumption or restoration through what is fitting or proper, as is done by means of the resumptive method. Beyond doubt old age and death can be retarded as long as after restoration the precepts of the conservative art are observed in the same instance. Never however whether gradually or suddenly when these precepts have not been observed with the resumptive or conservative regimen ought the old man therefore to pass over to the position that he is allowed to live according to his own will without these precepts for then his gerontocomia would be imperfect and weak. Sometimes nevertheless the resumptive method is accustomed to be employed instead of the conservative method. For, as Galen says,[138] that part of medicine named restorative has the purpose to preserve health insofar as it is possible; hence, as a science this part of medicine is attributed to Taurus and Venus just as is also the conservative part, and as that part of medicine which is curative they say is subject to Mars and Scorpio and is part of wisdom. First of all, knowledge of medicine was considered a part of wisdom, as Celsus[139] writes. Further, they call such a restorative method by the name preservative insofar as due to its use old men are preserved from their decline to a worse state of health such as the nature of old age entails. For conservation will have to be min-

[137]Galen, 1. 319; 6. 330, 331; 10. 650.
[138]Ibid., 6. 1.
[139]Celsus, *De Medicina, prooemium.*

gled with the preservative method in those bodies whose health is faulty, as is the case with old men. They instruct us correctly who say that the regimen of old age is composed of both conservative and preservative methods, as Averroes and his followers say:[140] it is very difficult to tell one from the other by specific differences. One must know, however, that also by means of the resumptive method life is somehow slowed down by resistance to the swift course of old age and by defending it in every way against the causes which accelerate old age and by preventing the natural humidity from being quickly destroyed, thus obviating also the corruption and accidental alteration which proceed from the causes of illness. By means of the resumptive regimen the body is not protected from extrinsic harm which is casual nor does it prevent a natural death nor any effect which precedes old age nor is the body brought to the ultimate length of life which is absolutely due to a man by this method, but that service which it renders the individual man insofar as he is a man has been set down in the preceding chapter IX.

[140]6. 94v.

Chapter XII

The Care of the Aged By Use of the Six Non-naturals in General

The bodies of old men and their members are not only essentially cold and dry as well as weak but also of little blood and spirits; they are accidentally humid. These facts have been referred to somewhat in preceding chapters; it is worth analyzing the causes for these defects point by point more carefully in the present chapter. First of all, old age is cold because the blood of old men in its natural disposition of constituents although it may be good and commensurate insofar as it is congruent with that age is not however absolutely good because of its frigidity which occurs through the weakness of innate heat. In old age this heat is rendered impotent to such an extent that it converts less than usual from the food into blood. For this reason the three spirits, vital, animal, and natural, are weaker. Hence by the deprivation of much blood and spirit the bodies of old men are rendered frigid and likewise weakness of nature is dominant in them. To speak further of the cause of the dryness which occurs in old men because of their age, there is no doubt that it is due to excess frigidity. For the members are nourished by a warm humor which is blood. They are dried out by the absence of their nutriment and frigidity follows their dryness, for a dryness greater than it should be quickly renders the body colder than it should be, as Avicenna[141] tells us. That dryness is dominant at this age is easily discovered by experiment from the hardness of their bones and their roughness of skin as well as a judgment from the great length of time and distance from the beginning of their generation in which there were sperm, blood, and a vaporous spirit. The cause of the dominant dryness in old age is continuous in old men through a long dissolution of the humidity

[141]Avicenna, I, 53.

contained in them and a drying out made by the natural intrinsic and extrinsic heat, for an old man is not dry, as Galen[142] says, except because of the fact that a boy is humid by reason of the solid and radical members which become dried out in old age. These are bones, ligaments, membranes, pulsating veins, nerves, tunics, and flesh. All of these according to the course of nature proceed into dryness and earthiness in which life is at last completed. An accidental superfluous humidity dominates in old men because of the collection of an overflow of superfluity as shown by their eyes which are constantly full of tears, as Galen[143] says, and their nostrils are filled with mucous secretion and their mouths with phlegm; therefore they frequently spit and cough. Thus it happens with all this by the weakness of nature and the predigestion through innate heat of the food which enters the body a very great superfluity and raw humors are collected in their bodies. The coldness and dryness which are thus abundant in old age must be corrected by an opposite temperament, warm and humid, by the teaching of the resumptive art and by applying to old men those things which assist the swift and perfect nutrition of the aged body. The nutritive digestion of old men is deficient in two respects: it is slow and diminished. The cause is the dominance of coldness in the old, which among all the qualities which are at the service of nutrition and life is considered the most inconvenient. In second place after cold is dryness because it is necessary for all old men who are thus deficient to maintain themselves in proportion to the nature of each one. Before all, however, one must know the nature of the body of old men, since some are slender, others are fat, others hot, others cold, some humid, others dry; some have a spare taut stomach, others have sagging stomachs. Rarely does anyone, as Celsus[144] says, not have some weak part of the body. All however tend toward accidental cold and humidity but essential dryness. One must make every effort to prevent the aged body from becoming dried out, to compensate for coldness by the use of whatever provides heat, that is, which has the power to heat and to relax and dissolve by the equal heating from food and drink, motion and rest, by the use of that which softens or mollifies the dry-

[142]Galen, 6. 357; 15. 186; 16.101.
[143]Ibid., 10. 316; 17. B. 651.
[144]Celsus, *De Medicina, prooemium.*

ness and resolves it as well as of substances that humidify with equal effect. The weakness of the body must be repaired by every means which will restore the heat of the entire body and power to the veins since old men are of slight blood and heat. All these means retard the advent of old age just as their use increases the strength and security of their bodies from whatever chills and dries them out. For, as Galen[145] says, older men and boys are destroyed and weakened more swiftly. Thus their power is diminished due to the same cause as in boys, that is, the airy humidity which is more quickly evaporated and their thinness of spirits; hence in those who are decrepit there is a deficiency of power because of extreme dryness. This condition is to be combatted as they tell us by more frequent rest, moderate exercise, frequent warm baths especially after meals, a soft bed, a sound sleep but not too long so that it may make the shadows brief, not too much cold, with security of mind without worry, in tranquillity, with the consumption of food and drink which is most suitable to human nature such as foodstuffs of moderate sweetness, somewhat fat and especially cooked. "Cooked" comes from *cogendo* as they say because by *cogendo* coercion is exerted so that the food may be brought to the proper condition for eating. Bodies increase with sweet and fat substances and with rather frequent food and drink, as much as it is possible for them to be prepared for digestion especially to absorb the foods which come from cold and rainy regions and which make the body humid and liquid, the use of which is increased by good odors, moderate joy, the frequent mention of pleasant subjects of conversation, and the avoidance of sadness with those whom old people like. By the use of these elements in general and singly the old man grows humid, his powers increase, and his life is extended by fleshiness. Let him eat and drink sufficiently and let him abstain from business affairs and everything which may provide worry for his mind. Let him sleep well and avoid overloading his stomach and at the same time avoid both the sun and the cold. Food is especially important among all these means of restoring the strength of a weak old man because it alone as part of the nourishment of the body is assimilated into its substance. It is one of the accidental means of humidification because it prevents similar

[145]Galen, 17, A. 32; B. 574.

members from drying out or because it increases and extends the humidity which is contained in the midst of the members. Morbid and languid old age abounds in superfluous and accidental humidity. As a salutary remedy it is useful to draw off this humidity and the crude humors which are congested in the old man for digestion so that the aged body can be made whole insofar as it is possible. In order to attain this condition old men should be guarded from all those materials that stop up passages which are then quickly converted into putrid phlegm by evacuating and consuming the aqueous undigested matter approximating the heat of that putrid phlegm as well as the first particles of the aged body which make it cold and dry. The body may become easily filled with serous and phlegmatic superfluities because of the weakness of the power to expel them when it tries to do so. Insofar as it is possible to do so these superfluities must be warmed and humidified in a proper manner. All of this process will be discussed at greater length in chapter XLIV. The observation of all these suggestions is so much the more necessary the more troublesome old age is to the individual. Thus by a moderate, adjusted, and suitable regimen that part of medicine called dietetics by the Greeks teaches us the administration of the six non-naturals, sometimes with a rather light discussion or application of medicines just as that part of medicine they call pharmaceutics advises us they bid us in this manner to extend that life which is so much sought after. Galen has reminded us of this fact in his *Sanative Method.* Book I [or *De Sanitate Tuenda*].[146] His words are: "He who wishes to be long lived and healthy must live with himself alone, free from every necessary occupation, and be of a good disposition." In the administration of all these parts of the regime a gerontocomos must be in charge.

Just as one wishes to prop the tottering ruin
And tries to throw up some supporting timbers
Right then long time destroys our careful efforts,
Brings down the building with the props we fashioned.[147]

[146] Galen, 6. 62.
[147] Maximianus, *Elegies* 1. 171–74.

Chapter XIII

The Usage to Be Observed in the Recovery Process of Old People

By the term regimen most people understand medication; it also includes the observation of customary care. Therefore in taking care of old people by the resumptive art they tell us to make as important a place as possible for such care, which is completed by the activity of the physician whose task it is to oversee and regulate the care of the patient, as Galen says.[148] Old men teach us therefore that they must be restored by means of their accustomed interests even if these are hurtful and they should not be distracted from these interests nor be transferred to interests which are strange to them. For custom or habit is correctly defined as a kind of second nature acquired gradually by usage and associated with natural things with the mediation of complexion. It consists of the frequent and continuous repetition of the same act which gradually becomes uniform or even; on account of its long-standing effect it attains what they call the force of nature. Therefore no attempt to change the customs or habits of old men should be made, as Galen[149] advises, for this they think is difficult and harmful. For even if the danger of change can be undergone in youth and those things which harm the body become a habit in childhood a strong power tolerates without difficulty that change which has taken place with moderate use. Then also because in succeeding stages of life that which is beneficial to health still persists the body is brought back to a better condition. But to change an old man from bad to good habits is not without grave danger and should not be attempted even if by continuous and gradual efforts the old man could be drawn away from his bad habits, for such a sudden

[148]Galen, 6. 135; 7. 294; 10. 389; 17. A. 148.
[149]Ibid., 4. 452; 15. 556.

change will be futile and harmful. Then there is the lack of time required to induce a good habit when the bad one is abandoned. All habits, customs, and vices have brought about callousness in old men; even if it is valuable to soften it sometimes it can never be completely removed. Thus it is troublesome to change a habit, especially one which is ingrained and in an old man just as that which does harm through the habit itself whether soft or hard, to such an extent that what one is accustomed to for a long time even if it harms is usually less painful than that which has not yet become a habit. Thus we can see old men who have become weak nevertheless are able to bear accustomed labors more easily than stronger young men who are unaccustomed to them. An indication of this fact is the delight which arises in old men from that which has become a habit with them, for delight is a sign of a habitual quality especially by reason assumed from habit although it is proven that what is accustomed may sometimes disturb old men because those parts of a habit which are continuously offered as replenishment allow no vacant space nor faculty for reception. Those who write on this subject say that animal life is to be measured not only by motion but also by quiet when all animal motion is at rest from all action. Hence it results that often that which is accustomed does not delight one greatly. An indication of this is that listeners are disturbed by what is frequently repeated, according to Aristotle in his *Topics,* Book V.[150]

[150]Aristotle, *Topics* 5, 130.

Chapter XIV

The Conditions and Duties of the Gerontocomos and His Assistants

The person in charge of the aged must be a man whose chief function is their restoration, for this is his prime duty. Let him be liberally educated so that he can be instructed in the resumptive art as a diligent observer of its rules. Let him be frugal so that he can urge his assistants or servants toward frugality, and of middle age for his assistants will obey him more willingly in their service toward the aged. These assistants must nevertheless be of proper age so that they can carry on their work without any hampering effects and yet not old men, nor should they be boys who cannot easily bear the difficulty of wakefulness nor the burden of labor which must be borne by those who bend to the task of caring for old people. The gerontocomos must be experienced in both the affairs of a family and those of a physician, for many things are difficult for an inexperienced person which are very easy for an expert. Not only must the gerontocomos give orders but also carry them out so that his assistants will imitate him as he does so. The resumptive method is no small part of the science of medicine, as I have said in that part of this book devoted to it, chapter XI. Hence his duty will be to examine the urine of the old gentleman daily. If it is white in color or somewhat yellow or pink or red this will be a sign that the old man is in very good health. For one signifies that a concoction is present and the other that concoction has taken place. Let the gerontocomos be endowed with good habits, skilled at his work, of long experience, sympathetic, solicitous, and a frequent visitor of the old man so that by all these services the latter will then reach the goal of restoration which is desired. The purpose of the care of the aged is restoration. Religious service is established to lead the old men to the cult of the divine at whose will human life is extended. Let him be very zealous in regard to cleanliness and elegance of surroundings in which area he should not be unskilled on behalf of the old man who is to be restored in the practice of living whether he has followed a life of labor or of rest in the past, with luxury or with frugality. With these and similar means a new regime of restoration is to be maintained. Let him watch out lest the old people or his assistants become chilled, nor should they become too warm or thirsty. Let him finally be dedicated and intent upon his duty in the restoration of old age, for one task is more perfectly completed toward one end than toward many, as the poet says: A purpose directed toward many ends is less intense than when directed toward one.[151]

Whatever is brought into the house for the restoration of the aged the gerontocomos should carefully inspect, receive it, and take custody of it lest (as they say) a year's expenses be spent in a month. As to his physical appearance, the gerontocomos should be modestly dressed, of cheerful mien, clean, well-dressed, without fetid odor or sweat, so that he may be more pleasing to all the old men whom he should never deprive of the hope of extending their lives. Let him employ assistants who are zealous and keep them very frugal. He should remove the lazy and stupid. Among the assistants there may be men or women. Off duty or on duty they are ordered to behave politely. Let the gerontocomos impress upon them that they should be easily available for restoring the old people. Their duties are first of all not to disturb the functions of health-care since not all the assistants are equal to all services involved. This situation is not helpful to the man in charge, less helpful to the assistants, and least helpful of all to the elderly. Thus no one of the assistants should think that any task is his own particular province nor seek to escape the labor of all involved in common since of the total number of assistants some may be accustomed to do their work more diligently and others to do so more slackly. People consider that number of assistants to be most convenient for taking care of the old people in accordance with which not too large a group believes this task pertains to them as single

[151]*Bedae Prov.*, in Migne, *PL* 90. 1106. See Hans Walther, *Carmina Medii Aevi Posterioris Latina,* II/3; Göttingen: Vandenhoek und Ruprecht, 1965, 842, no. 29, a proverb widespread in numerous collections: *pluribus intentus minor est ad singula sensus.*

individuals nor should the old people have a just complaint due to the improper number of assistants. They say this form of administration not only stirs up competition but also apprehends the lazy workers. Let the workers strive to carry out the orders of the gerontocomos properly and not think they know more than he does; let them be most obedient to the old men whose orders they listen to. It is most urgent that they should remain in the house entirely or most of the time in order not to miss the hours of restoration required by the old people. They should not be greedy or such as the ancients used to call *catillones*[152] [plate-lickers] or *degulatores* [gluttons]. Let them be chaste, self-restrained, and let not the cups or food of the old people be touched by any servant except by one who is not a grown man or certainly one most abstemious in sexual activity. If any of them has indulged in sex, be he man or woman, he or she should before they touch the drink or food wash themselves in a river or a running spring within the hour as was the custom of the ancients because they wished this service to be carried out by boys or virgins at whose hands whatever was required for the old people should be prepared. They should be the first of all to rise from their beds; the servants of the bedchamber especially should be the last to go to bed. They should speak to the old men politely and carefully prepare both night and day those things necessary for their comfort. Often they should spend the night near them and not allow their bedrooms to be deprived of light. Their beds should be provided with soft covers, pillows, and mattresses as well as hangings, valances, and whatever things of this kind are needed which will furnish comfort for the daily care of the old people. They should take off the old men's shoes, dress them, and see that urinals and chamber pots are available for them. Let them also arise sometimes at night if there is need of assistance for the weaker elderly. Let the attendants be trustworthy so that no one can persuade them to give food to their charges which the Greeks call *deleterion,* or poisoned food. Let them be sober so that sluggish with intoxication and too heavy a sleep they do not hear the calls of those who require their services. Let them be close-mouthed, not talkative or loose in talk, and always alert to spring to their duty, completely free of idleness so that absolutely

[152]Paulus ex Fest. 44; 90 Müller; Lindsay 39, 80, note 2. See also on *cossus,* ibid.

nothing shall be lacking to the task of extending life. Attendants ideal for the care of the aged should be selected, strong and swift, agile and without impediment in their arms and legs, strong enough to assist, serve, and bring help to the aged both day and night, ready to run up and down according to the service needed. Let not their duties be entirely sedentary. They must oversee the kitchen and those who prepare food for the aged. Not every nation is fitted for this work. The English are men of immense pride, the Swiss intolerably suspicious, the Illyrians foul-mouthed, the Hungarians hostile to the Italians of all people. Ideal for this kind of work are the Bretons, Germans, some of the French, those Spaniards who are more similar to the Italians. Best of all the Italians are the Lombards. Care should be taken to see that no one is an *ambro,* that is, a man of evil life, nor a *cossus,* a man of wrinkled body. Finally, their duties are not to be left entirely in their own care; these should be so selected that the gerontocomos can keep an eye on them as they are performed. They say the attendant will be more diligent if he remembers that there is some one to whom he must render account frequently. If any one either of the aged or of their attendants begins to be afflicted with bad health it is the duty of the gerontocomos to bring him back to health as comfortably and quickly as he can. From this care benevolence will grow toward him and no less obedience. The attendants will desire to serve him more faithfully than before since he has been solicitous toward the sick man who by the master's diligence has regained his health.

Chapter XV

The Atmosphere Most Suitable for Longevity

The experts say that after an observation of the conjunction of the sun and moon and of the opposition of the other stars necessary for the resumptive regimen those dispositions of the airs or the atmosphere which are suitable for the resumption and care of the old people and most certainly fitting for all ages must be observed, that is, cleanliness, clarity, and purity. All of these factors reveal the salubrious quality of the air. Its excellence and clarity are shown if it is not polluted with some putrefaction of vegetables, dung, legumes, or animals and such like, free of clouds at night nor troubled by stagnant water or thick vapor nearby nor enclosed in any region, and free from low valleys, for a hollow region surrounded by high mountains receives no change of air. This suffocation of putrid and muddy vapor makes the spirit sad. The purity of the air must be observed so that it is not infected by evaporation from stagnant water or swamps nor that it receives a poisonous breeze from a sewer or a stream used as a sewer or from the sewage flowing from some large city or an army of many men. For such a corrupt air flowing about brings many causes for trouble to the old men as is shown by bodies of the inhabitants when carefully inspected. Columella[153] says that if their color is not healthy nor their heads firmly upright nor the light of their eyes dim nor their hearing sound and their throats are not blocked for the clear passage of the voice then the absence of these signs of serious damage shows that the individual is in good health. Beyond these qualities of the atmosphere which bring comfort to whatever age they are helpful to human nature as convenient for the old. Great praise has been given to a type of air equal in prime qualities, tending somewhat to the warm and humid without too much flow.

[153]Columella, *Res Rustica* 1. 5.

It is well for the air flow to be reduced since old age is cold and dry. But if the air is changed in whatever other way into a quality proper to these dispositions of the aged it will perform its proper operation for them. Therefore they tell us to avoid the transference from a healthy location to one that is burdensome because such a transference will not be at all safe, nor will the reverse move, from burdensome or heavy atmosphere to the healthy. If the move must be made it should be carried out in early summer, and the move from the salubrious location to the burdensome one should be made in early winter, as Celsus bids us.[154]

THE HABITABLE PLACES, CLIMATES, AND REGIONS IN WHICH OLD AGE IS RETARDED

They tell us that the place, climate, and region chosen as a dwelling place for the resumption of the aged must be those which combat the causes which bring about a swift death and which assist the extension of life by their qualities. Among these the location facing toward the north is not the best for the purpose since that location must dispel by resumption the defects and weaknesses of the body. Avicenna[155] is authority for the statement that in northern locations on account of the prevailing cold those who have weak complexions suffer from cuzem, which is a kind of spasm. Nor are those places which face the south conducive to the prolongation of life, for in them there occur paralyses of the aged on account of catarrhs of which old men's heads are filled. Similarly they are afflicted with asthma, epilepsy, and fevers in which heat and cold are combined, as well as long winter and nightly fevers, for the proper mixture of their humors in men's bodies is removed by the nearest course of the sun which burns their bodies. It is best for old men to avoid the heat of the sun everywhere. Places open toward the east are more healthful as dwelling places for the care of the old. Their air is more salubrious because it is thinner and more temperate. They are even better if these locations face somewhat north and south, for the sun does not recede so much from such places that they are oppressed with cold nor

[154] Celsus, *De Medicina* 1. 3.
[155] Avicenna, *Canon* III. Fen II, cap. viii, p. 201.

does it approach so closely that these places are burned with its heat because the sun is elevated at the beginning of the day above these places and purifies their air and recedes when the air has been illuminated. When the sun in these places scatters its heat moderately it keeps the body temperature moderate. Hence it happens that the inhabitants of these places are of a temperate condition, sound of body, with stronger powers, of a white color mixed with red, with few diseases, fleshy, loud voiced between deep and shrill because of the mixture of humidity which makes the sounds of the voice heavier and its heat more sharp. They are endowed with prudence and are completely, as they say, people of health and quiet. Those who are experts add that old people should not dwell in places facing west. These are of more impure air, thicker and more humid; the latter is injurious both to body and spirit for it dulls the natural talent, blunts the perception, and distorts the affections. Turning to regions, of all habitable locations none is more adapted to extending life according to the judgment of almost all experts than that which lies under the equinox (if the experts think that region is habitable) for the sun does not recede too far from it nor delays too long in that direction. Hence it enjoys a salubrious sky, with a temperature not excessive in summer and winter. The days of the equinox are not of extreme heat. They say that in one year four crops are grown in the seasons of the year in great abundance of produce. Two crops are grown just as if in two summers, and the experts say there is a perpetual spring with perpetual flowers. The healthful sky is always like that of spring, and summer does not bring a burning heat. In fact, the quality of the air is always the same without any perceptible drawback of a harmful sort. To the people who inhabit this region there come no enfeebling illnesses, no sickly old age, as Lactantius[156] tells us. Their memory and all their dispositions are noble and similar. The experts add that there are climates and other regions whose quality is inferior. Of these the ones tending toward hot but by a slight excess turning toward cold are more praiseworthy, for in them heat and humidity which are the beginnings and the cause of life are preserved better and for a longer time and those exposed to such regions have a longer life than in the colder climes. Such

[156]Lactantius says nothing of the kind.

regions are chiefly India, which stretches from the Mediterranean sea to the rising of the sun, as they write. On the north the Caucasus mountains and on the west the Indus river bound this region, which lies next to the Red Sea. It is filled with islands rich in gold and silver and it never lacks fruits, with two crops in summer and winter of cinnamon, pepper, sweet flag *[calamus aromaticus]* and lotus [date plum]. St. Jerome[157] says there are in those parts golden mountains which on account of dragons, gryphons, and monstrous giants one cannot approach. The upper eastern part of the region is measured by the first climate between the equinox and the tropic of Cancer; astrologers say its inhabitants are dominated by Saturn. Therefore, they are so long-lived that many of them die only in extreme old age. Isigonus[158] says the Cirni are an Indian people who live two hundred and forty years. There are also in India people called Pandorae living in valleys who they say live two hundred years; in youth their hair is white and it grows black in old age. Nor should the eastern region of Chaldea be passed over in silence in this place. It bounds Arabia on the north side and extends to the Persian Gulf; here natures have been invigorated, prophecies and sciences invented, as the experts report. Albumasar, *Introductorium* IV, says:[159] Noah the prophet who must be venerated when he fled the corruption and cold of the air went to Chaldea from the mountains of Armenia in which the Ark rested in the seventh month (as Moses says in Genesis viii) in search of warm air. Our first parents dwelled in Chaldea down to the time of Abraham, who, having been born there, was led into the Promised Land by the Lord. Moses writes that those parents lived there a very long space of life. This longevity could by some means result from a perfection of complexion and a proper regimen of their life as well as from the excellence of their nourishment before the flood, also by reason of the praiseworthy aspect of the stars which dominate in that region. But since it is impossible to test the matter by way of documents it must be regarded as a miracle for the greater extension in the hearts of the faithful of the crea-

[157]Jerome, *Epist.* CXXV.
[158]Isigonus: cf. Pliny, *N. H.* 7. 27, who quotes him.
[159]Albumasar: Abu Ma'shar of Bagdad, the Greek Apomasar (Abū Ma' šar), *Introductorium Maius;* Venice, 1489; *Dict. of Scientific Biography,* s. v.; *Encyclopedia of Islam,* I (1960): 139–40. Circa 787–886 A.D.

tion of the world, which (as Rabi Moses says) the pagans in great part denied. Before the flood all people were of very long life, but only those of whom sacred scripture makes mention. Lamech, father of Noah, was a contemporary of Adam himself. Abraham, whom they say was also a principal person in the preaching of the faith, was sixty-three years old when Noah died, and so they say the testimony of the creation of the world was sufficiently continued by the length of their lives from the time of Adam down to the time of Abraham. That this region with adjacent places was the region of the wise men is the statement of Jerome, whence also the magi, that is, the wise men who came from the east to Bethlehem to adore Christ we hold in faith were from Arabia in their origin. The temperature of those regions tends to be hot by reason of the swifter passage of the sun under the equinoctial region and its change in the first climate as it moves with greater velocity; the intensity of its heat in those regions is broken by the blowing of many winds which temper the air and restrain the refraction of the sun's rays. Thus they assist the same purpose by creating lofty vapors which come from the sea, rivers, or lakes. The same thing happens by reason of the signs of heaven which dominate every zone to all those living elsewhere, whatever the disposition by which they are afflicted. The first zone is rendered harmless to the Indians, first inhabitants of that region. Their color is saffron or dark, in order that I may add features which pertain to the body. They are not black as are the Ethiopians who dwell in the second climate (or zone) and are farther south than the Indians. Hence the former become darker because of the more violent attack of the heat. There are other regions beyond the first zone with their inhabitants whom the expert astrologers and medical men regard as more fortunate because of their long life which the gerontocomos would do well to select just as those situated at the end of the third zone passing thence to the fourth zone and properly, as the Conciliator[160] says, that region which lies between Chindia, which is located opposite Constantinople, facing east and between Choum. The experts add that some regions of the sixth zone are more conducive to longevity and that in them a better temperament of bodies is found, like Greece, which is among the Greek physicians

[160]Pietro d'Abano, *Conciliator Controversiarum* etc.; Venice: Giunta, 1520, 67.

considered well tempered; most well tempered, however, is the homeland of Hippocrates. Greece is in the same zone as Rome, which once possessed the boundaries of the whole world and every region, situated in the middle with its adjacent regions. Italy is also numbered among the southern peoples which are nearest the meridian axis and the peoples who live in the second zone; since these are oppressed with burning heat on account of the swift depletion of their natural humidity they become old in the thirtieth year, as Avicenna[161] says, which of course is a very brief period of human life. These are the Ethiopians, some part of whom according to Pliny[162] lives only on locusts hardened with smoke and salt for annual food and do not live beyond the fortieth year. Their hair is curly and black; their teeth shine brilliantly. Their bodies are rather short, their eyes black, their limbs are strong and due to the impact of the sun their blood is thin. Therefore they are rather timid and suffer from heat and fever. The middle of Italy is another area among those where people dwell in the extreme northern and colder regions such as those in the seventh zone and beyond. They are the first people of the Arctic polar region and far away from the equator. A swift death occurs among them not only violent due to putrefaction and the choking off of respiration which comes from a stoppage but also due to a natural consumptive death. For the natural heat propelled into the inner parts of those who inhabit colder regions penetrates the innermost area. When the humidity therein is overmuch consumed there ensue corruption and a consequent destruction of the living being. Nor does the abundance of humidity which is visible from their fat assist the extension of their lives; in fact, it is adverse to it for that which is aqueous, not airy, is in comparative relation to the heart, not to heat. Those in northern regions also live a shorter life because of an inordinate regimen, for it is characteristic of them to be gluttonous, fat, corrupt, vile, and brutal of face. They have huge bodies, white color, straight red hair, blue eyes, sometimes gray, a heavy voice and much blood, with wild behavior, stupid mind, and lack of reason. Those peoples are foolish, as Vitru-

[161]Avicenna, I, 32.

[162]Pliny, *N. H.* 6. 195; Galen 19. 344, also says the Ethiopians grow old quickly.

vius[163] says, because of the heaviness of the climate, the obstruction of the air, and the coldness of their humor. For just as a warm air makes people more sharp in intelligence it does not by any means burn their minds, as is possible to see in Spain, where, being cooled off considerably, the people sustain slower accesses of heat and rarer fevers by their abundance of blood and resist bravely with the sword. Hence they are bold and virile, very confident in themselves; guided by no reason they attack boldly with great ferocity and are a people without restraint who consider it justifiable to rush into any kind of crime to such an extent that they may even eat human bodies. They say that the Scythians or Parthians are this kind of people. Passing from Róme with its adjacent regions such as Latium, Etruria, and Campania, to Italy especially are ascribed fields green the entire year, in fact, to all Italy, which has the median type of habitable climates, tending more toward the north which is a more salubrious region than the south, as Varro says.[164] Without doubt the peoples of Italy will be longer lived since they are most temperate in respect to each part of their bodies with vigorous members and spirits. Many examples make this clear. Marius Valerius Corvinus, the Roman, lived one hundred years, and of the Roman women Cicero's Terentia, they say, lived one hundred and seven. Between the northern and the southern temperate zones with minglings or overlapping on each side Italy receives due praise, cooling off with its counsels the ferocity of the barbarians and the wiles and cunning of the southern peoples so that no part of Italy lacks praises. Thus caring for human affairs God has located the noble and temperate monarchy of Rome in this region, as Pliny[165] says, where the hills are most salubrious and a convenient river by which the products of the southern region are carried down to the sea and overseas supplies are received. The ocean is conveniently near nor by being too close to it is the river exposed to the perils of foreign navies. The middle of Italy is ideally located for the growth of a city so that the people there are able to live a longer life after all their enemies have been driven off; the location is of advantage to the safety of

[163]Vitruvius, *De Architectura* 6.1.3,4.
[164]Varro, *De Re Rustica* 1.2.4.
[165]Pliny, *N. H.* 3. 39; cf. Manilius 4. 694–95; 773–76.

the human race. Not only are regions dissimilarly disposed for the longevity or brevity of life because of their climates but the same region is dissimilarly disposed according to the variation of water supply, winds, and mountains or of other factors for the extension or shortening of human life. Hence it results that peoples live a longer time in some places of the sixth zone and the beginnings of the seventh especially in mountainous regions. Avicenna[166] is authority for the statement that those who dwell in high habitable places are healthy and strong and live a long time while enduring much labor. For those places where the sky is clear and windy are ventilated by the blowing of healthful winds, as is fitting, and are especially exposed to the eastern winds and protected from the western and southern winds as long as there are no other impediments such as swamps and valleys nearby. Thus in these elevated open places men grow old slowly, preserved from putrefaction by the purity and clarity of the air and by its frequent renewal. There are examples and proofs of this fact in some places of Italy, such as Parma, Piacenza, Faenza, Bologna and in their hills, and in the region of Riperia the Lago di Garda in Veronese territory, whose air is very healthful for the city of Verona, among its other gifts of the gods. No less attractive is the region of Bergamo, in which it is possible to find very many men of long lives. They say also that the constitution of flowing air is most adapted to the longevity of men; an ancient tradition holds that human life at Bologna is greatly extended. Pliny[167] tells us that Titus Fullonius of Bologna lived one hundred and fifty years. This happens also in other regions and places in Italy, as in the realm of Galicia and Valencia. Lincolniensis[168] reports that near a certain pole the mountain dwellers due to the uniform and regular reflexion of the sun's rays which creates an equality of the air those who have become old are affected with boredom because of undue longevity and jump into a river near the mountain with the intent to commit suicide. At the top of Mount Tmolus which they call Tepsis men live one hun-

[166]Avicenna, I, 32.
[167]Pliny, *N. H.* 7. 159.
[168]Robert Grosseteste, *De natura locorum,* in *Die Philosophische Werke,* etc., ed. L. Baur; Münster i. W., 1912, 69.

dred and fifty years, as Mucianus[169] says. Likewise, on the island of Taprobane they say that a lifetime of one hundred years is moderate. In fact, on that island Artemidorus[170] tells that the longest life is lived without any bodily suffering. One should note also what Columella[171] says about the healthfulness of regions, that is, there are certain places which grow less warm at the solstices but shiver intolerably from the cold in winter, as they say of Thebes in Boeotia. There are also places which grow warm in winter but heat up very severely in summer, as they say of Euboea in Chalcidice. People seek an air tempered by heat and cold which is to be found in the middle of the hills because it does not become heavy when pressed down by winter frosts or grow hot in summer with vapors nor lifted to the top of the mountains by very small movements of the winds or rage with rainstorms at every time of year. The best position is in the middle of hills; it is best adapted for the extension of human life when it faces directly east since this is preferable for tempering the summer heat and because of the pleasantness of the situation. A place where streams of sweet water issue forth in the midst of hills is useful for the carrying of water, that is, an aqueduct if the terrain allows this. Hence these are called river cities, that is, situated beside a river, because although at a rather long interval from the sea they are preeminent for the healthfulness of their location. They add that places situated on the middle of a hill and near the sea as well as near islands and a country area provide a longer life for their inhabitants than those in wild places, as Averroes[172] says. Marine animals, as they say, have a longer life than those in the wilderness. Some have therefore praised warm lands near the sea for the longevity of life which they bestow with the heat and humidity of their air, such as Venice, the noblest city in Italy. It happens that either this fact or the saltiness of the air preserves the bodies of men from putrefaction or by reason of the equability of maritime regions, whose complexion, as must be more truthfully believed according to Avicenna,[173] is equally

[169]Pliny, *N. H.* 7. 159.
[170]Ibid., 7. 2. 30.
[171]Columella, *Res Rustica* 1. 4. 9.
[172]6. 91r.
[173]Avicenna, I, 32.

warm and cold. The tendency is toward humidity with the absence of any injurious breeze and vapor and without any detestable quality in the air such as is found in the vicinity of a swamp from which insects armed with injurious stings arise and fly against us in very dense swarms. Hence there arises a pestilential poison, infection from water snakes which often inflict unidentifiable diseases whose cause physicians are unable to detect, as Moderatus[174] says. An example of the extended life of island dwellers is provided by Gorgias of Sicily, who, they say, lived one hundred and eight years.

PRIVATE DWELLINGS SUITABLE FOR THE CARE OF THE AGED

Dwellings for the care of the health of the aged such as cubicles and libraries and similar housing are to be chosen in the most healthful part of the regions where the old people live, facing to the east, not to the south, north, or west, since the air on the eastern exposure is more healthful, easier to breathe. They should not be closed in nor covered or arched over like a turtle shell and by no means built underground where the air is heavy and humid, creating constriction of the chest and heart, heaviness and sluggishness of the head, and drowsiness and dullness of the senses with induration of breath and difficulty of respiration which results in the loss of voice. Private dwellings quite open to the four corners of the world are preferred. The eastern exposure is best with open access on all sides; such places are called by those who are acquainted with them by the name *conflages,*[175] that is, places where the winds blow from all sides. If the dwellings are elevated they will be too hot in summer and rather cold in winter so that the aged bodies cannot be defended from cold or heat. They should be sunny so that the sun and the eastern winds may approach the homes of the aged and that these may enjoy a pleasant view, for the sun improves the air and is a good preserver of life. There is no life for living things except gods except by means of the sun and moon, as Albumasar[176] says in *Sadan* [al-Sa'dan: Jupiter and Venus, the

[174]Moderatus (Columella), 1. 5. 6; Varro 1. 12. 2; Quintilian 3. 1, 8.
[175]Paulus ex Fest. 40, 10 Müller, Lindsay 35; Isidore, *Orig.* 14. 8. 27.
[176]Albumasar: see note 159.

lucky stars]. The sun clears up the clouds of the human spirit, as Pliny[177] writes. They say that a well-mixed or equable air in the dwelling with light and warmth is the best. Thus it softens and tempers the suffering of old age, for a shining light relaxes the body with its warmth, as Galen[178] says. A cold, dark air constricts the body with its excess. The dwellings should be made bright with white wash, that is, polished with lime. For the protection of the old people who are cold by nature in the chilly time of the year and in cold regions, especially mountainous ones, the winter dwellings should be prepared so that they can receive almost all of the movement of the winter sun in order to cheer the old people. The serviceable floors should be if possible of wooden planks of Italian oak or larch or such like so that they may resemble in the heat the temperate disposition of spring, for powers that have become drowsy can be stirred by the coolness since they also induce thirst, as Abulkasim[179] says, and they cause the undigested food to descend and must be rectified by the northern air. If the old person happens to have a habitation facing this air they tell us that we must guard against it by proper bedsteads or rectify the situation by a fire which heats and dries moderately, with a flame that is not smoky but pure made from dry grape-vine stems, laurel, cedar, cypress, or olive wood. We must also purge the air of this place with fumigants of aloes, incense, myrrh, storax, juniper, and such like medicinal plants or compounds, especially in winter. The summer dwellings should face the eastern solstice and the northern exposure, with doors and windows open so that some breeze may also approach. The floors should be earthen, tessellated, or of mosaic, which can receive marble or square tiles by which it is made smooth with the corners joined with bricks, or if these are not available then you should scatter rock dust over the marble or sand mixed with lime to soften it or to interpose planks[180] between the tiles and not to water it. The old man's bed should be located in that part of the dwelling where the air can pass in and out more freely. You should scatter sandalwood scent, roses, or green plants

[177]Pliny, *N. H.* 2. 13.
[178]Galen, 15. 369; 16. 359, 391.
[179]Abulkasim: the appropriate section of his Kitāb al-taṣrīf has not been published; see Introduction.
[180]Paulus ex Fest. 16 Müller; Lindsay 15.

which have a sweet odor around it and scent all the bed clothes and pillows. These perfumes purify the air of the dwelling, increase the vigor of the brain, bring delight with their odors together with other stimulation to the senses; they also drive off vapors which pollute the air. These preparations should be varied to suit the four seasons of the year. Thus if the cold increases the old man should be heated with a fire not too close to him nor should he remain too long beside it especially after he has eaten a meal and with his face toward the fire, for the weaker spirit of the old man is more easily impaired, his digestion hindered, his sight less keen, his blood grows thin so that he often becomes dizzy. He should make a moderate use of the fire with his back turned toward it. Some defence of his eyes should be placed between him and the fire's heat. His room should be heated with a fireplace in the winter so that it will be as warm as in summer. It will be more healthy for him in the winter to be placed in a protected room when there is no fire and where the old man can be rubbed down both winter and summer after he has emptied his bowels. In the summer old age requires lodgings in which he may spend the season in pleasant surroundings for the summertime environment where it is deeply shaded can make some old men of soft and delicate constitutions complain that they are living in a winter home. Locations which encourage head colds and catarrh are especially to be avoided. Celsus[181] recommends a building that is flooded with light, well ventilated in summer, with access to the sun in winter. One should beware of the midday sun and the morning and evening chill as well as breezes blowing from rivers and swamps. One should also avoid exposure to a cloudy sky and the full force of the sun lest the old people become alternately hot and cold. This care should be maintained even more in places where heavier air can create pestilence. Sheltered by this sort of care, aid, and precaution Antiochus the physician described by Galen[182] lived to the age of eighty hale and hearty in every sense and limb. These dwellings moreover should be kept free of all excrement and mouldiness and be perfumed with good odors lest they stink with foul and fetid smells, according to the experts. Rabi Moyses [f. 29r] says it is

[181]Celsus, *De Medicina* 1. 2.
[182]Galen 6. 332–33.

good for pigeon nests to scent the homes of men and for the pigeons to dwell there also because they help to protect human beings from nervous ailments, paralysis, twisting of the mouth, spasm, and trembling. It should be observed, however, that the pigeon droppings should not be allowed to pile up since they putrefy and befoul the air.

CONCERNING THE SEASONS OF THE YEAR CONDUCIVE TO THE RESUMPTION OF OLD AGE

Certain accidental changes of the air occur which are called seasonal weather. Those which are equable in temperature are extremely useful to old age, both cold and warm but those which tend rather toward warmth. The worst changes in the weather for the elderly are those which vary sharply. Most salutary are the clear, bright days since they are better than those which are misty or cloudy. It is useful to know not only these changes but also those which precede them. Other natural shifts take place during the four seasons. They begin from the time the sun passes from one quadrate to another in its orbit. These are especially observed in the resumptive regimen, for among all the changes of weather those caused by the stars are quite important. They induce from their quadrates a great alteration in the bodies of living creatures. Among the four seasons of the year thus divided for the resumptive benefit of old people whose innate warmth is slight, as was said, there is the summer season, salubrious because of its superfluous accidental humidity. Summer's first day occurs when the sun is in the sign of Taurus on the seventh day of the Ides of May [May 9]; summer contains ninety-four days, as M. Varro[183] says. Old men feel better in summer just as young men feel better in winter for old men's cold nature is aided by summer's heat. Avicenna[184] proves this by experience in these words: In summer you will see old men and those who resemble them become stronger, for the cold weather is hostile to the old thin man although it is advantageous to young men and all who are full bodied. Hence summer days are the more healthful to old age the more the west

[183]Varro, *De Re Rustica* I. 28. 1.
[184]Avicenna, I, 30.

wind blows. They say that winter is more unfriendly to old age. Its first day occurs when the sun is in Scorpio on November 10; winter has eighty-nine days. If there is much water in this season it generates catarrh in the old people. The beginning of autumn is regarded as healthful for the old. In summer and early autumn it is agreed among the authors that old men are in the best of health although they regard the end of autumn as harmful to them. Although autumn somehow resembles the nature of old age yet it is clearly bad for it at all times, causing pestilence and acute mortal diseases. For every period and every nature in every region it is uncomfortable, accursed, and very dangerous although less so to those of hot and humid nature. The first day of autumn when the sun is in Leo falls on the seventh day of the Ides of Sextilis [August 11]; autumn has ninety-one days. It is not called autumn because it increases health *(augere)* but because at this season the crops and fruits of mankind are harvested. Yet it is not considered as hostile to the old people as winter. Whether the nature of spring is warm and humid, as many philosophers have taught, or temperate and mild nevertheless at its beginning it is humid and not far from temperate, as some of the physicians declare. It is also moderate to such a degree that it brings a mixed temperature and strength to the operations of nutritive power and innate warmth; it is very healthful to the human body. Springtime is most opportune for the cure of all ills but not moderate according to the proportion of primary qualities. The first day of spring occurs when the sun is in Aquarius on the seventh day of the Ides of February [February 7]. Spring has ninety-one days.

THE WINDS TO BE SELECTED FOR THE SAME PURPOSE

Since the dispositions of the wind vary not only do they affect man with diverse alterations but they should be carefully observed for the protection and use of old age. The east winds which have an equal mixture of hot and cold, blow over grassy places, and are cleansed by passage over water, are very suitable for old age as for other periods of life. They increase and strengthen the spirits, but since they also generate ophthalmia and coryza according to

Abulkasim[185] the harm they do can be removed with rose or violet water. Since the west winds have a mixture of warm and cold, if they shift to the north they are not particularly pleasant in the spring for the resumptive regimen; they excite the digestive power. The west winds are a bit more humid than the east winds but the northeast winds are not quite as humid as the western winds which blow over the sea. Then also because the sun diversifies them with its movement they resemble in many dispositions the winds of spring since in spring it happens that weather changes to a certain salubrious temperature. When the west wind blows (known as both Zephyr and Favonius) since it is most clear and brings delight "gentle Zephyr brings back the leafy branches which Boreas bears away," as Boethius says.[186] However, the west wind also brings cold and shivers which are ills to be combated with a created heat. The south winds are warm and dry. If winds pass over the regions described as favorable they are considered by the experts as especially beneficial to old people of advanced age and cold and dry in nature both in autumn and in the northern region. They bring assistance to the chest, but they make the weather heavier, slow the hearing, produce headaches, loosen the bowels, make the entire body sluggish, humid, and languid, disturb the senses, bring on dizziness and slow movement. Useful remedies for these discomforts are rose water and camphor. The winds have different effects according to the nature of places and regions and especially of the variety of mountains over which they pass by reason of the air, the sea, stagnant waters, swamps, valleys and the like. They differ as well because of deserts or burned areas or those areas close to the place of origin of the winds. They say the wind from the Mediterranean land is salubrious, that from the sea is heavy and has an opposite effect. The south wind at Rome they call the sea wind among us, for it disturbs and makes the weather rainy. They call it *auster* because it draws up *(haurire, auster)* the winds, attracts clouds and water, and creates many ills.[187] Among the Scots, Dutch, and Norwegians it is healthful and clear.

[185]See note 179.
[186]Boethius, *Con. of Phil.* 1, M. 5. 19: *Ut quas Boreae spiritus aufert/Revehat mites Zephyrus frondes.*
[187]Isidore of Seville, *Etym.* 13. 11. 6.

This wind, however, is detested as far as preserving and restoring health is concerned. In a similar way Boreas, the north wind, performs an opposite function for us and those nations mentioned since wind *(ventus)* is said to come from coming *(veniendo)*.[188] Because it is vehement and violent continuously the more it blows the more it is purified by its motion and made thinner. But when it begins to blow it is thick and turbid and creates humidity. We, however, are located closer to the south than are those northern nations and farther from the north from which Boreas blows; the situation is vice versa for them. I know a district in southern Bologna exposed at right angles to the south whose inhabitants, suffering from a defect of hearing, are almost all deaf, and no wonder, for a southern exposure creates heaviness of hearing, according to Hippocrates.[189]

ON THE CLOTHING SUITABLE FOR THE CARE OF THE AGED

The external appearance and clothing of the aged should be seen to by the gerontocomos and made as stylish and useful as possible in accordance with the season and the old people kept diligently from the cold of wind and rain. He can prevent all discomfort to them by means of skin garments whose sleeves and tunics are made double as well as by the use of garments made of pieces of fur sewed together and cloaks with hoods. The gerontocomos should provide covering for the head and the entire body suitable for protecting the old people from the winds and inclement weather by whose attacks they may suffer and become chilled. He should take care that there will be no day so intolerable that the old man cannot walk or remain a little under the open sky.[190] Clothing should be adjusted to the nature of the old man as well as to the condition of the winds, regions, climates, constitution of the air, seasons of the year, and similar factors worthy of mention. The old man whose nature is temperate, sanguine, or choleric may wear in summer a linen undershirt or tunic and should wear it at every other season as well as a basic garment. The nature of linen is cold and dry and a garment made of it is cooler than all others

[188] Idem, 13. 11. 1: *Dictus autem ventus quod sit vehemens et violentus.*
[189] Cf. Galen, 16. 412; 17. A. 33; B. 570.
[190] Columella 1. 8. 9.

and clings less to the body, as Abulkasim reports; likewise Averroes [6. 90v] says the nature of linen is temperate, moderating and containing the body's heat and condensation of moisture on the skin, preventing the escape of vapors through the pores and presenting a shining brightness or sheen and a softness of texture. Hence they say *linen* is from the Greek because the linen-weave is soft and smooth. Of this kind also are garments made of cotton, which is a very white and soft kind of linen, or a variety of thicker silk. Garments of this kind they call cotton (or a fine kind of linen). Silken dresses have been made for women's luxury clothing woven in the manner of spider webs, which Pliny[191] says Pamphile, daughter of Platea, first discovered. She ought not to be cheated of the glory of making a silk dress that covers a woman but reveals her charms. Silk garments interwoven with cotton are more delicate, softer, and finer for old men to wear, since the old men are delicate as though they were dedicated to luxury. Such a garment is more easy on the body than a linen garment because it is not so cold and is also less cold than a garment made of silk alone. It does not inflame the blood or make it hot and it will guard old age from the attack of the winds. But the glory of a silk garment above that of linen is to be recognized thus: the silk garment increases the body and makes it smoother. The natural power which has been lost and its operations are restored; the memory increases, and thus the black bile is brought forth from the capsule of the heart, on the authority of Rosarius.[192] It happens that silk garments vary greatly as to heat and cold for those made with a nap that is not shaggy which Pliny[193] calls *rasas* [scraped] are less warm. The hairy surface of cloth fabrics which are best united to the body and adhere to it makes them warmer. Of this sort are garments whose nap is curled like citron. Silk clothes are soft and warm. Serapio the son[194] says that silk is warm and humid and provides both warmth and humidity in a garment preeminently and all clothing of silk provides warmth in moderation, but clothing of other materials is of a flat texture, not woolly or velvety, while linen is cold.

[191]Pliny, *N. H.* 11. 76.
[192]Rosarius: I have not identified him.
[193]Pliny, *N. H.* 8. 195.
[194]*Liber Serapionis de simpli. medi. sumpta a plantis, mineralibus et animalibus, etc.;* Lugduni: Jacobus Myt, 1525, f. 25.

The same must be said of whatever cloth so woven that it remains thin. In winter the old man must be covered with woollen garments for they are warmer than those of other materials. Wool is less warm than humid but rather rough to the touch for the more delicate old man. They clothe him in silk quite shaggy and shiny, as being more praiseworthy. Clothes woven with both wool and silk are warm and dry and keep one moderately warm. They are recommended as warm and helpful for old men cold by nature in winter and in mountain locations. However, they induce inflammation when the material is mixed with linen. It is recommended that old men wear these clothes with a rather loose girdle at times and tighter at other times so that the restraint thus provided by their weight is lighter in summer and heavier in winter. In the latter season old men should be protected by three or four tunics and woollen coverings for chest, thighs, and legs. This sort of dress should not be regarded as strange for the custom proceeds from the wearing of a breast plate, as Pliny says,[195] so lavishly made that the clothing constituted a burden. Fur garments have a diversity in nature corresponding to the diversity of the animals from which they are obtained. They should be worn in the resumptive regimen by old people. Sometimes woollen and silk garments are augmented by skins or furs. Their Greek names indicate that for the greater part they were not in use and thus failed to receive names in Latin. From all these the most adapted for keeping the human body warm are the best. Some of these skins are those of the animal physicians call the beaver, others are hyena or pig, which is very warm. Next to it is the fox, which is lighter in weight and more suitable for garments; it provides a good heat although many people regard it as harmful and prefer sheep skin. The skin of the hare is admirably adapted for old men; it warms and strengthens their bodies as well as those of the young and provides aid in illnesses of the joints, giving strength to the nerves. The same judgment is made of rabbit skin, of *dosseri, varri,* and *armerini.*[196] They differ little in warmth and possess lightness and smoothness, suitable for temperate bodies. The skins of animals called in Italian *zebellini, maturelli,* or *fovini* are known in Latin as

[195]Pliny, *N. H.* 8. 197.

[196]Du Cange, *Glossarium* s. v. *dorsus, doscis,* Fr. *petit gris,* It. *dosso,* skins of little animals; s. v. *vares,* squirrel fur used as trimming; cf. vair in heraldry: *sibelini, armelini, dossi, vares, vulpes* all used for their fur; It. *armellino (ermellino),* ermine.

fales and *meles*.[197] Like the lynx and leopard they are highly valued and more praiseworthy than others, especially the fox. Lamb skins increase bodily strength and are adaptable for the protection of the kidneys. Rabi Moyses [f. 23] says exposure to the bodies and skins of cats induces phthisis, consumption, and emaciation. They say also (if we can believe it) that putting on the right shoe before the left preserves one (if it is credible), although marvellous to relate, from diseases of the spleen.

THE PROPER BED FOR THE AGED

They say that an old man who lies on a smooth, soft bed is thereby humidified in heart, liver, and the entire body, among other advantages. A soft bed contributes to fat and corpulence. A feather bed is more suitable for this purpose, which they call cushion-stuffing *(tomentum),* like a soft sack of feathers. So pleasant to the human race is this kind of bed that without it the spine and the body cannot endure. It is even better if made of swan's down, next best if of duck or goose feathers. Then comes a bedspread of cotton rather than wool. Silk or wool such as those into which threads are woven to form designs[198] or cotton varying in smoothness and weight to fit the season of the year and the nature of the old individual, with other considerations, are also desirable. So sensitive does the weaker old man become that the complaining poet says:

> Soft couches are like hard and jagged rocks[199]

No less variety is required in bed curtains and coverlets, sometimes of linen in the summer (the Greeks call them *peripetasmata*), curtains which hang down and shut off the place where the bed lies as well as for decoration. These are to be selected according to the needs of the bedroom and the means of the old man who is being cared for, some of silk or cloth dyed purple or scarlet with oak dye *[Quercus coccifera]* or cochineal in winter. The quality of silk is excellent in warmth and dryness, creating a fine substance for the spirits to which it has a great affinity. It also assists the vision and memory and the spirit in the liver. A sign of this fact is that silk contributes to fatness.

[197]Varro, *De Re Rustica* 3. 12. 3: *ne faelis aut maelis* (weasel and badger); *TLL* s. v.: cat and bear.
[198]Cf. Pliny, *N. H.* 8. 195.
[199]Maximianus, *Elegies* 1. 253.

Chapter XVI

The Proper Exercise for the Aged. Baths and Rest

The advantage of exercise in the resumptive regimen is shown in its assistance in the preservation of health by extending the body's powers after the old man's general decline has set in. Its necessity consists in the marvellous results it produces, as Averroes says [6.93r]. Before taking food and drink by which old age is restored exercise and rest are prescribed so that exercise always precedes meal time. This sequence must be maintained in order to keep the inner or innate heat stirred up, not checked by the consumption of food. Thus the abundant superfluities caused in the old body by its weakness of digestion, especially of the third one which is completed in the members, require their evacuation lest these superfluities obstruct the operation of the members, reduce the body's heat, and thus prevent the distribution of aid to the members. This evacuation is accomplished most effectively by means of exercise more than by a reduction of food and drugs, for exercise is by nature an ideal instrument for driving the superfluities to the skin and thence expelling them through the pores of the body or at least preparing their expulsion. This is the doctrine of the experts on the evacuation of the humors which move down to the skin since they are thin and readily disposed for expulsion. The process is completed by bathing and a rub-down, which are especially conducive to good health as long as they are temperate and moderate. They facilitate the removal of the excess humors, restore the body's balance in this respect, and nourish it. They restore the color to a rosy glow and send the blood to the extremities with its dilatation and dispersion. The gerontocomos must be a good judge among all these aids to health, especially of exercise, to lessen instead of increasing it, lest the old men come to grief and their strength be exerted beyond their bodies' powers and they suffer from aches and pains. There are many kinds of exercise for old people adjusted to each one's strength and ability. Thus the stronger among the old men should exercise at first by apprehension [grasping objects][200] and walking, but not violently, for just as the structure of the body is best adapted in youth to all very strenuous efforts of this sort so it is adapted in old age to all moderate efforts, as Celsus observes.[201] Just as in an illness exercise must be used carefully so it must be used in old age for the same purpose, to promote health. The types of exercise employed for the resumptive regimen and suitable for the aged are gentle, soft, and light, and they are of many kinds. Some are adapted for every one; these are called common because they extend to the entire body.[202] They include suspensions, that is, being carried about, or riding, of which there are many kinds; the easiest is done by being rocked on water or in a cradle, by standing, lying or sitting in a boat in a port or on a river, or the high sea, or in a litter or a sedan chair or more rapidly in some vehicle, either a litter or a wagon. More active forms of exercise are walking about, hunting (which is more strenuous), playing with a small ball: this depends on opportunity and should be done with restraint. Whichever form of exercise is chosen should produce pleasure. Thus walking is the most ideal for the elderly. Hunting or ball playing may be difficult or impossible. Horseback riding is sufficiently moderate since its motion reaches the entire body and is very helpful to the stomach and coxae, especially riding on a male or female mule. Each sex of this beast goes straight down the road, as Columella[203] says, and covers the ground comfortably, although the male is more adapted to saddles and is more agile. In regard to agility, gentleness, cheapness of maintenance, and general thriftiness, the mule is better than the horse and is more frequently used by priests at Rome as they go about their duties for the papal court. However, although exercise by some kind of carrying about is rather difficult for old people yet they should use a litter or chair or an *arcera* to be carried about gently and without injury. In this fashion that old physician

[200]See Galen, 6. 125 (chaps. 8–10) and 140–41 on types of exercise such as lifting weights, climbing ropes, etc. Also Avicenna, *Canon,* I, 56v.
[201]Celsus, *De Medicina* 1. 2. 3; 4. 9. 12.
[202]Ibid., 2. 15.
[203]Columella, 6. 37. 11.

Antiochus used to take exercise. As Galen[204] tells us, he used to go long distances to visit his patients and was carried in a sedan chair, but sometimes he rode in a carriage. An *arcera* is a carriage covered on all sides and protected like an ark, provided with bed clothing, in which the very sick or old people could be carried while lying down. But if none of these conveyances is possible due to the exceedingly weak condition of the old man his bed should be suspended on ropes and moved back and forth. If this also is impossible a rope should be attached to one leg of his bed and thus he can be pulled about here and there by hand, as Celsus prescribes. Such a shaking is suitable when done with a cradle, as Avicenna states. In the regimen of the elderly sick people who are convalescing and sit about without being able to move on their own feet this process if carried out gently entices sleep, discharges flatulence, is an aid in forgetfulness, stimulates desires, and excites the general nature of the person. The gerontocomos should have his plans for persuading his patients to have their beds suspended in order to alleviate their illness or to induce sleep. But if none of these things can be done the old man should be rubbed down once or twice since rubbing can be a good substitute for exercise in building up a man's strength when carefully administered as to quality and quantity. Such rubbing when done with soft cloths in hand brings much relief, they say; if done without the use of oil it warms the body greatly and dries out the patients who are of a humid nature in winter and in the northern regions, as Abulkasim says. It dispels and liquefies the superfluous humors, opens the pores, makes the members more solid, and aids expulsion of those humors which remain in the third digestion. When bothor [an abscess or tumor] is generated it must be treated with bathing. Rubbing with oil, however, has passed out of frequent use in our time for old people since it is more adapted to those who are ill than for the time at which exercise is taken by those who are healthy. Exercise should take place in the morning, for such early exercise or walking tempers the body, as Theodorus Priscianus says.[205] It is very helpful for the head and eyes and makes the stomach easy for all old men. When suitable exercise for at least an hour takes place

[204]Galen 6. 332–33; also Celsus, *De Medicina* 2. 15.
[205]*Experimentarius Medicinae: Theodori Dieta;* Argentorati: Joannes Schott, 1544, xix.

the body is purified of its internal superfluities from the intestines and from the bladder without any cacochimia [corrupt humors] remaining in the inner parts and in the veins. These corrupt humors are spread throughout the body by exercise when food is taken before it is digested in the stomach, liver, and veins, also hastening the time for taking further food. The cacochimia can be diagnosed from evidence of the digestion which appears in the urine both in substance and color. But if the old man is rubbed with soft hands and turned over and massaged on many different parts of the body in turn such as the muscles or if he is rubbed thoroughly with a soft towel it is of great assistance to him. A massage with abundant warm sweet olive oil either in the sunshine or near a fire softens the roughness of the skin and disperses the superfluities; it also makes the massage swifter and softer, thus reducing the tensions in the body. The skin is kneaded and made soft and pleasant. Olive oil is of particular value for the old and especially for those of advanced age, as Averroes says [5.79r; 81r], because of the weakness of the power of attraction in the members as long as its use upon the members is only to furnish them with aliment and no more. A prolonged use of the oil upon the members greatly relaxes them and alters the body. Furthermore, the towels chosen for the massage should be soft and smooth lest their roughness harm the flesh; the massage should be gentle. If the friction is rather harsh it will be painful and difficult, but if it is gentle it will be more effective nor will a large part of the oil evaporate: a too vigorous massage tends to dissipate the oil. If done in moderation it soothes, softens, and adds to the body, beginning from the top and going downward, from side to side and transversely, gradually increasing so that the pores may be opened everywhere. There is no determined frequency for the massage of old people, as Celsus says.[206] This must be judged by the varying powers of the individual to be massaged. If the old man is quite infirm fifty times can be sufficient. If he is more robust he can be rubbed down two hundred times. Between these limits the proportion should be determined on an individual basis of hardihood. Women should be massaged less frequently than men and a boy less often yet or an old man than a young man. But if the afore-

[206]Celsus, *De Medicina* 2. 14.

mentioned forms of exercise by motion through pulling or the use of animals or other means are too strenuous for a weak old man such as riding or being driven about then a loud-voiced reading will comfortably exercise him.[207] Cicero[208] also says the bodies of older men grow sluggish with the fatigue of exercising but their minds are refreshed by it. Which and what sort are the exercises of the mind will be described in the following chapter XLII. There are furthermore other kinds of exercise which are devoted separately to different parts of the body. Each of the organic members requires its special exercise which must be taken into account in the resumptive routine. The chest, lungs, throat, uvula, tongue, and mouth require exercise by means of the voice for sometimes it is deep and heavy, at other times sharp or shrill and covering a range of tones between these two extremes. These organs bring a splendor to the individual's skin coloring and clear the chest, as Avicenna says. Exercises of the hands and feet are not unknown. The back is exercised by standing, for the back is that part of the body which is borne downward. The vision is exercised by gazing at visible objects less than moderate in size and becomes keener in the process of seeing lighted things. The hearing likewise improves in response to sharp and sometimes loud sounds, and so with the teeth and similar organs which can be exercised. But if some one of these parts becomes weak it is due to some ill, such as gout in the feet or hands, upon which occasionally some tubercules grow out from callouses, varicose veins in the legs, polyps in the nose, and so forth. The organ which is afflicted must be administered to and must by no means be violently shaken. The old man whose care is the purpose of this book is one who has his organs in sound condition to begin with. Those apprehensions or worries of the mind, as they call them, should be rendered more moderate by moderate exercises for the aged. Such exercises benefit the spirits, dissolve and expel the superfluities of the nutritive members, and render their substance softer. The old man's hair

[207]Celsus, *De Medicina* 1. 2; 6. 8. An appropriate exercise. Reading in antiquity was done aloud. See J. Balogh, "Voces Paginarum," *Philologus* 82 (1927) 84–109; 202–40; G. L. Hendrickson, "Ancient Reading," *CJ* 25 (1929) 182–96; W. P. Clark, "Ancient Reading," *CJ* 26 (1930/31) 698–700; E. S. McCartney, "Notes on Reading and Praying Audibly," *CP* 43 (1948) 184–87; B. M. W. Knox, "Silent Reading in Antiquity," *GRBS* 9 (1968) 421–35. See also Avicenna, *Canon* I, 57r, on reading as exercise.
[208]Cicero, *De Sen.* 36.

should not be neglected; it is good to comb it daily, especially when he has risen in the morning and before he has emptied his bowels and urinated. Aristotle to Alexander is author of the statement that frequent use of the comb averts the vapors upon the head which impede vision. It draws the vapors to the upper regions so as to move them from the area of the eye, says Avicenna.[209] Therefore daily and frequent use of the comb is ideal for old age, for it wipes away the mists or obscurities of the eyes and brain, thus purifying the organs of cognitive power and swiftness of understanding and acumen of learning.

ON BATHING

They claim that bathing, just as exercise, is very useful in the resumption of old age for it revives the innate heat no less than exercise does with its movement and more than any other form of exercise its moderate use humidifies the body, especially a bath in fresh water which they call *lavacrum.* Since the word bath *(balneum)* comes from *valaneyom,* from the Greek *valo,* which is "I place or put" there is a similarity between a bath which causes one to sweat with hot air and the *lavacrum,* which humidifies, and about which I am speaking now. The *lavacrum* is properly recommended in the regimen of old age. It involves the total immersion of the body in water which preferably is fresh. A hot bath is suitable for boys and old men, as Celsus says.[210] It is not so hot a water as that used in what they call a *caldarium* since the latter by heating the fresh water has the power of heating the body's force too much and not humidifying it; hence it is not suitable for old age. But if the heat of the bath is of the proper temperature it warms and humidifies the old man equally. The body is thus renewed, the pores are opened, the dirt that has collected on it is washed away, repletion is reduced, flatulence dispelled, sleep provoked, lassitude removed, and appetite is excited. It is more suitable for the protection of the old man of frigid and humid nature in winter and in the northern region, as Abulkasim reports. It thins the phlegm, increases the body, moves the urine, removes itching and scabies, and carries off the rheum and catarrh of the brain. If oil is added to the bath

[209] Avicenna, *Canon* 3. 204v, 214r.
[210] Celsus, *De Medicina* 1. 3.

the mingled oil and water are especially beneficial to the stomach, according to Theodorus Priscianus [xvii]. If the bath called a *tepidarium* is used it cools off the body and humidifies it greatly. Its particular function is to guard the aged body from hemorrhoids as Judeus [f. xr] says. However, so excellent are the warm and humid baths called *lavacrum* with their moderation of strength in the regimen of the aged that they are eagerly sought for and not only benefit the warm and dry bodies but cause the thirsty to thirst no more, for the bath works on them like wine. Not only does this kind of bath function to cool off the hot body or to warm the frigid one but it brings on sweating by drying out and humidifying. Hence they say that a bath and a moderate drink assist in a disease and are proper for treating a disease. The proper time to be chosen for taking a bath to aid resumption of the natural disposition in old age[211] is that after the food has been completely digested (or concocted) in the stomach and liver. Then the food is already absorbed in the veins and the time is at hand for another meal. Thus beyond the purpose of resumption there is also the purpose of adding flesh to the body. Hence, the most convenient hour for bathing is after the time of saturation of food, since as Avicenna [I, 58r] says a bath dries out, renders thin and weakens those who are empty of food or fasting but it fattens those who are full of food and in addition draws the humidity to the surface of the body. Nevertheless, the bath can also create an obstruction or oppilation because it draws the undigested or not thoroughly concocted food from the stomach and liver to the members. It is best therefore to bathe at the end of the first digestion before the advent of hunger once more; thus the bath contributes to a moderate increase of fat. They say old men should engage in a vigorous and brief exercise before bathing until they are completely tired and when they bathe they should be calm and silent, as Celsus says.[212] They should desist from activity while some one pours water over them, followed by a rub-down. There are many uses for the bath in the first and last stages of old age. For those old people not completely decrepit a bath is necessary three or four times a month on account of the little exercise they take. Baths may be taken over a more extended

[211]Cael. Aur., *Tard.* 5. 10. 95; *Acut.* 4. 2; *Veget.* 1. 25. 1; 3. 6. 11; 3. 45. 5; 4. 4. 2.
[212]Celsus, *De Medicina* 1. 2, 3.

period and thus less frequently by old men in their prime. For the weak and prostrate bathing is strictly forbidden. In regard to bathing they divide old age into three parts. The first includes those old people who are not yet removed from domestic and civil duties nor from an association with other people. The second refers to those quite aged men who are led about or directed as if they were children. The third part is divided into those who are unable to sustain themselves and cannot bathe on whatever day they wish without assistance. In bathing one must keep account of the strength of the individual nor must the old man be neglected whose energy is low because of exposure to the heat of the day. He should be bathed more quickly, taken out of the bath and wrapped up in a gown, as Celsus says.[213] Cold air should not blow on him and he should be rubbed with oil, especially a weak old man of dry nature in the summertime. When he is humidified he is preserved from apostemata [abscesses] and his general bearing becomes lively. His body should then be mildly soothed with the sprinkling of chervil and rose water. Thereafter he may resume his meals. It has been said: After you have bathed, eat or go to sleep, for sleep after bathing is good for the health of older men. So long as nothing is being digested or dissolved, as they say, which should be digested or dissolved sleep after bathing is very helpful. We should remember the procedure in this respect followed by Telephus the grammarian, as told by Galen.[214] He maintained an excellent health for almost one hundred years. In winter he bathed twice a month, four times a month in summer, and three times a month in each of the other seasons. On the days when he did not bathe he was rubbed down lightly around the third hour. Then he ate a meal of spelt grits[215] cooked in water mixed with pure honey of the very best kind. This was a sufficient breakfast for him at the first hour of the day. He dined at the seventh hour, or a little earlier, first on vegetables, then on fish or chicken, but barely tasting them. At evening he ate only bread dipped in diluted wine.

Bathing may be used for any particular bodily member which requires it in accordance with the habits and strength of the indi-

[213]Ibid., 1. 3.
[214]Galen 6. 333.
[215]Pliny, *N. H.* 22. 25. 61. 128; Celsus 6. 6.

vidual, as, for example, the head and the feet. Bathing is good for the brain with a mixture of warm water, spelt, camomile, laurel, and leaves of senna. An application of this mixture strengthens the brain and nerves; in fact, according to every manner of administration it increases the viscosity and aids the hearing. Mesue[216] says: For those afflicted with a morbid or sickly old age a frequent fomentation of the feet is helpful for repairing the memory of old men and very helpful for their vision. It is ideal also at the same time to go to bed without eating. It likewise helps to bring on sleep, assists the brain and the instruments of the senses, dispels the vapors which arise to the upper parts of the body unless there is something which may prevent this. The old man's beard should also be shaved, especially for those old men whose nature is cold and humid in winter and in the northern regions, as Abulkasim says. Thus nothing should be overlooked which may be of help in the resumption of the old man's health. Every care should be taken also to keep his private parts and anus clean and free from filth. His nails should be cut according to those who are anxious observers of the days of the week; this should be done on Wednesday (Jove's day), for if the nails are cut on that day their breaking apart is prevented. Care should be taken, nevertheless, not to cut the nails when the moon is in Gemini. They say that the nails of the toes should not be cut when the moon is in Pisces and especially when it is in conjunction with Mercury or Jupiter.

ON REST

As much quiet rest as possible is advantageous for old people who are troubled by the weakness of their powers of locomotion. Rest should follow, as has been said previously, a rubdown moderate in quality and quantity with olive oil, for a rather rapid and gentle rubbing loosens tension. Moderate rest is recommended for old people especially of a warm nature who have wide pores in a particularly hot summer and in hot regions. It provides relief to pains of the chest, as Abulkasim says. However, rest which is inordinate creates phlegm which is dissolved by motion, for old people

[216]Mesue, d. 857, *Aphorismi* = Yuhanna ibn Serapion = Janus Damascenus, *Therapeutice Methodi* (Basle: Henricus Petrus, 1543), f. 42.

do not require rest at all times. They say the cause of this state is that their frigidity lacks the heat which is created by motion. The heat of the aged deeply desires to be fanned since it is in small amount so that it may be cherished and become greater. Large flames do not need to be fanned but are sufficient in themselves so as to survive and grow stronger. A balance must be sought in the matter of rest and exercise in the resumptive regimen so that the suspension of the routine of exercise should not afflict the old man while too lazy a life is not helpful to him either. Excess exercise swiftly ages and sickens him.

Chapter XVII

Food and Drink in General Recommended in the Care of the Aged

After the discussion of motion and rest appropriate for the elderly we must come to observations concerning their food and drink. Since exercise stimulates hunger you must restore the emptiness of the body with food. Exercise wears down the aged and excites appetite in them, proclaiming the necessity of aliment. Since food is necessary for restoring the body to its wholeness according to the experts by increasing it the loss of food in the body's dissolution is repaired insofar as is possible. The body's balance should not be altered in any way nor should it have any superfluous quality inharmonious with its nature such as pungency, ponticity [a special flavor in foods from the Black Sea: Pontus], and sharpness. Therefore the gerontocomos must observe certain matters in the process of resumption and its administration. Food and drink must be chosen according to certain conditions or qualities they possess in order that the blood created from more excellent food should be converted into excellent blood. The special advantage of food consists in the fact that it is easily digested, descends more quickly and is sufficiently completed with a viscosity and thickness which do not exceed a proper measure. Too much viscosity of food in the veins, capillaries, and narrow passages of the body prevents the blood from being carried to the extremities. Thus a moderate amount of food causes it to adhere more perfectly to the members. An excessive amount of food because of its density is especially harmful for the resumption of the strength of the old people for the old man who has little heat in him cannot change the dense food into nourishment. Extreme thinness of food is also not recommended since it evaporates more quickly from the members. A moderate amount of nourishment provides strength, as it should, to the aged body since it is the closest form of material for making blood. This process is accomplished by three stages of nutrification: adhesion, union, and assimilation. In addition, a moderate superfluity is required for proper nourishment together with the aid of the individual innate strength of the aged body proportionate to that kind and amount of food which is determined for the nourishment of whatever species of animal and appropriate not only to its nature but also in accordance with reason, such as the warm and humid nature of the human. Likewise, the substance of all the food appropriate to the cold and dry nature of animals provides for them what they call their hidden power. Thus for cattle the bitter vetch,[217] grass for donkéys, squinanthia for camels, acorns for pigs and so on for each species there is a particular food which they either dislike or prefer. There is no small variety of choice for each distinct individual although sometimes appetite is rather weak and desire for food flags. This preference for certain foods is often restored due to the fatality of the stars. Astrologers say that when the planets that forbode ill are in the ascendency of their horoscope or nativity people will relish foods of insipid and bitter flavor. The contrary situation prevails according to a more favorable horoscope when they will delight in foods of pleasant odor and such like. The foods suitable in the regimen of old age under these conditions are humid and tend to be somewhat warm, for they are thus more quickly conveyed to the members and converted into flesh since the nature of old age is dry and cold. Old people live longer when they are restored by such food, as determined in chapter XII. The experts warn against a great excess in the heat of foods, however. Galen[218] says that a long-standing correction of the foods which are dried out can be made through humidity and it is less deceptive than through frigidity. The experts insist that foods used in the regimen of old people should be most flavorful and of pleasant odor, for thus their effect upon human nature and especially upon that of the aged is more gratifying. Those foods tending toward a certain sweetness are particularly pleasant. They are not to be eaten, however, while

[217]Cael. Aur., *Acut.* 2. 19. 113.
[218]Galen 7. 258; 15. 289, 412, 416.

fasting nor after meals [i.e., between meals] but during the regular meal, as Theodorus Priscianus [xvi] prescribes, since all sweet foods create flatulence and indigestion. Sweet smelling foods are no less attractive to human nature; they are very nourishing. For this reason they say that a good smell is the food of the soul because it revives the spirits and lengthens life. Thus it is said in the Book of the Apple[219] on the death of Aristotle that his life was prolonged by the odor of an apple. The commentator on Galen, *De Sectis,*[220] also reports the marvellous story about Democritus, who when he was about to die, while still making fun of mankind, was an inhabitant of the city of Aldiris at a time when a solemn festival was being celebrated there. When the citizens asked him not to die until they had completed their festival and its banquets Democritus asked: "How many days do you wish me to wait before I die?" They said three or four days while the festival lasted. Then Democritus told them to bring him a cup of Attic honey and he remained four days still alive, smelling the honey. Others say that Democritus noticed an oven being opened in which loaves of bread were being baked and thus survived on the smell of the baking bread. Pliny[221] also says that on the extreme boundary of India on the east near the source of the Ganges there lives a race of people who have no mouth; they live, however, by breathing an odor brought into their nostrils. They have no food or drink, only the various odors of roots and flowers and of the wild apples which they bring from a distance so that their smell may not be lacking. They are easily killed by an odor which is somewhat stronger.

The experts recommend the flesh of chickens and partridges and the extremities of young goats for these are most easily digested in the stomach because they are light food and more easily converted into blood in the liver and veins and thus more assimilable by the members of old people. They produce less stinking feces, as Avicenna says, and in every way this type of food is good

[219]*Liber de Pomo et Morte: The Book of the Apple,* ed. D. S. Margoliouth in *Journal of the Royal Asiatic Society,* 1892, 187–252. See Diogenes Laertius (Democritus) IX. 43; H. Diels-W. Kranz, *Die Fragmente der Vorsokratiker* II (1956): 83–84; 89 (28. *Anon. Londin.* c. 37, 34ff; ed. H. Diels, *Supplementum Aristotelicum* iii pars 1; Berlin, 1893); Cael. Aurel., *Acut. morb.* II, 37.

[220]The story does not appear in C. D. Pritchet, ed., *Iohannis Alexandrini commentaria in librum De sectis Galeni;* Leiden, Brill, 1982.

[221]Pliny, *N. H.* 7. 2. 25.

for old people. A small quantity of it has great nourishment, as for example the yolks of sucking eggs, rooster testicles, and the flesh of recommended animals such as kids, small sucking calves, year-old lambs, pigeons, young turtle-doves, and wheat from which extraneous material has been cleaned out. The experts approve of all these foods. Bread baked carefully in ovens is recommended and foods which tend to be sweet together with wine of good odor. I shall discuss all these in what follows. If the old man is quite advanced in years and has grown weaker he must be restored with liquid foods for speedy digestion, such as gruel, juicy broths made of boiled chicken, and the like. If the old patient still grows weaker then his diet should be that befitting illness in old age, that is, ethical [i.e., a state of emaciation, the fever of debility, from *ekteko,* "I am exhausted" in Greek].[222] This diet is humidifying and creates substance, as the physicians call it, easy of penetration, swift in descent through the human system, without viscosity, such as the water of flesh made by sublimation or reduction of the flesh of fowl or four-footed animals to a fine consistency more suitable for digestion, as well as sucking eggs fresh and quivering and fine wine of good odor and golden color but in small quantity. Old age requires less food than do people of other ages since its heat is small and weak; it needs little to survive. The food for old age should, however, be strong and very nourishing.[223] In this way the strength of the old man's members is not overloaded. Old men should be thus restored by their food nor should this be deleterious nor dangerous to their health *(delecteron)* nor easily spoiled *(deisperion)* nor of a kind which induces black bile or phlegm. Above all, his food should not be very hot or piquant nor dry, such as are some foods flavored with vinegar and salt. Nor should pungent hot aromas be used excessively; these are to be used only by way of medicine. Otherwise, the gerontocomos will shorten the life he is trying to extend by the resumptive art. Further advice holds that spoiled foods should be avoided as well as whatever cooked food makes the patient cold or any food altered in smell and everything acid, for acid hastens old age, as Avicenna says. If the old man eats salted meat or game or fish of hard flesh such food should be

[222]R. Dunglison, *A Dictionary of Medical Science,* 1860, s. v. hectic fever.
[223]*alibile;* cf. Varro, *Res Rustica* 2. 11. 2.

eaten together with melons or cucumbers. If this food is flavored with salt and vinegar one may eat it without the melons or cucumbers. If the gerontocomos determines that the old man is suffering from cacochimia [depravation of the humors or bad juice] he should be fed with a reduced diet from which the humidifying elements have been removed since they are not helpful in this situation. However, if discomfort results from this procedure they say it is safer for nourishment to be given in liquid form rather than in that of solid form in order to avoid nausea; thus thick nutriments should be removed from the diet. Such a revulsion causes pains of the joints and kidneys, dyspnoea, gout, hardening of the spleen, jaundice, and the ills of melancholy and phlegm. The experts furthermore disapprove of many courses at the same meal especially of those which stimulate the appetite for those who eat frequently suffer from an unconquerable and powerful gluttony. In order to avoid overeating and thus the surfeit which accompanies it Augustus Caesar used to dine on only three courses although when he offered a lavish banquet he allowed six courses, as Suetonius[224] tells us. The courses of a meal are more advantageous when composed of foods which have particular food value in strengthening the stomach and its digestion by the ingestion and then full digestion of food. When food is added to the stomach while it is digesting the food previously eaten digestion is impeded and assimilation blocked. Gluttony with its blandishments of different delicious flavors and foods entices the appetite so much that the stomach accepts more food than it can readily digest. This would not happen if less food were eaten for then appetite would decrease. When various foods of different consistencies are swallowed, some easy to digest, others hard, the result is an imperfect nutrition of the members. Also when one type of food is digested before that type which is swallowed on top of it a mixture occurs and the digested food precipitates the undigested food downward and spoils it if it remains in the stomach awaiting complete digestion. A variety of foods prevents the completion of digestion since it causes the old man to drink more frequently. This impedes his digestion just as the bubbling of boiling water is decreased when water is frequently added to the pot whose water is just coming to a boil, as

[224]Suetonius, *Divus Augustus Caesar* 74.

Rainaldus says.[225] Thus a longer period of mastication of the various courses is hindered. Between the first and last course the process of the digestion of food which is just beginning to be digested is hampered by overloading the stomach with more food. This practice must be avoided in old age lest the very attempt to prolong it should result in shortening the individual's natural life. A proper order should be observed in the choice of foods, humid and smooth being preferred to that which is dry and constipating, sweet flavor to acid, cool to hot, and so on, with thick and soft foods judiciously mingled. Care should be taken that the old people eat at the last course of a meal something astringent such as coriander flavored with sugar, a pear or citron, and similar foods to prevent the ascent of vapors to the brain.

HOW OFTEN OLD PEOPLE SHOULD BE FED EACH DAY

Since there are very many critical decisions to be made in feeding old people it has been set down as a precept concerning both natural and non-natural elements that an account must be maintained in their regimen not only of the number but of the quality and quantity of foods; it is not easy to measure the latter. Averroes [6.94r] says that their regimen is partly made up of food and partly of exercise; as to the other six non-naturals there is a wide latitude of choice according to the age of the individual. First, it must be understood by the old person that too much food is not advisable for every overloading of the stomach is very similar to a sheer waste of food and is as unhelpful as is an excessive abstinence from food. Boys and old men are least able to endure hunger.[226] Hence the gerontocomos must exercise very diligent care in regard to food and drink so that the more lively of his charges should be seldom fed with many rare or unusual foods. The distribution of food should be selectively made to those old people who are weak by nature, not simply age. Those who are in the first stage of old age are warm and humid, of a prepossessing bearing, endowed with firm, compact flesh, a broad hairy breast, good liver and stomach, and are well filled with blood. They are

[225]Rainaldus: unidentified.
[226]Galen, 1. 597; 17 B. 401; on the quality and quantity of food, 6. 331.

not burdened with external cares and possess what is necessary for life in moderate locations, seasons, and dispositions. They are able to eat as much food as is sufficient and can thus eat and drink to their satisfaction. They rarely have excessive raw humors in their stomachs or veins which require digestion. In contradistinction to these more healthy old people are those with wide pores and thin humors; these must eat more sparingly but more often, twice or three times a day. Those people who range between these two groups can be fed three times every two days since their powers are better preserved. The age of the individual must be carefully observed, for a more lofty purpose is based upon strength, as Galen says.[227] In the determination of a man's strength it is necessary to take account of his age. Furthermore, the older the men are the weaker they become. They should be fed with more frequent and smaller meals so that the food will be digested more quickly and so that their small natural heat should not be overwhelmed with too much food. According to their power of digestion and their state of weakness their nourishment should be carefully given at the rate of two or three times daily, to be increased as they require more. Their nature is like a lighted lantern, as Galen says,[228] ready to go out; when almost extinguished it is restored with a little oil but its flame dies when too much oil is added to it. Thus old age in its extremely weakened final stage requires only a little food nor is it inclined to eat much. Not much food but frequently should be given both night and day so that the amount of it should not overburden the stomach, which is adapted to food of the finest consistency such as a weak person requires. If old people make a slight mistake in either the quality or quantity of the food they eat they suffer not a little, as Antiochus the physician rightly observed. In his old age and already weak he ate three times a day and thus restored grew old in great tranquillity.[229] This practice of moderation is by no means to be neglected; if a man abides by it at other stages in his life so much the more should he do so in old age when people should not be drawn away from their established habits. The cause for this maintenance of pre-

[227]Ibid., 6. 19; 15. 582 sq.; 16. 598.
[228]Ibid. 17. B. 413; 7. 673–75; 1. 660.
[229]Ibid. 6. 331–32.

vious habits is discussed in chapter XIII. So much power does habit have in the regimen of the human body that when we abuse it by deviating from it in our eating and drinking and choosing to abandon the course which has kept us healthy we shall find it dangerous to make such a sudden change. Old people should be fed oftener in a mild climate than in a more rigorous one, oftener in summer than in winter, and they should take more exercise rather than less and be fed more with light foods than with heavy. It is also more necessary to hasten the frequency of the meals since they tolerate hunger less easily. These are the people to whose more sensitive stomachs the yellow bile customarily descends even if the physician recommends heavier food. Furthermore, it is of course understood that those old people who earn their living with their hands should have additional food. Our present care of the aged [gerontocomia] does not extend to them. They prefer to live contented with plain fare.

THE HOUR FOR MEALS

Since it is agreed that old people can in no wise endure prolonged hunger an appropriate time for meals must be chosen. This time should be that which follows a complete digestion of the food previously consumed. This can be recognized in those who have a normal appetite when they feel hunger and the stomach feels the veins sucking. The veins suck when the emptied members draw from the veins the nutriment which they carry. This happens when the innate heat of the members as it dissolves their substance creates a lack of nourishment. This process is carried out in order that the heat and nutriment may continue to exist and to fulfil the increased need of restoration, thus serving by nutrition the natural strength of the members which they can thus make stronger for their function just as it happens among the other natural powers which may also operate more vigorously as they serve some necessity. It is more imperative in the resumptive than in the conservative regimen that the old man whose appetite has not completely disappeared should not eat except when he is hungry nor should he be delayed in his meals since his hunger is genuine. As was said, old men and infants and all those who cannot endure hunger during the day should be fed at the first hour of the day, as Avicenna thinks, or at the third hour or at the latest at the fourth hour, as Galen reports.[230] When exercise and massage have expelled the superfluities which gather in him the old man should be given his meal. The inner organs of those who do not have a midday meal grow old more quickly, as Pliny affirms on the authority of Hippocrates.[231] At this time some of the measures which purge the stomach may be used. I shall speak of them in chapter XL. At the meal something which is especially helpful to the eye and the brain should also be served for the old people who are ill, a food which is valuable for its excellent chyme and not easily spoiled in the stomach, such as the flesh of chicken with its simple decoction or broth. It is always helpful for the old people to rest after dining nor to distress the mind with any worries nor to walk about nor to be moved even gently but to be soothed with a quiet conversation. It happens that old men are stimulated by a great variety of factors which include the season of the year, their location, and the changes in temperature. In summer the places where people stay become somewhat cooler in the shade of trees or other shelter and the hour of the day less hot and uncomfortable, for external heat makes the innate heat of the old men weaker, according to Averroes,[232] just as the sun does when it shines on a fire, which however is kindled and strengthened when it is placed in the shade. At the time of the setting of the sun they say the same foods of old age should be reduced to a small amount. Care should be taken in the warmer seasons of the year not to eat the flesh of animals with firm substance. One may eat vegetables and varieties of milky food and coriander flavored with vinegar and sour grapes. There are many old people whose appetite has entirely disappeared and who are able to taste nothing. Their diminished or lost appetite must be stimulated insofar as is possible; the importance of simple pleasure in their food is by no means to be disregarded in the regimen of the aged. That food which is more tasty is more valuable since the stomach and the power of nutrition are more strongly stimulated by it and will result in an increased production of substance in the body. Delight in food has so much influence in the feeding of old

[230]Galen, 10. 544; 15. 195, 552; 17. B. 417, 484.
[231]Pliny, *N. H.* 28. 56.
[232]1. 8; cf. Galen 11. 663; Aristotle, *Probl.* 875a6.

people that of two kinds of food they will choose that which is of less nourishment although more tasty. Nevertheless, people say that the less tasty should be chosen since among simple as well as compound or mixed foods good for the stomach there are many which are less tasty. These excite the appetite by warming it. They will be discussed in chapter XXXVI. The following recipe is in use for old people who have almost lost their appetite and is recommended as helpful in reviving it. Take three dragmas [one = the eighth part of a handful] of the best cinnamon, a half ounce of galanga, one ounce of the most fragrant rose water, and as much sugar after its third stage of refinement as is suitable. This mixture is without doubt of value in exciting the appetite if taken by the old people who have lost it. The time for taking it should coincide with the regular meal time of those who need it and they should be fed before they get obviously hungry. Their feeding should be adjusted to their needs and food given them in moderation so as not to increase tension and heaviness in the stomach. One must carefully observe the condition of their weak stomachs so that the gerontocomos can restore that which time takes away from them. The digestive tract of the elderly as well as their weak appetite requires assistance by the use of agents which promote digestion *(peptica)*[233] or foods which are easily digested since the corruption [or spoilage] of food in the stomach is the mother of many illnesses and the origin of chronic infirmities, as Avicenna says in the previous chapter IV. For the old person who has just begun to digest his food rest is prescribed; for him who has not digested at all complete rest from everything, work, exercise, and business. In addition, for his renewal antidotes from among special medicines are to be selected for him by the experts, for if that rumor or fame which many people call fame is not utterly lost, as Aristotle says, how much the more that which many wise men regard as fame. Lest its low esteem deprive him who desires it of this remedy Galen says in *On Simple Medicines,* Book V:[234] "I at any rate do not know anything more helpful in aiding the digestion of food in the stomach than the body of a man which comes up close to it and

[233]Cf. Galen, 11. 779.
[234]Ibid., 11. 724; 14. 1, 13, 19, 90, 163. Zerbi may have *N. E.* 1124a in mind in referring to Aristotle.

touches it on the outside. Some men therefore cling to boys and embrace them at night, finding them of great comfort since the natural heat of the boy warms the man's stomach if the boy gets close to him." Avicenna agrees with Galen on this point. The boy should not be one who sweats or has a hot breath. There are some men who embrace puppies or a black male cat, which is also quite helpful to the stomach. A complete mastication of food should be carried out by those old people whose teeth are still powerful enough to tear and chew their food for by this means the food acquires some digestion. The bowels are loosened when the food is made finer by thorough chewing. In the discussion *On Simple Medicines* it is said that almost every food which is hard to chew is also harder to digest. If the old man lacks teeth and lest the hapless man injure his gums he should be fed with soft bread and liquid nourishment or at least food ground up fine by some means nor should he devour his food greedily. Food which is voraciously swallowed is imperfectly digested and those who do so grow old more quickly. A sign of this is the fact that you rarely see voracious eaters who reach a natural old age and this is one cause why those who have few teeth frequently have a shorter life. Since the entire resumptive method has two avenues of approach, by food and by medicine, they have their respective faculties and often simple medicines are as effective as those which are compound; it seems appropriate in what follows to list their names, properties, and mixtures.

Chapter XVIII

The Benefits of Wine in the Recovery of the Aged

The resumptive regimen especially requires a particular use of wine in order to make a proper mixture of food in the stomach and to transfer it through the members, as experts agree. This process must be assisted in old age by some liquid so that food may be swallowed without mastication and more at that age than at any other. On account of the contraction of the passages for the food due to cold and dryness among old people food is not assimilable by them unless it is moistened so as to render it more able to penetrate those passages. If such a liquid has also the power of resumption it is all the more suitable for use by the aged, as experts prescribe. Let every other form of drink, such as beer, used at meals in place of wine yield place, for there is no liquor or juice which creates so much strength and is more adapted to human nature for bringing this aid to digestion about than wine. The experts list two liquors as most pleasing to the human body, oil and wine.[235] The best wine is made from the juice of ripe grapes and is therefore endowed with excellent quality of penetration of food and as a carrier of it throughout the body to the greatest enjoyment of the human especially one broken with age so long as it is moderately used. Just as wine is judged to be very bad for boys so it is most friendly to old people, as Galen reports,[236] since blood, flesh, and innate heat are increased by its use. It will help nature in its operations and its power for digestion is strong. It assists the easy expulsion of the superfluities, the urine and the perspiration. It induces sleep by which everyone's strength is restored. It contributes to good health and retards old age. Young people whose heat is strong should not use wine except in small quantity and

[235]Galen, 11. 487, on the medicinal use of oil; 19. 761.
[236]Ibid., 4. 809; 6. 54, 319, 334.

only for the sake of nourishment. For old people, however, as much wine as may revive their strength but not reduce it is recommended. The heat of wine restores their small heat. Heat and strength are thus increased and returned to the veins of the entire body and the blood gains in color. Therefore they say that wine *(vinum)* is so named because when it is drunk it fills the veins *(venas)* quickly[237] with blood. It works against the frigidity of old age and in the resumptive victory its effect is like that of medicine, for wine with its heat not only combats the weakness of old age but also with its humidity it provides a gradual heat and moisture by way of refreshing sips. Thus it thoroughly humidifies the substance of the old man's members dried and withered due to his age and quickly restores it, thus providing the best assistance. It leads the yellow bile to the urinary ducts so that it may be more easily voided from the bladder. It attacks the viscosity of the phlegm which is created by cold and moisture, breaking it up and ripening it, and dissolving it with heat. It acts in the same way on the black bile as it does on cold and moisture, removing its dark vapor and turbidity. It makes the blood clearer by purifying its warm and humid constituents. Although there are many kinds of food which can fill the place of wine in restoring weakened bodies nonetheless they do so less efficiently and more slowly than wine. Of all foods wine is the swiftest and most immediate (as they say) to such an extent that nothing thus far has been discovered to replace it in cheering the soul, as Avicenna says. For a good wine not only fortifies the body's strength in old age but also that of the soul, which it makes gay and jolly so that one is thought to smile without cause when the contrary is true because there is no impression as he says without something to produce it. Wine makes the spirit copious by generating a strong glow for man's nature and flesh. Thus it disposes the soul, of which the spirit is the instrument, as much as possible toward hilarity and joy. A moderate amount of wine is extremely helpful but when used more freely it harms the nerves and the eyes. It is good for the stomach, excites the appetite for food, drives away sadness, dispels the urine and the chill of the body, brings on sleep, stops vomiting, cures imperfect or inhar-

[237]Isidore of Seville, *Etymologies* 20. 3. 2: *Vinum inde dictum quod eius potus venas sanguine cito repleat.*

monious operations of the body's parts *(vitia),*[238] and entices the soul to extend its powers. As Isaac Israeli[239] says, wine turns the soul away from impiety, avarice, pride, sloth, fear, idleness, taciturnity, and cowardice and toward piety, liberality, humility, solicitude, boldness, cleverness, eloquence, and talent. Rufus[240] says that the Persians in disputation were accustomed to say that the causes of knowledge were to be sought in the collaboration of reason and that those who wished by the process of taking counsel to govern the state should always make use of wine since it provided a salutary method of conducting business, restoring strength, and demonstrating rectitude and veracity. The Greeks also when about to compose verses and to play music drank wine, having learned by experiment and reason that it made their minds more quick and supple for understanding, more skillful and shrewd in learning, increased their ability to reason, and extended their powers of action. Just as the moderate use of wine increases the strength of the body and soul to that extent Asclepiades declared[241] its power was scarcely equalled even by the power of the gods, thus going so far beyond the limit of the powers of the soul and body as to result in an unrevealed damage to them. From this source, i.e., excessive use of wine, he draws the ills of the brain and the liver which arise in the ultimate frigidity, as Galen says,[242] apoplexy, paralysis, subeth [coma], lethargy, epilepsy, spasm, and tetanus. Hence arise defects of the nerves, for wine fills the nerves because it is warm and heats them when unmixed and quickly penetrates the body, especially if the wine is thin. Hence arise pallor and hanging cheeks, ulcers of the eyes, trembling hands that pour out the contents of full vessels, as they say, nightmares, restless nights, and fetid breath.[243] Hence arise the great stiffness of chills in the elderly because their natural heat is cooled off and extinguished when they are overcome with wine, just as a fire's flame is accus-

[238]Cicero, *T. D.* 4. 13. 39: *vitium, cum partes corporis inter se dissident, ex quo pravitas membrorum, distortio, deformitas.*
[239]Isaac Israeli, *De diaetis universalibus,* etc.; in *Opera Omnia;* Lyon: Bartholomew Trot, 1515; f. clv *(Diaetis particularibus).* See Pliny, *N. H.* 23. 38.
[240]Not by Rufus of Ephesus: see Herodotus, I. 133 and Tacitus, *Germania* 22.
[241]The famous physician often quoted by Galen and others but whose works are not extant: Pliny, *N. H.* 23. 38.
[242]Galen, 1. 661; 201. 14; 14. 737; 17 B. 541. 548, 649, 787.
[243]Pliny, *N. H.* 14. 142.

tomed to be extinguished when many pieces of wood are added to it or a lantern's light when much oil is added to it. Then too since the bodies and brains of old people are weakened with an illness of the nerves their nature is not able to resist the harm done them by wine nor to tolerate a far less quantity of it than young men can. Old men who have an empty stomach are also harmed by much wine, for as Pliny[244] reports, new wine drunk on an empty stomach is most injurious. When Tiberius Claudius was emperor forty years ago, says Pliny, it was decreed that those on an empty stomach might drink wine and that it could precede the taking of food, according to certain opinions of some foreign physicians who prided themselves on the novelty of their decision. The Parthians sought glory for this virtue for themselves. Celsus[245] disapproves of this practice when he says: The body is made thin by the custom of drinking not too cold wine upon an empty stomach. It brings on spasm rather quickly and mental illness, as Galen[246] says. As far as the effect of wine upon the soul is concerned, it is well known that drinking too much wine sometimes deranges the mind, extinguishes the light of reason, and increases the irrational force of the soul; they call this the state of drunkenness. The thick raw vapor which rises from the wine is carried to the brain and stops up its passages. As a consequence sometimes that part of the soul with which we understand and are intelligent undergoes an obscuration and perturbation of its animative operations. The result, as they say, is that the body remains like a ship without a helmsman and an army without a leader. This state of being is very readily brought about in a weak brain for the mark of a strong brain is that it is not injured by the fumes of wine, as Avicenna says. It happens that the effect of wine when drunk heavily or sparingly is different according to the individual nature. Thus they say that wine makes those who have been cooled off taciturn and sober at first. Then when they have drunk a little more they become more talkative; after drinking still more they become positive, audacious, and eloquent, and later become harmful to others. With more wine yet they become maniacal, stupid, and epileptic and

[244]Ibid., 23. 41; later, quoted verbatim from *N. H.* 14. 141–43.
[245]Celsus, *De Medicina* 1. 3.
[246]Galen, 14. 64; 170.

suffer *angina vinaria.*[247] That is, they are suffocated with wine. Wine is similar to a great theriac [an ancient alexipharmic electuary used against snake bite] in that it warms those who are cold by nature. It also cools those who are warm, moistens the dry ones, dries those who are moist so that we may agree with Pliny when he says: There is nothing more useful for the strength of the body than wine nor anything more pernicious than its pleasures if it is not used in moderation.[248]

THE SELECTION OF WINE

That type of wine is greatly praised for its beneficial effect upon old people which by its nature from the earmarks apparent in it is most suitable to the temperament of old folks. This suitability can be recognized first in part from its color, that is, if it is *helvolum,*[249] or of a color midway between reddish and white or yellowish or red, of abundant odor, clear, of subtle essence or body. It warms the members and provokes the urine, thoroughly purging the serum of the blood.[250] The hotter and more diuretic it is the more valuable and helpful to the health of old people. The gerontocomos should find that variety of wine between new and old, for new wine is regarded as useless for old people.[251] If it is warm in its first stage of vintage it is full of lees, vaporous, and creates flatulence. It fills the body with gas as must does and that wine which has not aged. As Celsus says[252] it is squeezed-out wine, that is, issuing most recently from the wine-press, and being entirely musty is useless to the stomach, although it is pleasant to the veins and quickly inebriates because its watery part is more penetrating. In fact, it leads to that ill they call hepatic dysentery.[253] Old wine has heat and dryness to the third stage; even though it creates less flatulence yet it is very harmful to the old man for it excites the

[247]*anginam vinariam habere dicuntur, qui vino suffocantur:* Paul. ex Fest. 28 Müller; Lindsay 25; Galen, 14. 29.
[248]Pliny, *N. H.* 14. 58.
[249]Ibid., 14. 32; 23. 47.
[250]Galen, 6. 336.
[251]Celsus, *De Medicina* 2. 20; 27.
[252]Ibid., 5. 26. 19; Galen, 3. 270; 6. 55, 319, 336; see also Pliny, *N. H.* 14. 130; Cato, *R. R.* 23. 4; Columella 12. 36; Cael. Aur., *Acut.* 3. 21. 217.
[253]Cael. Aur., *Tard.* 4. 6. 84; Pliny, *N. H.* 26. 45; 28. 128.

senses, which is very injurious, as Galen says.[254] He tells the story of the servant of a certain notary. When his master had gone for his daily bath in the company of another servant the first one remained at home. At times he became thirsty. Not finding any water with which to quench his thirst he drank a great deal of very old wine. He became utterly sleepless, fell into a fever, became deranged and died.[255] Older wine is more powerful in its ability to harm; its age varies greatly in different climates. The Spaniards say no wine is old unless it has aged a year and a half, according to Averroes of Cordoba [6.94v]. Other people put the proper age for wine at two or more years. Among all wines, however, a pure clear appearance shows it has been cleansed of its dregs and has a white or bright reddish or yellowish color; such wines are very good for old people since the color is an indication of a uniform quality and even more if the wine has a very good aroma; this word will be explained in chapter XLII. The function of such a fine wine is to purge and cleanse the stomach and to promote the process of digestion. It lends boldness to the heart, revives the natural body heat, and improves the strength of the individual. Wine of a sharp odor is not forbidden to the aged when it is pure and unmixed especially if it is yellowish, clear, and one year old. It should be diluted with water, however, particularly for those old people whose nature is cold in the northern regions in the springtime. Wine which has been heavily diluted is suitable for boys; a pure unmixed wine is, however, adapted for old people. A diluted wine is quite watery whether it is such by its nature or by the mixture of a great deal of water with it. The tasteless wine which Lucilius[256] calls *crucium* is useless for old men since it is cold and inflates the stomach injuriously. I confess that a wine is more praiseworthy to me whose nature tends toward an even quality so that it is not very strong even when unmixed; this is the wine more preferable for an old age. It may be drunk either mixed or unmixed with water. Let the wine finally be one which does not display any un-

[254]Galen, 4. 812; 11. 646, 655; 15. 702.
[255]Ibid., 15. 702.
[256]Lucilius, 419, in *Remains of Old Latin,* III <*vinum*> *crucium,* pang-wine. Paulus ex Fest. 53, 5 *crucium quod cruciat;* Lindsay 103. A nasty wine, says the editor, E. Warmington (LCL). Isidore of Seville, *Etymologies* 20. 3. 9: *Crucium vinum est insuave quod servi potant.*

usual color which as by a sign will indicate any *dyscrasia* [distemperance or lack of proper mixture] in heat or cold or humidity or dryness. Of these features of the wine none is more properly perceived as indicative of its differences in body and strength than its odor. The color of the wine itself has no effect upon the old man; in fact, this feature is far less important than taste and odor because colors exist only as an external feature and this is more or less true also of odor although it serves somewhat as food value in wine for old men. It is not possible to judge hastily the exact differences of wines as to body and strength, but it is quite easy to distinguish them by taste or flavor. The dry wine shows its dryness in this way, the tart wine its heat; although the sweet wine is not revealed by its degree of heat or cold nevertheless its sweetness is betrayed by its consistency. They say old people should avoid sweet wine except as a laxative and especially a dark sweet wine before meals and not much of it at any other time since nothing which is panchimeron, i.e., of full body, is useful for the old, as Galen reports.[257] By nature it becomes hot in the second stage of its manufacture but dry in the first. It obstructs the liver, the spleen, and the kidneys although it depletes the chest and lungs of the heterogeneous humor which is quickly mixed with other putrescences which are convertible to the nature of yellow bile. Indeed, some people become hydroptic for this reason; some incur lithiasis,[258] that is, the formation of stone in kidney or bladder, if they drink much sweet wine except old people of a cold nature in winter and in a frigid region. These people may be allowed sparkling dark red wines of full body and thoroughly cleansed of dregs. In summer old men may drink a very diluted wine to quench their thirst and not to heat the body, especially a somewhat watery white wine. It is closer in its thin simple body to the evenness of heat. It should be drunk through a tube and is good for quenching thirst. They also praise that wine which is mixed with a third part of rose water. It produces hilarity of soul and an expansion of the spirits, increases the strength of the stomach and does not result in drunkenness nor attack the brain. The best mixture for an old man is one ounce of golden oriental wine with one half ounce each

[257]Galen, 6. 276, 339; 11. 449; 14. 457; 15. 638.
[258]Ibid., 6. 338; 19. 424.

of rose water and of bugloss, drunk every ten hours or thereabouts. Excellent wines for the use of old men, as Galen writes,[259] are among Italian wines first the Falernian, not too new or old; then Tiburtine of Tivoli, then that of Signia[260] [the astringent wine of Segni], which is of indubitable effectiveness for the bowels, and then the Sorrentine, a wine of great quality grown only in vineyards. These wines do not burden the stomach nor attack the brain. They check rheumatism of the stomach and intestines. When old, however, and when they remain a long time in the stomach they bring about a griping of the bowels and do not provoke the urine. Of all these the Hadrian, Sabine, and Alban wines are more helpful for the nerves, as well as the Gabian, Trifolinian, and those around Naples, and the Tuscan, especially the Trebilian.[261] Of those wines which are not too new a moderate use is allowed by old men of weak brains. Falernian is for those with strong brains and has the best food value, as M. Varro says.[262] The Rhaetic wines around Verona have some that are good. Suetonius[263] says that Caesar Augustus took a particular delight in these wines. The Rhaetian wine is less valued by Vergil[264] than the Falernian and the Sorrentine, which are especially approved for the convalescent on account of their fine body and salubrious quality. Tiberius Caesar[265] used to say that the doctors agreed in giving the palm of nobility to Sorrentine wine. Therefore it is allowed to old men when convalescing in the resumptive regimen. The less pungent type should be chosen for the pungent is astringent or costive in the bowels. Of the Greek wines he praised the resinated wines, as Celsus says,[266] when grown in good rather than thin soil and in a temperate climate rather than in one too wet, dry, cold, or hot. These wines are good to drink at meals both in the resumptive and conservative regimens. They are helpful in

[259]Ibid., 6. 334–38.

[260]Celsus, *De Medicina* 4. 5. 19; 4. 12. 8; Pliny, *N. H.* 14. 6 on Signian wine as astringent in diarrhoea.

[261]Galen, 6. 334; 14. 15; Pliny, *N. H.* 14. 64–69; 23. 35–36.

[262]M. Varro, *De Re Rustica* 1. 2. 6; 1. 65.

[263]Suetonius, *Divus Augustus Caesar* 77; Pliny, *N. H.* 14. 16; Columella 3. 2. 27.

[264]Vergil, *Georgics* 2. 96: Falernian is described as *severum, ardens, vehemens, forte.*

[265]Pliny, *N. H.* 14. 64.

[266]Celsus, *De Medicina* 2. 18. 11; 4. 5. 29; 12. 8; 26. 9; Pliny, *N. H.* 14. 120, 124, 129; 16. 54; 23. 46.

increasing weight or softening the bowels, as Pliny reports.[267] *Vippa,* which is bread dipped in wine, is recommended. Galen[268] praises the practice of Telephus the grammarian in Book V *On the Sanative Method [De Sanitate Tuenda]* who at evening ate bread alone soaked in diluted wine; he lived almost one hundred years. This sort of food is adapted to old age for with its heat and humidity it resists the frigidity and dryness of the aged although it seems to cool the stomach more than wine alone. It happens that the moisture of the wine soaked into the bread in the form of *vippa* adheres to many parts of the stomach; thus its actual frigidity is more preserved because it appears to refrigerate and moisten more. Wine by itself without being soaked in bread does not thus adhere to the walls of the stomach and more quickly passes through and warms it. Although *vippa* is praised to this extent yet it is regarded as *vappa,* which is an inferior wine which has lost its strength by evaporation.[269] Old men who by their nature or whatever other cause are nauseated by wine are bidden to drink hydromel in its place. This potion is good for the stomach, creates appetite for food, quenches thirst, and lends assistance in illnesses arising from chill and especially those affecting the brain and nerves, which particularly afflict old age. It purges the chest of thick phlegm and is good for the kidneys; it also prevents stone. Nor should *aqua mulsa*[270] [honey water] be passed over in silence for it has the highest value in assisting the extension of life. Pliny[271] says many people have lived a long life by drinking honey water chiefly and no other food. We have the example of Pollio Romilius,[272] who lived more than a hundred years. When as a guest of the divine Augustus the latter asked him how he maintained such a vigor of body and mind, he replied: "With honey water on the inside, oil on the outside." *Mulsum* [mead] is made of wine and honey; others make it with vinegar.[273]

[267]Pliny, *N. H.* 14. 64.
[268]Galen, 6. 333.
[269]Pliny, *N. H.* 14. 125.
[270]Ibid., 21. 129.
[271]Ibid., 22. 114.
[272]Ibid., 22. 114, 150.
[273]Ibid., 22. 110.

Chapter XIX

The Selection of Water

Water[274] has its place in the regimen of old age just as it has at any other age, says Galen, which is not true of wine, food, exercise, wakefulness, sleep, and sex, which are not suitable for all at all times but only on a selective basis as to individuals and ages. Therefore that water by which we live has been condemned when drunk unmixed with anything in the resumptive regimen, especially by those whose nature is cold. However, mixed with wine, sugar, or honey and drunk at meals they say it is good for old people as long as it is light and clear and not completely bad in taste and odor. Its excellent quality will be quickly apparent as pleasant when it quickly descends while it is drunk and it seeks the lower part of the abdomen. Such a water is very praiseworthy for the regimen of old age, for it liquefies the food, thins it out, rectifies it and furnishes an easy penetration of its humidity. With its coolness it checks the rise of natural and accidental heat if there is any in the old people and extinguishes the fire in the heart. In addition to all these virtues it is by nature of assistance in bodily activity. Such a prime water will first of all not be stagnant, for they say that found in swamps is always pestilential. In winter when it is made softer by rain[275] the effect can be recognized; rain water is particularly salubrious for it dilutes away even the pernicious element in poisoned liquid. Black water should not be drunk; it is properly condemned. Ice and snow water[276] must not be drunk lest, as Pliny says, we turn the hardships of the moun-

[274]Ibid., 31. 39 on the quality of water; Galen, 6. 817; 11. 390; 15. 697; 17A. 336; 17 B. 155; 815.
[275]Galen, 16. 438 on rain water; also 17 B. 184; Celsus, *De Medicina* 2. 18. 12 on water in general; rain water is the lightest.
[276]Pliny, *N. H.* 31. 32, 33; Galen, 19. 689.

tains into the pleasure of our gluttony. Nor should we drink water which originates from metals, that is, ores, unless by chance it originates from a gold or silver mine. Rain water, which is called heavenly,[277] is agreed by authors to be most ideal for the health of the body especially if it is led off into a covered cistern through clay pipes.[278] It is thus the safest for drinking purposes. Next comes water from a fountain issuing from eastern springs and especially of a clear color and not spoiled in taste or odor which moderates its chill even in winter and cools off the heat of summer as it comes out of the earth, very pure, without thick sediment, not sandy nor too sluggish or slimy, i.e., brackish, but of medium consistency so that it can make a quick change from hot to cold and vice versa. This water is the most approved. Then there is the water which comes splashing down from the mountains through rocks; it is not easily mixed with impurities. After spring water, there is the river water from large streams, highly praised especially when running openly and free from sediment. The sun's rays purify this water more than it does spring water so that the thicker particles of sediment are more easily separated from the smaller ones. Waters are of different levels of quality because they issue from diverse locations. Many rivulets come together and much water cannot collect except in summer when these reach the larger streams and when rains fall and the snows melt on the mountain heights. When these waters combine they become turbid. They say a sign of this is the fact that when waters as pure and free from sediment as possible are collected and preserved in vessels a part of them resting on the bottom of the container is sand or sediment, denoting the impurity of the waters. In quiet water a certain thick substance is found at the bottom, although this happens more rarely and with less substance in the springs already described. For this reason they believe that river water is the more impure the farther it has flowed from its source. Others deny this and believe that river water is of better quality in proportion to its distance of flow because it is agitated and disturbed by much movement and hence is made more pure and clear. Next there is well water from a hill or water which is not found at the bottom of a valley. Water safe for the

[277]Pliny, *N. H.* 17. 14; Columella 3. 12. 2; 3. 13. 7; 7. 4. 8.
[278]Pliny, *N. H.* 5. 128; 16. 224; 2. 33.

health is recognized, as they tell us, first by its lightness, which is established by its apparent weight.[279] Of waters of equal weight that one is better, they say, which heats and cools more quickly and in which vegetables are more quickly boiled or if scattered in a shining brass vessel it does not make a spot on it, or if boiled in a brass vessel it leaves no sand or slime at the bottom, or if of a very translucent quality it has no moss and any kind of pollution, or if two waters are poured into two clean pieces of linen cloth or silk they say that water is the lighter of the two whose moistened cloth is more quickly dried, remains cleaner, and retains less weight. The remedy for polluted water is to strain it, boil it, and to reduce it by half. In this way a residue of some fine particles will result by the rarefaction and dissolution of the thicker part of the water which was congealed, or, at least, being propelled to the bottom, the water is separated from its thicker parts. This process may be carried out by sublimation, as Avicenna describes the rectification of water. Water sufficiently pure in itself does not require any of these treatments. Such are the waters at Rome, which are highly praised by Johannes Alexandrinus, the commentator.[280] Theodorus Priscianus [xiiii] writes that boiled water is of very great value for the health of the body. The indications of bad health resulting from bad water, they say, can be judged from the health of the inhabitants of a region since those who drink impure water suffer from ills of the throat, lungs, and thorax but not the head.[281] If the head is ill and the illness runs down to the lungs or stomach the air rather is to be blamed. If bad water also with its frigidity remains a long time in the abdomen it produces a rumbling[282] in the bowels, gurgling in the stomach, flatulence, and sometimes colic. It diminishes the strength of the stomach, impedes digestion, and assists the food greatly to depart from the body. Good water, they say, acts in a contrary manner in the body.

[279]Celsus, *De Medicina* 18. 12–13.
[280]See note 220. He does not mention the Roman waters, but Galen 17. B. 159 praises them.
[281]Pliny, *N. H.* 18. 27; Galen, 16. 435.
[282]Aur., *Tard.* 32. 4. 7; Jerome, *Ep.* 22. 11.

Chapter XX

Bread

Almost all who are acquainted with human nature have regarded bread as the fundamental item of food and for this reason it has been called *panis* since it is served with all food and because every living creature desires it.[283] They command that its use in the resumptive and conservative regimens should by no means be omitted and especially that bread which is made from unspoiled grain. Nothing has been discovered by experiment or reason more praiseworthy from which bread may be made conducive to the health of man than *frumentum,* as the Greeks and many of the barbarians have concluded, according to Galen.[284] *Frumentum* is more nourishing than all other grains and of first rate heating value in its nature; it is equal in humidity and dryness and produces a more temperate blood than do other grains. *Triticum* is of good juice, *panicum* of bad juice, *legumina* and *hordeum* the same, although *hordeum* is more close to *frumentum* than to other kinds of grain.[285] Bread made of *hordeum* is astringent and cools one off, Theodorus Priscianus [xv] declares. In ancient times it was rejected for human use and given as feed to animals.[286] Bread made from *panicum* (or *panicium*) is rejected although it is called so as being as it were *panificium,* the process of making bread,[287] because many are fed by it in place of bread. It is good for those who are the overseers of the old people in the process of caring for them that we should not distinguish kinds of grain for bread baking as veterinaries might do. Thus the preference is given to *frumentum* because when bread is baked from it its food value is the highest,

[283]Isidore of Seville, *Etymologies* 20. 2. 15.
[284]Galen, 6. 508; 11. 733; 18 A. 473; see Isidore of Seville 18. 3.
[285]Celsus 2. 20–21.
[286]Pliny, *N. H.* 18.74; also 62,72.
[287]Varro, *L. L.,* 5, 105; Celsus 2. 18; Isidore 17. 3. 13.

as Celsus[288] says. The stronger grain among the kinds of *frumentum* [grain in general, especially wheat] is hard and dense, difficult to chew, and scarcely divided by the teeth. Its color is between white and red, [i.e., pink] it is large in the kernel, plump, quite fresh, for freshness is more quickly contributory to fat and corpulence, as Avicenna reports, although when it is freshly harvested it is of a more viscous and phlegmatic nutriment and stops up almost all of the liver. The ancients also condemned it severely as being of a dryer and inferior form of nourishment. It should be full in body, heavy, quite ripe, gathered in a good harvest, stored with care, and cleansed of extraneous material. It is best grown on a hillside rather than in a field for hills yield a more hardy *triticum* although less in quantity. M. Varro[289] says that the best food value is given by *triticum* raised in a field. Bread made from such *frumentum,* with salt and yeast added, kneaded and baked, is white in color, light in weight, not compact in texture, and moderate in size of the loaf. It lasts for a day or for three days when it is baked as well as possible, according to Galen. The experts including especially Averroes [5.80v] agree with him since the better of these foods grown in the soil for man is *triticum* prepared with skill. For it is more quickly turned into blood with brightness and good consistency, very close to the best kind between thick and watery, as Galen says. Bread made from *triticum* thus prepared gives more heat and strengthens the forces of the body so that one can lead a tranquil life. It restores the digestion in older people who are deficient therein. Nor should yeast *(fermentum),* said to be from the word *fervor,* be omitted in baking bread. A sufficient quantity of it makes the bread stronger, gives it pungency and hence sponginess whereby it is more quickly and easily digested as being more adaptable to alteration with its humidity and airy lightness. Hence bread baked with yeast is listed among those foods which stimulate the bowels to action.[290] Salt likewise mixed into the dough in moderation is recommended. With its heat and dryness it removes the humid and aqueous element which is in excess and prone to bubble up and

[288]Celsus, *De Medicina* 2. 20–21.

[289]M. Varro, *R. R.* 1. 6. 5; see also Pliny, *N. H.* 18. 48 on the various kinds of grain discussed thus far.

[290]Galen, 6. 342, 486, on bread suitable for old people. See also 11. 882; 16. 661; Pliny, *N. H.* 18. 102, 104; Galen, 6. 481; 480–524 on grains used in bread baking.

putrefy causing it to evaporate from the bread dough keeping it free from putrescence. Salt also makes the bread lighter, more digestible and tastier when joined with yeast. For if the bread has little yeast and salt and is not properly baked it will acquire viscosity and density. If it abounds in these defects it will be too dry for the old people to eat. Bread should be kneaded with care and patience for frequent and prolonged kneading during the baking process will make it easier to break up and to be eaten while its humidity is removed. In the baking it should not be carelessly burned because burned bread stops up the bowels. They call it sailor's bread if it is thus baked twice.[291] Nor should it be under baked for toughness or stickiness and viscosity arise in this way from its humor and produce a hard food. They also condemn the eating of hot bread because it creates thirst and its vaporous humidity swims around in the stomach, as Avicenna reports; thus it is more quickly saturated and although more swiftly digested it descends slowly from the stomach. Its white color and lightness are signs of the purity of bread. A substance that is light in consistency due to proper kneading contributes, they say, to the creation of a large, thick, nourishing loaf full of much crumb, which is relaxing to the bowels. When there is little or no crumb the bowels are constipated and expulsion of the feces retarded. A medium size and power of nourishment are recommended, and especially a loaf of that shape which allows the fire's heat in the oven to bake all parts of the loaf uniformly. The crust-parts are to be rejected for they have little nourishment and are difficult to digest; they dry out the feces and constipate the bowels. The crumb in contrast inflates itself (or rises in the process of baking) with its humidity, dense and viscous, creating a humid phlegm. Old people should not eat unleavened bread, for they say it is very difficult to digest, has very little nourishment, is evacuated very slowly, and contributes to stoppages and flatulence. It is entirely unacceptable for use except by laborers and harvest hands.[292] From this discussion one may understand that every other kind of bread except that made from *triticum* is to be rejected as being easily corruptible when ingested, such as *hordeacum* [barley], *siligineum* [winter wheat], *fabi-*

[291]Pliny, *N. H.* 22. 138; its propensity to stop the bowels is increased.
[292]Galen, 6. 486.

ceum [from beans],[293] *castaniceum* [chestnuts], *orobiceum* [chick peas], *sorricium* [?], *miliaceum* [millet], or *paniceum* [panic grass]. Grains similar to these create black bile and types of little cakes such as soldiers' cakes dry out and make the body thin, as Theodorus Priscianus says.[294] Likewise bread from Picenum made by milling although it is very strong made of *frumentum,* honey, and cheese and is in frequent use nevertheless should not be used in the old people's diet.[295] Broth, gruel, pan cakes, starch, and barley water since these are soft and of good juice are considered ideal for old people. *Similago* [*simila,* the finest wheat flour][296] is also among these foods. Even more praiseworthy is a food made from *triticum* pounded very fine so that it resembles something between farina [ground wheat] and spelt. Bread made from this flour is highly regarded and is like *similago;* a juicy serving of it is more nourishing and more highly regarded than that made of starch or any other kind of flour and more adapted to the resumptive regimen.

[293]Celsus, *De Medicina* 2. 20. 21 on the good or bad juices of these grains or legumina. See Galen, 6. 529–32, on beans.
[294]Theodorus Priscianus, cap. ii.
[295]Macrobius, *Saturnalia* 2. 9.
[296]Celsus, *De Medicina* 2. 18; Pliny, *N. H.* 18. 89.

Chapter XXI

The Meat Preferred and First That of Domesticated Quadrupeds

Flesh *(caro)* although it is said to come from creating *(creando)*[297] has not been included in the resumptive regimen except insofar as it is suitable for eating and nourishing the old man and properly the flesh found in blooded animals. For although blood is the true material of flesh, in a wider view flesh also exists in animals which lack blood, that is, it is relative to flesh properly so called. Flesh is a food which, according to the experts, restores the human body to which it is more akin so that by its conversion it will nourish and make blood more powerfully than do other foods since it has more food value. It restores strength and builds up fat as its end product just as it usually does according to their species and their members for those animals whose flesh in turn is eaten by humans. It is especially suitable to be added to the diet of old people in the course of their care. It is pertinent to the facts of old age to know the properties of animals to be used as food. Some are land animals, others are of the air, and others live in the water. It is best to begin with the footed animals as being more perfect and more in use for human consumption. Their powers are considerable as well as their differences both as to their parts and as to what is contained in them and generated by them, such as eggs, milk, blood, cheese, and butter. Not all of these products have the same food value just as with the individual parts of the animals which also vary in this respect. The flesh of the domesticated animal regarded with especial favor in the regimen of old people is whatever flesh is closer in its nature to that of humans, more easily digested, and the best for making blood. The flesh of these animals differs greatly in regard to their natures, ages, colors, sexes, habits,

[297]Isidore of Seville, *Etymologies* 20. 2. 20.

times, places, pasturing or food supply, methods of preparation for table use, roasting, etc., and the preservation of their flesh after the animal has been killed. The flesh of an animal of various colors is of less food value; nevertheless, the flesh of one that is red or black in color in every species eaten is more tasty than the white because red and black colors attest to their heat since it is abundant according to the nature of the flesh, perfects the digestion in the members of the body, and renders the flesh tastier, softer, and sweeter to eat. The flesh of an animal closer to its infancy is more humid and the flesh of those animals which are growing is more perfect since the flesh of all growing creatures is better and more easily cooked although it furnishes less nourishment, such as every animal which is not yet weaned, as Cornelius Celsus reports.[298] The flesh of animals of a dry nature such as young kids of male and female goats is more suitable for old people to eat. For every fetus is humid; the closer it is to its birth the less food value it has by nature and proportionately the more remote from its birth the more food value. Its chief characteristic is that it is dry by nature; therefore the flesh of the old animal and of the one near to birth is disapproved of for eating. The flesh of males is considered better than that of females in many respects, for every female flesh produces bad blood with the exception of she-goat flesh which is disapproved of less than that of he-goats. Likewise, most authors have approved female chicken flesh more than rooster flesh; hence also that of a castrated animal of each sex both fowl and footed creature is considered better than that of the non-castrated because the innate heat is reduced by castration. Thus it turns out that this animal the more it is fattened the more burdensome it is to the digestion. Therefore the flesh of the majority of non-castrated animals is more recommended in the resumptive diet than is that of the castrated. It is both fat and lean in moderation. Very lean flesh especially of a domesticated animal is of bad juice although less unsuitable for the stomach than fat flesh. All fresh flesh is stronger than the salted and recently killed than the stale flesh in its food value and when killed in the spring than that killed in the

[298]Celsus, *De Medicina* 2. 18. 7; Avicenna, *Canon,* II, 104v, on the relative value of colors in animals which are eaten.

fall.[299] Wild game among animals which live in deserts is of more and better food value than that of domesticated animals of the same species and of less supervacuity although the flesh of a tame animal is more humid. Every wild animal is of lighter food value than a domesticated one and whatever creature is born in a humid climate rather than a dry climate is also weaker, as Celsus says.[300] Where the pasture is by nature and form specifically adapted to the particular animal its flesh is more praised than if it is fed with food not adapted to it. Those who feed in mountain pastures have pure air and fragrant herbs on which to feed, such as wild thyme, oregano, mint, pennyroyal, poly-mountain, brook willow, sweet Benjamin, and such like herbs. The flesh of animals who feed in valleys, swamps, and muddy areas they say is better, and in those places also which are wetter in summer as well as dryer in winter. Matters vary completely in respect to food from creature to creature and season to season as to methods of preparing it. Boiled meat is better than roasted and is more beneficial to old people, for whatever they eat that is roasted or fried provides a dryer nourishment to the body. Meat boiled in water is more humid; that boiled in oil is in the middle between these two, i.e., dry and humid, as Galen reports. Similarly, whatever is seasoned with wine dries the body out and nourishes and warms. Sour sauces nourish well enough but heat the person less. Broiled meats flavored with salt and cooked nourish less and dry out bodies and make them thin although they sufficiently satisfy the stomach, as Theodorus Priscianus[301] says. When they are boiled they are more satisfactory in the regimen of old age because all flesh that is juicy is numbered among those foods that heat. Boiled foods receive humidity from the water, which is the wettest of the four elements. Resumption is achieved through humid substances as noted earlier. Thus boiled meat is more suitable and more nourishing as food just as juicy meat nourishes more than roasted, roasted more than fried. Hence boiled food is more recommended in the resumptive regi-

[299]Celsus, *De Medicina* 2. 18. 9–10; Galen 6. 63 on castrated flesh bad for the elderly; 660–88 on meats and parts of animals; 11. 530 on the use of oil; 15. 186; 17 B. 403 on diet for the old.

[300]Ibid.

[301]Cap. vi.

men. Juicy or boiled fat meat stimulates the bowels of the old person. If old men happen to eat the flesh of large animals especially of those which are thin they are advised to eat it boiled and steeped in flavors. It should be thoroughly cooked after the animal is killed and preserved for some time before cooking in the winter, especially if it is an animal which walks around. Thus the meat will be more easily broken up and digested. In the summer the flesh of animals killed at dawn should be used after sunset. It seems best to begin my survey of edible meats with those quadrupeds which are domesticated because they are of the strongest kind.

GOAT FLESH

In regions of the sixth climate the flesh of all tame footed animals while still sucking is recommended for the diet of old people and is preferred for those who are convalescing since the reductive art is the same for both groups. When bodies which have suffered particularly severe illnesses are convalescing they are treated in the same way as old people and the same nutrition and strengthening measures are employed for each. Hence Galen[302] in the fifth book of his *Sanative Method* affirms that goat flesh is not without use for the old as being uniform, especially that of a male goat not more than forty days old without any mixture of a bad quality, that is, kids still sucking, not females. The flesh of both sexes which are older is more difficult to digest and has bad chyme [i.e., the pulp formed by the food on its way to digestion]. But the flesh of a little male kid *(edi)* so called from eating *(edendo)*[303] is more recommended than that of any other domestic footed beast in pleasantness of flavor, nourishment, ease of digestion, and in the generation of good thin blood. This is the opinion of almost all the experts. Celsus[304] says pork is the lightest (or weakest) of flesh, beef is the strongest. Avicenna says goat flesh should be eaten cold because in this way its vapor is reduced. In warmer or drier climates lamb is held to be better than goat meat.

302 Galen, 6. 340.
303 Isidore of Seville, *Etymologies* 12. 1. 13.
304 Celsus, *De Medicina* 2. 18. 7.

LAMB

The flesh of lamb which is not sucking and has been exercised in the flock and carefully fattened in stables with flax seed or farina or whatever other food is regarded as good for old age, for although the flesh of a sucking lamb is very humid it is blamed for its viscosity and phlegmatic quality. However, the flesh of a one-year-old sucking lamb is better than that of a non-castrated exercised ram. Avicenna says lamb should be eaten warm because its bad odor is thus dispelled.

CASTRATED RAMS

These also are good to eat for old people if they are castrated, have moderate fat, and are fed in good air in feeding places which Varro[305] calls *pastiones,* i.e., around the farm house. In hilly and rocky places where there are few gentle slopes their meat is thinner, weaker, and more full of flavor for they say such rams resist the melancholic humor.

VEAL

This too is acceptable in the resumptive regimen if the meat is that of a young bullock or a suckling, fat, one to three months old or between fifty and one hundred days old. It furnishes much ideal nourishment for old age; it is easily digested and provides good blood. It lacks that toughness and frigidity which abound in the flesh of oxen or cattle. Therefore, veal is by nature not far from being warm and humid although the female calf is much more uniform in this respect but not so well adapted for old people in humidity and toughness. Both male and female calf meat [veal] is said to be of a green age, and thus like goat meat it uses a moderate form of activity and old people eat it with good results.

[305]Varro, *Res Rustica* 3. 2. 13.

Chapter XXII

The Meat of Walking Wild Beasts and First of All the Meat of Wild Goat and Deer

Although the flesh of wild quadrupeds is stronger [i.e., has more nourishment] and of whatever creature is larger, as Celsus[306] says, all of their flesh generates the melancholic humor, as they say. Nevertheless, in the resumptive regimen because all game meat is of good juice and creates the least flatulence some of their flesh is not forbidden, such as that of the little female kid which Avicenna calls gazelle, sucking or just being weaned. Its flesh is more temperate than that of all other woodland game, useful to old people, more easily chewed, easy to digest nor superfluous in fat which causes nausea, of delectable flavor and in every way superior to the flesh of tame animals. The flesh of young wild boar is also praised or that of one closely neighboring to those who are tame since that is called a wild beast who is impelled by its own desire for a certain natural freedom. The continuous motion and effort of such animals purifies their blood to a greater extent and thins it; their pores are opened by which they expel superfluities. The flesh of the wild goat has a peculiar quality, says Judeus [f. cxxxii], since the water used for boiling and softening this flesh strengthens the force of the soul in case of a sudden loss of power or syncope brought on by a too violent purgation; this is a unique remedy. The flesh of larger wild goats is dryer than that of smaller goats and constricts the stomach, as Theodorus Priscianus [vi] tells us. Therefore, it is to be rejected in the resumptive regimen along with deer flesh.

[306]Celsus, *De Medicina* 2. 18. 2.

BOAR

The flesh of a young wild boar or of a tame one, that is, of an animal born of both a boar and a domestic brood sow is recommended in the diet of old age. It is very nourishing nor is such flesh of an animal very close to the time of birth difficult to digest as is that of a boar who is older. Nor since it is a wild animal does it have as much humidity as the domestic pig however young or old. Theodorus Priscianus [vi] writes that boar meat is more nourishing than deer or goat meat of the larger animals and dries out the person more. All this is to be understood of the flesh of boars that are grown.

TURTLE

Turtle meat is held to be very nourishing and healthful for those who require physical restoration. It expels superfluity from the body. Turtle flesh is composed of matter in which the four elements are equally mixed, both heavy and light, as Isaac reports, although such a mixture they do not say is the same as that of the human body, a minimum of one and the other.[307] The mixture of elements in the turtles is a juxtaposition of parts. For fattening and restoration of the thinned and weakened body it is particularly ideal if it is cooked in the proper manner. Its nourishment is similar to that provided by chickens or quail.

RABBIT, HARE, DORMICE

Included in the diet of old age is rabbit meat from animals living in the woods or groves in burrows in the ground. Some people call them hares. They receive their name *(cuniculus)* from their underground home. Other people call them *cunicus.* Varro[308] calls *cuniculus* an animal similar in part to our hare but with short legs which he says is native to Spain. Old people are urged to eat sometimes the flesh of these animals as being properly nourished and fat. It provides a viscous aliment such as the flesh of the hedgehog,

[307] f. cxxxvi.
[308] Varro, *Res Rustica* 3. 12. 4–7, 15.

bear, and dormouse. Hence a rather frequent use of it is not recommended. The flesh of the dormouse and *spiriolus* which is a creeping semi-wild creature of the breed of mice although not much in use for food is not altogether ruled out. The inhabitants of Carinthia eat a great many of them since they are in good supply. Dormouse meat is abundant in oiliness; they are made fat by sleeping for to swell up *(gliscere)* is to grow *(crescere)*.[309] It induces nausea more when eaten although it is humid and savory than does the flesh of *spiriolus,* because of whose sweetness the censors once upon a time removed from the dinner table no otherwise than snails or birds imported from abroad, as Pliny relates.[310] The flesh of the *spiriolus* is sweet, a delight to eat. It feeds on fruit and nuts.

HARE MEAT

Elderly folk cold by nature in winter and in frigid regions should eat hare meat especially of young and growing animals captured by the sagacity of dogs and by hunting, says Abulkasim. The hare is rated in the middle group of animals for moderate nourishment and for combating the qualities of frigidity and accidental humidity of old age. It is more recommended for good chyme than the flesh of sheep and cattle as well as that of young male or female goats, as Isaac reports [f. cxxxv]. Therefore he advises that it be given to those who wish to have dry natures. To those who follow a slender diet he denies it as adverse to their purpose. Abulkasim says hare meat is warm and dry, but Avicenna says it is cold and dry. It checks the bowels, gives thicker blood, and is more likely to produce melancholy than other flesh. It induces wakefulness, as Abulkasim reports, although Cato[311] believes when hare is eaten it brings on sleep. Hare is not entirely approved or disapproved of in the diet of old people. As to what Martial[312] thinks of it, he ascribed the chief glory among quadrupeds to the hare. Theodorus Priscianus [vi] writes that hare meat

[309]Isidore of Seville, *Etymologies* 12. 3. 6.
[310]Pliny, *N.H.* 8. 223.
[311]Cato apud Diomed. p. 358 P.
[312]Martial 13. 92. 2; Z. read *gloria* in his text rather than *mattea.*

stimulates the stomach, dries the members, and provokes the urine.

SALTED MEAT

Salted meat especially when boiled is not forbidden nor is salted fish if it is quite lean. It makes an appetizing dish and strengthens the powers of the stomach particularly if cooked with a bit of salt; they say it is very suitable for the stomach. The same is true of ham, morsels of pork, bacon, and sausages *(tomacinae),* which others call *tomacula. Taniacae* are a food made of pork which resemble in shape a travelling hat; they call this food salted shoulders of pork[313] [*petasus,* travelling hat].

[313]Varro, *R. R.* 2. 4. 10.

Chapter XXIII

The Meat of Birds, Especially Domestic

The flesh of almost all birds is ideal for human consumption and in relation to that of quadrupeds is of a dryer nourishment. Theodorus[314] declares that birds do not have bladders for use in gathering their urine nor do they emit saliva. Bird flesh is of a slighter and weaker food value and is more easily digested so that all wild fowl and game birds are listed as ideal for the stomach and as producing very little flatulence. Both roasted and boiled flesh descend rather quickly in the stomach. They say it is of a temperate nature because of its low heat although there is nevertheless some tendency toward heat in it. The flesh of all species of birds who use their legs rather than that of those who fly is stronger among the median class and that of those which are larger than that of small birds like the fig-pecker and the thrush. The flesh of those which do not live in water furnishes a lighter food than that of birds which know how to swim, as Celsus reports.[315] The flesh of castrated birds is more useful than that of walking animals. The flesh of domesticated birds which hunt for food in the fields is more praiseworthy than that of birds which feed in enclosed places such as a coop or *ornithoboscion* [poultry house], which is a place for feeding chickens,[316] both because of their continual exercise and because they seek the food they require at their liberty. The flesh of all these birds before they grow feathers generates humors which easily vitiate the stomach and produce nausea. The boiled flesh of domestic fowl is recommended in the resumptive diet for it gives a more humid nourishment to the body. The more recommended flesh, they say, is that of fowl which do not live in swamps, stag-

[314]Theodorus [vii] borrows from Aristotle, *H. A.* 2. 16. 506b25.
[315]Celsus, *De Medicina* 2. 18. 6.
[316]Ibid., 3. 9. 2.

nant places, or rivers; it is more prized in dried form than fresh, as Galen says in the fifth book of his *Regimen of Health.*[317]

CHICKEN

The flesh of a rooster of moderate fat just beginning to crow and before it copulates and similarly the flesh of a hen which has not yet laid an egg are regarded as preferable among all tame fowl. It is of a temperate nature, swiftly cooked, of easy conversion into good blood, has few superfluities, softens the bowels, and strengthens the appetite. Averroes [5.77v, 82v, 94v] says pullet flesh with its certain marvellous property equalizes the human complexion and the humors in old men of cold nature in winter and in the northern region. It is most useful for all ages and natures although it furnishes less nourishment the more tender it is. Some prefer rooster flesh to hen, others vice versa. Mesue bids us to choose the black ones especially;[318] others prefer black or yellow. White chickens are to be avoided since they are gentle and less lively and cluck similarly. Chicken flesh is not converted into bile or phlegm especially if it is that of a healthy fat young hen which has not yet produced offspring and is a pullet not yet one or two years old. Pullet is regarded as better than other fowl or winged creature in its ability to equalize or moderate the human complexion. It is better for the stomach if it is boiled than either lamb or kid, Avicenna reports, for thus its humidity is preserved. Since every woman knows how to raise chickens and since it is the function of the chicken-stuffer *(fartor)* to make them fat it is enough at present to say that chickens are best fed in the shadows with farina or half-cooked barley. The castrated roosters which some[319] call capons and others call[320] *papons* are called half-males or *capi* by Columella and are castrated for the sake of destroying their sexual desire. Whatever they are called, if they are moder-

[317]Galen, 6. 351, 700–702.
[318]f. 38.
[319]Columella, *R. R.* 8. 2. 3.
[320]Albertus Magnus uses the word *papons,* which Ulisse Aldrovandi says he dreamed up since it occurs in no ancient author: see my *Aldrovandi on Chickens;* University of Oklahoma Press, 1963, 407. Avicenna, II, chap. 296, p. 119, quotes Rufus on the rooster and hen before copulating and crowing or laying eggs as preferable to eat.

ately fat and pick up their food freely they are the more healthful of all fowl, they say. Chicken meat is indeed more praiseworthy for its good nutrition and its slight superfluity. They say one should tire them out before killing them so that their flesh may thus be more digestible and easier to chew.[321]

PIGEON (OR DOVE)

The flesh of the pigeon squab when it first begins to seek its own food is lighter than that of the bird which cannot yet fly in which there is heat and a superfluous humidity which can be recognized by its heaviness and inability for flight which they lose when they begin to fly. At this time their flesh is more quickly digested and the strength of spirit increases, especially of those pigeons who are domesticated, are nourished more quickly, and come to their full size. Old men of cold nature in the winter months in regions particularly snowy should eat their flesh, according to Abulkasim, although Theodorus [vii] says a tame pigeon constrains the bowels; they are, however, more nourishing. Those who dwell in groves are of dryer nourishment since they feed on acorns. These are said to be useful for old men of cold and humid nature. Young wood pigeons have a wonderful ability for strengthening softened and relaxed members and for curing tremor in the entire body especially of those people who, as they say, drag their legs and feet behind them and those who are deprived of sense and motion and of those whose speech is cut off. Pigeon flesh is good for repairing bodies made weak and cold by a great loss of blood. It is also good for those who are choleric by nature and hot in the brain; it is also good for the eyes, removing migraine. The neck and the head are particularly effective when roasted for the human brain. In this opinion Rabi Moyses [f. 26r], Abulkasim, and Avenzoar agree.[322] These ills are relieved if the flesh is seasoned with vinegar, coriander, or agresta, and the inner part of a melon.

[321]Avicenna, II, chap. 296, f. 119.

[322]Avenzoar, *Theizir Abynzoar, Morbos Omnes,* etc., printed with Averroes, *Colliget;* Venice, 1542. He also wrote on kidney stone: *De curatione lapidis;* Venice, 1508. Cf. Zoar at note 338 = Avenzoar. Note the symptoms of poliomyelitis or stroke described in the passage above.

TURTLE DOVE

Most of the experts including Avicenna think the flesh of the turtle dove is better than that of other birds both in lightness and excellence of nourishment. It also has a wonderful quality for sharpening the wits, increasing imagination, and strengthening the memory and every force of the sense. These virtues make it a fine protection for old age especially since they call old age itself the mother or home of forgetfulness. The turtle dove is so commended perhaps because in those regions in which it is most praised its use is so good; but other people prefer the flesh of many birds to that of the turtle dove. Its flesh is considered to be hot and very dry in nature but preferable to that of the pigeon. Very good is the flesh of turtle dove pullets which are well fed and especially of those which remain in their nests the longest. These squabs are ideal for the diet of old people. You should not select an old turtle dove to stuff with food but one about a month old and confirmed in its squab-hood.

Chapter XXIV

Wild Birds, Especially Pheasant

Although the flesh of domestic fowl furnishes somewhat more nourishment than that of wild fowl due to the moderate nature of their humidity and their physical effort yet people prefer the flesh of some wild fowl to that of domestic because all the birds of the median class are of good juice, such as pheasants, whose pullets are more praised than those of domestic chickens. The pheasant is so named from the Greek island of Phasis,[323] whence it was first exported. Avicenna calls it the woodland chicken. Its nature is moderately warm and dry and it constrains the bowels, Theodorus says [vii]; when young and fat, old men and convalescents like to eat it. Pheasants are by nature close to chickens in being almost of the same species. They furnish drier nourishment and exercise more. Abulkasim says their flesh is harmful to porters and laborers and especially to those who are fatigued by carrying heavy weights. It is not suitable for those who are in good health and especially for those who move about a great deal.

PARTRIDGE, FRANCOLIN, GRAY PARTRIDGE, QUAIL

The nature of these birds in relation to each other and to that of pheasants is very close. The flesh of all of them before they have reached pullet-hood and who leave their nests rather late is regarded as very acceptable for strengthening old people and convalescents. Their nature is on a par in respect to active qualities; however, they are less dry in the pullet stage. At that stage partridges are dryer, as Theodorus Priscianus [vii] asserts. The young ones furnish good blood and have fewer superfluities; they are easier to digest. Galen[324] says the flesh of birds is more digestible, especially that of partridges, francolins, doves, chickens, and

[323]Rather, a river in Colchis: Pliny, *N. H.* 10. 132.
[324]Galen, 6. 700, 435.

the rooster. Hence some declare that their flesh is more suitable for building up the body's strength. Some say this is true also of the bird they call the gray partridge, a creature of large body like a gray goose or one ashen in color but not that small animal discovered in Etruria which constricts the bowels. After this comes the flesh of the quail, so called from the sound of its voice, which is a bird similar in color to a large pheasant, with red feet and beak.[325] Abulkasim gives it special praise for strengthening old people of a cold nature in winter and in mountainous regions. Its nature is temperate with some tendency toward warmth although it is of a somewhat thinner substance and of good chymé. It is good for healthy and stable bodies and breaks up kidney stone. Pliny[326] writes that the seed of a poisonous plant [hellebore] is very pleasant food for a quail and therefore they are rejected for table use by humans. Likewise, because they are accustomed to spit out the disease of epilepsy to which alone among animals except man they are subject they are shunned. Others fear that from eating quail they may contract tetanus and spasm not only because these birds like to eat hellebore but because there is a power in their substance which is less than that of other birds so that they are not recommended as food. The experts say all this is to be understood of a little bird called *hortigo* or *quiscula* which although it is more full of flavor than other birds yet other people think it is worse. Since the flesh of the ortygia [ortyga, ὄρτυς] is of a warm and humid nature it is not completely ruled out of the resumptive diet of old men of a frigid and dry nature in autumn and in cold regions. It is good for building up fat, very nourishing, yet brings on nausea if very much of it is eaten.

SMALL BIRDS, ESPECIALLY LARKS

These are little birds which live in bushes like the fig-pecker,[327] nightingale, tremula, lark, which the Arabs call zorag, finches, and the like whose beaks are rather slender. Those whose

[325]Isidore of Seville, *Etymologies* 12. 7. 64.

[326]Pliny, *N. H.* 10. 69, 197. The *Regimen Sanitatis* of Salerno has *quiscula* in line 52: *quiscula vel merula.*

[327]Gabriele Zerbi, *Libellus de Preservatione Corporum a Passione Calculosa,* f. 45, describes this bird. Avicenna, III, cap. xix, f. 141, calls it *tragulidos.* It is probably a wag-tail.

beaks are larger are not pleasant to the taste; in fact, they are bitter. If by chance due to the size of their gallbladder they are fat they are useful for old people, Abulkasim reports, especially for those whose nature is frigid. They are better eaten boiled and flavored with fresh almond oil and pepper, as the poet[328] elegantly bids us in these words: When a fig-pecker, shining with its waxen flesh and plump sides, is given you by lot, if you have taste, add pepper. This applies especially in the winter in the northern region. Their food value is, however, less and they are less dry, as Theodorus Priscianus [vii] writes, and less useful for the stomach. Yet they drive away nausea and are small and airy. Thus somewhat dehydrated they fly more swiftly and are warm and dry. Their concurrence in this respect with their lightness and the food received from man causes them to create very much bile. They are not recommended for frequent use in the resumptive regimen unless by chance due to certain properties they possess they may be suitable for old people. Rabi Moyses [f. 26r] writes that the flesh of a young hawk or of a night owl is tasty; it strengthens the powers of the mind and is useful for one who is prone to melancholy and for the confusion of reason in the mind.

[328]Martial 13.5. The true name is motacilla f. Linnaeus.

Chapter XXV

Parts of Animals Both Four-Footed and Winged Especially Beneficial to the Health of Old People

The recognition of the particular properties (in order to indicate them according to each member of the body as these are in use for the nourishment of the aged) of those animals already discussed both in the conservative and resumptive regimens is regarded as very useful. Whatever part of an animal is used for food especially of a substance capable of feeling and subject to change is helpful to that member of man which is similar to it. For this reason they say that to eat liberally especially of lamb and goat meat with the milk contained in them produces an abundance of milk in the human being both because of the resemblance involved and the property found in them. They say that the more excellent and savory meat around the bone should be selected and from the right side rather than from the left side of the liver because since the latter is the basis of natural heat it flows into the part closer to itself and makes it more suitable for nutrition than the part more remote. The flesh of the anterior parts is preferred to that of the posterior parts because it is warmer and easier to cook; the parts closer to the heart provide a more temperate nutrition than those at a distance. The flesh close to those veins wherein the blood has been thoroughly prepared by the liver and the heart is not similar to that which forms part of the area from the middle of the umbilicus to the tail. The closest to these as they say is the flesh of the parts which are closest to the back, both because of their motion and their exposure to the sun and are separated by their state of rest and by the influx of the sun's rays from those which are closest to the abdomen and the flesh closest to the outer surface and skin of the animal as neighboring upon openings and pores. The flesh which adheres to the viscera is more preferable and flesh which is interlarded with fat both because it is healthful to the stomach and furnishes better blood, for all fat and glutinous flesh is of good juice, as Celsus says.[329] But too much fat softens the stomach, provides little nourishment, and is converted rather swiftly into bile and fume although it is more swiftly digested. They say that flesh midway between humid and dry such as that which has no fat as the flesh of the coxae because of its savory taste is of almost equal nourishment and of good digestion, especially if it is of animals whose nature is temperate as that of a kid or of a young unweaned bullock. They recommend in addition the flesh of those parts which lie close to the skin and the bones, especially of those parts not far from the source of natural heat if that flesh is rather tender and of moderate fat for it is sweet and easily digested both because of the great amount of superfluities dissolved from it issuing from the pores of the skin through perspiration as well as by the striking it undergoes from the bones which rub against that flesh. They believe that the flesh of the nates or buttocks is less good than fat flesh and not of good digestion and of bad chyme, hotter and heavier than fat. The flesh of the ilia they affirm to be bad and worse than that which is of the nates. The ilia are so placed as to provide movement and upon them we turn around. This is not true of the nates, which are so called because we rest upon them when we sit *(nitimur)*.[330] Flesh striped with fat and especially prominent in it is sweet to eat and furnishes a rather temperate nourishment. They say that the particles of flesh placed between the brain and the heart furnish useful nourishment; they are purged of their supervacuities by the natural heat of the heart to which it is a neighbor; it is also thoroughly prepared by the force of the heart and the liver with good blood. That flesh which is of the moving parts such as the upper arm is recommended in the diet of old age both because it is not excessive in humidity and because from the flow of blood from the liver and of the spirits from the heart it receives a good flavor which promotes digestion. The flesh of the posterior parts of pullets just reaching adulthood is regarded as better than that of the anterior parts because of its softer substance. The latter flesh is harder to chew. As the pullets grow older, however, the contrary becomes true. The reason for this

[329]Celsus, *De Medicina* 2. 20. 2.
[330]Isidore of Seville, *Etymologies* 11. 1. 101.

they say is that the posterior parts of the pullet such as the legs and coxae by which the body is supported and carried along are full of tendons and ligaments. Therefore they are dry and grow harder as the pullet grows older. The anterior parts because of their humid, viscous, and raw condition are not easily digested and serving as a protection of the spiritual members of these birds they are thus not easily digested. As they grow older their heat increases and as their humidity is drained off they are rectified or made more normal by their natural heat.

THE MUSCLES AND UPPER ARMS

They admit as ideal for the resumptive diet the flesh of the muscles, reddish without much fat yet not devoid of it, especially that of footed animals for it provides blood with little superfluities. The flesh of the muscular parts is better in their middle; since the extremities end in cords and are sinewy they are not so suitable as the middle part of the muscles for food.

THE BRAIN

Since the brain of birds is not extremely humid it is well considered as food more than that of quadrupeds. Of bird brains the preferable ones are those of the pullets of the starling, partridge, and especially of the chicken, to which in particular is attributed a brain resembling that of the human in its substance arising from a sharp intelligence. Then follow the brains of the rooster and the turtle dove for they furnish strength to the reasoning power, as they say. The brain of quadrupeds is not recommended since it is cold and humid and harmful to the stomach[331] with its greater excess, for it softens and relaxes that member, takes away appetite, slows the digestion, and is of bad and viscous chyme. All this is to be understood of large-bodied quadrupeds not of an equable nature in conformity with that of humans. The pig's brain is preferred to that of other domestic quadrupeds next that of the kid and of the unweaned calf. For the restoration of the spirits especially it should be seasoned with spices and salt when roasted; the

[331]Galen, 6. 676.

same should be done with chicken, Galen urges.[332] Of the quadrupeds especially lamb and kid the pettitoes and entire head are somewhat lighter than the other members so that they may be placed in the middle category of food, as Celsus affirms.[333] This is true both of wild and tame animals, especially of hare meat which is ideal in the care and protection of the nerves. Parts of the head with some exceptions and some muscles lying near the temples are not acceptable in the regimen of old age except perhaps those parts which are glutinous and light, as in the pettitoes and small heads of kids, calves, and lambs.

LUNG

Eating the lung is not entirely ruled out in the resumptive regimen, both because it is easy to digest and more quickly evacuated from the stomach and because of its good quality and thin substance; since it is like a fan for the heart it is called in Greek *pneumo*. Especially praised is the lung of a sucking kid among quadrupeds. The lung of other animals is useless because it has little nourishment and inclines toward the nature of phlegm; it is frigid and humid by accidental complexion. In its radical or basic complexion it is regarded as hot and dry.

TESTICLES

Abulkasim recommends the testicles of birds, especially of those which have been fattened, for old men of cold nature in the winter and in a cold region more than those of footed creatures. This holds true more for roosters beginning to crow. They are very good nourishment. Next come testicles of the partridge and of pheasants for they are warm and humid in nature and of good and abundant nourishment, with few superfluities and are swiftly digested. They are most praised in the regimen of stable weak bodies. Some people prefer the testicles of animals which do not engage in sex to those of animals which do, because they have an airy humidity the younger they are; therefore they have more af-

[332]Ibid., 6. 701.
[333]Celsus, *De Medicina* 2. 22. 2; see also 2. 18. 8.

finity for human nature. Others commend those who engage in sex because the exercise thus produced makes them furnish better nourishment as is the case with all exercised members of the body except that due to coitus they are rendered drier and more earthy with a very great loss of the innate heat and spirits resulting from the sex-act. The testicles of footed animals are prohibited from too frequent use because of the heaviness of their substance, with the exception of testicles of quadrupeds not yet weaned such as the sucking pig. Galen[334] praises them highly as a remedy in syncope resulting from the thinness of the humors next to the testicles of roosters boiled rather than roasted.

UDDERS[335]

Although many have listed udders as to their food value of frigid and dry nature because of the great number of sinews which exist in them nevertheless the udder of a heifer full of milk at her first giving birth is well digested when cooked with spices and is recommended for occasional use in the resumptive regimen since udders provide a nourishment close to that of meat.

FEET AND LEGS

These parts, especially of the anterior members of lambs and kids, are especially praised for they are warm and humid and swiftly and easily digested. They are situated close to the source of heat which is the heart. Since the posterior members are heavier and colder the anterior members which are lighter and warmer are preferred. The inner part rather than the outer part which they call the wild part is more preferable also. The motion in these feet and legs takes place more in the inner than in the outer part. Although these parts are of little nourishment because of their substance and thinness nevertheless they furnish good blood verging on viscosity, not thick, with few superfluities, of good digestion and good chyme, as Avicenna reports.[336] The proof of these

[334]Galen, 6. 675, 704 sq.
[335]Ibid., 6. 774–75.
[336]Avicenna, II, cap. 146, f. 104v.

praises is the speed of their expansion, especially of the feet, and their reduction to proper consistency when cooked thoroughly. They soften the bowels with their viscosity. Therefore they are sometimes used for food in the resumptive regimen after they have been steeped in vinegar; thus they excite the appetite. Of this kind of food are hoofs and claws, pettitoes, beaks, pig-ears especially as being glutinous, light, and ideal for the stomach.

LIVER, STOMACH, MILT OR SPLEEN

Although every liver *(iecur)* is of good juice the fat liver of a goose or duck is regarded as more savory, fed on milk and grain, than that of other birds and quadrupeds. Next comes the liver of a young fat hen, especially if it has been fed on farina and figs steeped in milk. They say it is of good chyme and very helpful in restoring the strength of the heart. The liver of footed animals is almost universally rejected because of its hardness; an exception is that of a sucking pig that is not lean, that is, scrawny, especially one that is fed on figs. In our time what Romans call the liver, the Latinized word *epar,* is thought to be very useful in the resumptive regimen and much praised in restoring bodies wasted with illness. The liver of other footed animals which is not at all more humid in nature gives a more solid sustenance, is more slowly digested and penetrates to the veins more tardily. The stomach of birds is more acceptable than that of footed animals and more nourishing than the lung. Goose stomach is more praiseworthy than others just as is goose liver because of its copious humidity. Next comes that of the chicken for these two stomachs provide better nutrition and more of it, as Avicenna reports, especially if it is a young goose cooked properly in water and salt. We should not pass over in silence the inner lining or skin of the chicken's stomach, which is used in medicine rather than as food, smoked, dried, and reduced to powder. It is a unique remedy for a disturbed stomach. The spleen of animals used for human food is cold and dry in nature; it furnishes a thick, bad nourishment, is of bad juice, and is slow to be digested. The spleen of pigs is more acceptable since it is helpful as a remedy for the stomach's astringency and acidity. In its medical use for stimulating the appetite in the resumptive regimen it should be used sparingly.

WINGS

Due to its almost continual motion and effort the wing of birds is more prized, with the exception of the testicles, than the other parts since the bird's wing is lifted into the air by its frequent use and thus the superfluities are dissolved from it, rendering it more savory and swiftly digested. It is highly recommended in the diet of old people and convalescents, especially the wing of the hen and the goose and of fat birds. The wing, especially that of the goose, is not made lighter except by frequent motion and exercise. The younger birds' wings are more preferable than those of older birds. It has, however, little nourishment, a low heat close to an even temperature, rather that part which extends the wing which they call white pulp. If it is of a castrated rooster it is very nourishing and more sweet and humid than a hen's wing. Everything being equal in respect of age, habits, feeding, place, time, and such like they say the wing is ideal for eating in the resumptive diet.

THE NECK

Of birds, the neck just as the wing is rightly included for old people and the infirm, as Celsus says.[337] Of all chickens the best is that of a plump heavy hen. It provides good nourishment they say because of its frequent motion as does the wing. The goose neck comes next although its frequent consumption is prohibited, for it is hard to digest and because of its viscosity like that of the head and skin is unacceptable. Zoar[338] is authority for the statement that the neck and the head possess a quality which creates blindness. If, however, one wishes to eat these parts they are thick and viscous and encourage the appetite and reduce the heat. They should be soaked in vinegar before eating.

THE TAIL

They say the tail is warm by nature. It is not restricted from the diet of old people except that it brings nausea to the stomach. If

[337]Celsus, *De Medicina* 2. 18. 9.
[338]See note 322.

it happens to be eaten by a person he should use something of those remedies which dispel nausea.

THE MARROW

The marrow of calves and deer is preferred as more nourishing than that of all others. It has much nourishment when digested. Nevertheless, it can be useless to the stomach, diminish the appetite, and disturb the stomach if it is eaten too frequently. It should be eaten spiced with pepper and seeds. Among the marrows the spinal marrow is preferred; it has the least fat because it is extended from the brain and thus drives away nausea. If it is well digested it gives no small nourishment to the body, as Galen writes.[339]

LARD AND FAT

These parts are listed as warm and humid to the second degree. These parts of an animal which tend toward equality are more recommended if as is fitting they are thoroughly cooked for the use of old men especially of frigid and dry nature in winter in the northern regions, as Abulkasim bids. But since they produce nausea because of their oiliness he recommends that they be eaten with salt and vinegar for these condiments assist in diminishing their thickness of texture. Famous physicians say that the nourishment they provide is useless and slight; they make foods lighter.[340] Too much use of them is frowned upon; they should be eaten in moderation, which may produce pleasure since the nourishment they provide is vaporous and oily with many superfluities. Hence they say that meat mingled with fat which they call striated or striped is more acceptable. If one eats these parts of the animal members they furnish a cold, viscous, and obstructive nutriment. They should be eaten with a mixture of something which separates and refines them, such as vinegar and spices.

[339]Galen, 4. 112; 5. 188.
[340]Ibid., 6. 679.

SUET, BOTH MILKY AND UNDER THE THROAT

The Romans of our time call the milky suet under the throat a little life or soul *(animula)*. There is no doubt that it tastes sweet although it is hard to digest since it is a kind of glandulous flesh [sweetbreads]. It is not excluded from the resumptive regimen.

BLOOD

Although blood is so called from the Greek because it invigorates and sustains[341] they say it is called *sanguis* in Latin because it is sweet. Nonetheless, due to its power of nutrition blood is listed among the obstructive foods. It is difficult to digest and is convertible into superfluities of small nourishment and is more delectable than valued as food itself, as Galen writes.[342] People have praised all quadruped blood, especially that of hares. Galen says it is very sweet and much esteemed even more than that of chickens and doves however they have been fed.

[341]Isidore of Seville, *Etymologies* 11. 122.
[342]Galen, 6. 699, 708; 11. 262, 675.

Chapter XXVI

Freshwater Fish

The nourishment provided by fish is by no means to be preferred to that of footed animals and birds nor can it be offered to old people unconditionally, for the nature of fish is cold and humid although a little drier than that of others, such as prickly sea fish *(Cottus Scorpio),* snails, another sea fish *(Trachinus Draco),* or a bluish colored fish,[343] as Theodorus Priscianus [viii] says. Abulkasim says that those who have a warm dry nature and are weakened especially in summer time and who dwell in a warm region should not be kept from eating these fish since they furnish a phlegmatic nourishment. They give little nutrition and are mild food with their watery temperate blood. Among less harmful fish are those which are freshly caught in a bay or a clear river or a rocky place in a stream for eating these fish in comparison with others they say furnishes a blood that is temperate between thick and thin. Those found among rocks are higher in nourishment than those found among sand and these are lighter than those in muddy waters, as Celsus says.[344] Thus the same classes of fish which live in a stagnant pond or lake or swamp or a dirty muddy spot such as gues or gubiones or a place where there are bad grasses or a river are heavier, and those who live in deep water are lighter food than those who live in shallows. The fish which live in waters flowing over rocks are praised most highly, as Galen says.[345] The nourishment they provide is not only easily digested but furnishes a very salutary blood of medium consistency not entirely thin and watery and yet sufficiently heavy. Thus they are more nourishing and temperate, more swiftly digested, and they move the bowels just

[343]Pliny, *N. H.* 9. 58.
[344]Celsus, *De Medicina* 2. 18. 9; Galen, 6. 718: gobio.
[345]Ibid., 6. 718–19. The gobio is the gudgeon.

as do all tender fish from rocky places. Their flesh is soft and fragile, sweet in taste, free from viscosity and heaviness. They have no thick putrefaction, nor is their flesh hard and dry, not fat or mucilaginous nor affected with a spoiled flavor. Marked with such distinctions fish is recommended no less for weak people such as old men are and convalescents than for those who wish to preserve their health and are given to exercise in proportion to their strength. They say that such people can more readily attain this goal even more if the fish they eat are neither tender nor hard but in between, such as the mullet and the pike (or wolf-fish), for they are of good juice. The fish they call *asini* or *aselli*[346] are not extremely small nor large although they are judged to be of better flesh, easier to digest, less harmful to the stomach but spoil more quickly, as Galen says. The big fish are detested and are very far from being temperate. Those fish which are in the median between extremes are more valued although they furnish less nourishment, as with fish of medium age and size just beginning to lay eggs. They are not overly fat or full of flesh. The scaly fish are similar to those which lack scales, for their flesh is purged of superfluities which nature converts into scales. As they are buffetted by storms and waves they have more solid and digestible flesh, according to Theodorus Priscianus [viii]. Celsus is authority for the statement that among all fish those which are least vitiated in the human stomach are the gilt head, scar, cuttle fish, lobster, polyp.[347]

SEA FISH

Although of the entire nature of things the sea is most harmful to the stomach, as Pliny says,[348] since it provides so many preparations for food, so many dishes, so many flavors derived from fish which are valued according to the perils undergone by those who catch them, saltwater fish ponds exhaust the purse rather than fill it, as M. Varro says.[349] As far as the gerontocomos is concerned the wisdom of the experts holds that sea fish are warmer

[346]Galen, 6. 721. The Greek *aphuē* is small fry.
[347]Celsus, *De Medicina* 2. 18. 7; Pliny, *N. H.* 9. 83.
[348]Ibid., 9. 104, almost verbatim.
[349]M. Varro, *Res Rusticae,* 3. 17. 2.

than those from fresh waters; they are also less humid and viscous. Galen does not entirely reject them in the resumptive regimen of weak and convalescent bodies especially if the fish swim in rocky places. Their flesh is more tender, more full of flavor, easier to cook but less nourishing. It is turned more swiftly into a temperate, not turbid, blood. It is not heavy; indeed, it is converted into a thin infusion and more quickly dissolved from the members or spread abroad in them. It leaves the stomach, however, rather slowly as well as the intestines due to its slight viscosity. From among many fish the *triglia* [Greek τρίγλη, red mullet] which the Venetians call *barboni* is prized. As Galen says,[350] the mullet is admired by epicures for its liver and the pleasure it gives. Others prefer mullet because it is drier and produces urine. The fish which an earlier age called *scarus [wrasse]* I think the common people call golden *fragolini;* their nature is drier and the inner parts constrain the bowels. The sole, plaice, sgombri [mackerel], parmulae, and pelamydes are other fish; the latter draws its name from the mud.[351] As they say it is at first a *cordyle* [young tunny] and then when a year old is called tunny. It dries and moderately constrains the bowels. There are fish of this same kind called *muscatella* [*musteli*]; Galen[352] says all of them are better when salted. The polyp and the white sepia are neither useful to the stomach nor nourishing. Theodorus Priscianus [viii] says they bring dimness to the eyes. Of them, the *viscella* compresses the bowels. Celsus[353] enumerates the ink of the cuttle fish among the remedies which relax the bowels. Those of large body among these fish are not acceptable.

FRESHWATER FISH

Sea fish are separate from freshwater fish. River fish they say are free from heavy marine odor and have thin spines. Those which grow in a bay and enter fresh water to dwell in are preferred to others, such as lupus [wolf-fish], spinola, sturiones, and the

[350]Galen, 6. 716.
[351]Pliny, *N. H.* 9. 72; 32. 49, 150.
[352]Galen, 6. 727.
[353]Celsus, *De Medicina* 2. 29.

like, for all sea fish like rivers, as Galen says.[354] In the regimen of old age fat crabs from ponds or springs and especially those who in form are called soft mollusks or *compatres* are especially praised when steeped in milk for a long time and cooked in barley water. Their flesh provides ideal nourishment to ill and wasted bodies. They increase the fat, are swiftly digested, and combat senile dryness. Many of these mollusks are found in seawaters. Crabs are in common use as food except that a few of the mollusks are prohibited. They dry the body although they stimulate the urine, as Theodorus Priscianus [viii] says, whether they are small sea crabs or large ones called lobsters. These are dry whether or not they live in fresh water and are hard to digest. If one eats them sometimes for pleasure they should be seasoned with wine and some salt water to which mint is added with parsley and spices. The intestines should first be removed through which they defecate; they are extended through the middle of the tail. After crabs come the fish which Celsus[355] calls rock fish who swim in rocky places although he lists them among foods of bad juice, unjustly however. All the more savory ones are fat and more salubrious such as trout and *timalus,* and even more the fish of ponds or rivers and of these especially *marsoni,* for their flesh is thinner and without many superfluities, of swift digestion, and providing a temperate blood neither thick nor thin in substance. Then there are *alatia* or *alosia* [shad][356] whom some[357] consider to be the wolf-fish of the Tiber. Its flesh is very fragile, sweet and fit to eat. It is completely forbidden in the resumptive diet. The famous river of Italy, the Tiber, has an abundance of most savory fish. They stimulate the urine and the stomach, according to Theodorus Priscianus [viii]. Nor should the fresh carp *[carpiones, murena ?]* whose rarity together with its good quality gives it a nobility among fish be passed over. This fish in the judgment of those who are keen students of the subject is found in Lake Garda in the region of Verona by a certain gift of nature. It is the most prized of freshwater fish, with few superfluities, and slow to become putrescent as is shown by

[354]Galen, 6. 714, 735; Pliny, *N. H.* 9. 97.
[355]Celsus, *De Medicina* 2. 18. 7, 9.
[356]Ausonius, *Mosella* 127.
[357]Galen, 6. 722–26.

the long time it can be kept in good condition after it is cooked. They say that nothing but golden sand is found in the intestines of this fish, indicating that it seeks its food around a gold mine deep in Lake Garda. After it comes the *themalus,* whose good quality is increased by its excessive exercise by which its mucilaginous component is removed, as with the tufted barbel and the *capitanus,* which they call *cavedanus,* of which the Reno River at Bologna has a supply, the golden trout and the spiny, resembling the *carpio* both in shape and in the nourishment it provides of which Galen[358] seems to have been speaking when he says the Nar River, which flows into the Tiber, has much better fish than the Tiber since it flows pure from high mountains and springs, with a sharp descent into the Tiber without the slightest pause in stagnant waters. Then there is *lucius,* the pike,[359] from ponds and rivers, which they call the king of freshwater fish as the dolphin is the king of saltwater fish. The pike and the trout are called the swiftest of fish. The trout exercises exceedingly as it ascends the descending waters at their waterfalls or cliffs. Nor should that fish which the ingenious glutton prizes so much be overlooked, the lamprey, which is also called *oculata* (furnished with eyes or shaped like an eye). It supplies non-mucilaginous nourishment without many superfluities since it lives in deep water among rocks by sucking like a leech or blood sucker. In its stomach they say nothing of fat is found. The same type of fish originates in bays and in fresh waters, among which is the salmon,[360] pronounced the most flavorful of all fish and especially the river salmon, which is preferred to all sea fish in Aquitania.[361] The ancients were accustomed to stock their lakes now and then with sea fish so that wolf-fish and golden trout were raised therein and other species which could tolerate fresh water. Some fish are preferred to others in different places and regarded as better, such as the wolf-fish in the Tiber between two bridges,[362] of which M. Varro says: The Tiber fish are best to eat. But among them the wolf-fish or pike has held first place. Some say it is the

[358]Ibid., 6. 722–23; 720, a list of soft-fleshed fish.
[359]Ausonius, *Mosella* 120.
[360]Ibid., 97–105.
[361]Pliny, *N. H.* 9. 68.
[362]Titius apud Macrobius, *Sat.* 3. 16. The quotation from Varro is obscure. See Galen, 6. 714, on the pike. *Labrax lupus* is the sea bass, known to the Greeks.

fish the Arabs call *sabor,* the Greeks *cobensus,* that is, *labrachi* or *laurachi,* the Genoese *lovatius* or *loratius,* the Venetians *variolus,* the Romans *spinola,* which Galen says he has not seen born in fresh water but has seen coming up from rivers or pools. Some call it *lucius,* others believe it to be the *sturio.* Others with more truth call it *alosia* or *alatia* or *chiepa* in the common language. It is the *lupus* which Columella[363] says grows weary in ascending the Tiber against the current. For they say the fish they call *alatia,* stimulated by worms and the itching it has in the head, swims into the Tiber against the current from the sea so that with the clash of the waves he repels the stimulus.[364] Therefore this fish is better in the Tiber than elsewhere, as with the turbot at Ravenna, the murena in Sicily, the elops at Rhodes, and other species similarly in different places. Humid oysters are ideal for the stomach for they minister to the bowels and the urine, according to Theodorus [viii], although almost all shellfish and especially their juice do so also. The snail and the shellfish *(conchylia)* although they cause little flatulence nevertheless constrict the bowels, have very little substance and thus provide very little food or nourishment. All fish are of bad juice (chyme) if they belong to the most tender species, are too hard, muddy, and of too large a size, as Celsus teaches.[365]

PARTS OF FISH

All parts of fish which have fat are not recommended although they are savory, for with their fat they provide a nourishment from their viscous substance and lubrication for the stomach and intestines which is difficult of penetration and easily vitiated within those organs. After the first eating of such fish it very quickly produces repletion and ruins the appetite so thereafter for many days we cannot tolerate the eating of fish, as Galen says,[366] especially if they are parts of a large fish. Of all the parts of the fish those around the umbilicus are more disapproved of since they are fatter, as well as the parts around the ears and near the eyes; the head too is rejected. They provide a food which floats in the stom-

[363]Columella, *De Re Rustica* 8. 16.
[364]Pliny, *N. H.,* 9. 169.
[365]Celsus, *De Medicina* 2. 21.
[366]Galen, 6. 713.

ach; with its oiliness and viscosity it is difficult to digest. Descending to the bottom of the stomach it destroys the villi [soft papillae and membranous tubes] therein, which being relaxed more quickly throw out the food, thus causing a heavy attack of diarrhoea. The larger parts of fish, especially those which are more mobile such as the tail, back, and fins, are of purer flesh; they have less fat, are swifter to be digested, and provide a more acceptable nourishment. The parts placed in an opposite manner to these are regarded in an appropriate way, that is, as less acceptable. The flesh of the tail, fins, and the bones of the back from head to tail is of softer substance, easier digestion, and good chyme in comparison to the other parts. Their nourishment is furnished by an almost continual motion. The frequent rubbing of the bones of those parts on the bones close to them creates a fragility, softness, and good flavor in them. The judgment concerning the ribs is midway between that regarding the tail and fins and the fact that the belly has good flavor, viscosity, and mobility. Fish eggs are harder to digest than their flesh. There is a great variety of methods for preparing fish according to whether it is boiled, fried, or roasted. Vinegar helps to lessen its viscosity; spices do the same for its frigidity.

SALTED FISH

Just as fresh fish, since it administers to the body, is suitable for the resumptive regimen likewise occasionally salted fish is also suitable. Since due to its hot and dry nature it dissolves or liquefies the phlegm with which ailing old age abounds it is useful for old people of a cold and humid nature in the winter in southern regions. Since its too frequent use induces itching, black morphea or scurfy eruptions, impetigo, and scabies the experts say it should be eaten with red honeyed wine. The best salted fish is the most recently salted, the more recently the better. Then it is seasoned with vinegar and other suitable condiments. Eggs *tarica (botargo),* which the common people call *botarica* by corruption of the word, is forbidden except for use in purging the bowels. They have a soothing effect on the lower abdomen, just as capers has according to Avicenna.[367]

[367]Avicenna, *Canon,* II, cap. 142, f. 103v. For botargo see R. Dunglison, op. cit., 136: the salted eggs and blood of the mullet.

Chapter XXVII

Milk, and, First, Mother's Milk

The experts say the regimen of old age should not lack human or mother's milk, which is especially ideal at the time she has given birth. Milk is an additional humor, white in color (the Greeks say *leukos,* the Latins *album*), of a double decoction generated in the breasts, of median quality approaching frigidity and humidity, however. It is quite beneficial in the restoration of the powers of those who are sick and old. It nourishes with a good light nutriment, restores and repairs the body, increases fat, and produces a lively complexion, especially when it is drunk with sugar.[368] As Marcus Varro reports, milk of all the liquids we take for sustenance is the most nourishing.[369] It corrects the vitiated humors by drawing them off from the abdomen to such an extent that nothing seems better than milk in the treatment of tabes, or wasting away [atrophy or emaciation], as Galen says.[370] It has the best chyme of almost all the foods we eat. It counteracts dry, cold forgetfulness, sadness, and alienation of the mind so that some old people by continuous use of milk have lived longer than a hundred years, safe and sound with the greatest advantage. Some observations have been made concerning the effect of its use on old age as to its food value and function in strengthening the old person. First, milk is composed of a substance partly serous water, whether warm, dry, cold, or humid in nature, partly from a substance thick, earthy, and cheesy in nature although while it is fresh and soft it inclines toward humidity. In part it is also of a warm, humid, buttery, and airy substance. Milk is more acceptable if it has these three substances in proper proportion in it. For although

[368]Avicenna, II, cap. 444, f. 121v.
[369]Varro, *R. R.* 2. 10. 11.
[370]Galen, 7. 701.

milk is swiftly digested, the thinner portion of it more quickly dominates the other parts in its composition; the part which is more earthy is more slowly digested. Of the kinds of milk the middle kind is airy and is better insofar as its watery and cheesy parts are equal. Of all kinds, human mother's milk is more preferable, more temperate than any other, since its superfluity is that of a temperate animal; the more similar other milk is to human milk the sweeter and more nourishing it is. If the mother's milk is that of a woman between twenty-five and thirty-five years of age it is the best, for the experts report this age is one of health and completion, especially if the woman is of good color, muscular, of solid flesh, not fat nor too thin, for they believe her milk is akin to her temperament in substance and quality. In addition, if the milk is of even nature and of unmistakable whiteness which when dropped upon a finger does not drip down and not a fluid or watery white, which does not incline toward dark green, yellow, or red, is of sweet odor without a tendency toward the acrid or tart, with a good flavor in which bitterness, saltiness, and acridity are not perceived, the woman's milk is of the best. The medium between watery and thick is cheesy, whose parts are similarly not far distant from foam from the time at which it is not convenient for the woman to have a miscarriage; she will bear a male child according to the natural length of time required within one month and a half to two months. The regimen of a woman who is giving milk is required to be temperate. She should abstain from exercise, rich food, strong drink, and sex. The milk should be drunk as soon as it is drawn from the breasts lest in any way it should suffer any change upon exposure to the air. Thus Euryphon and Herodicus[371] praise milk in the resumptive regimen, as Galen says. For they write that if anyone chastely places his mouth to a woman's breast and sucks there is nothing more ideal for him. They say that the old man who drinks milk does not suffer from brain fever. For anyone with ample veins whose flow through the viscera is easy the quality of milk is suitable. It is unsuitable for stoppages of strong abdomina, cases of strong istimbria, or indurations of tissue, fasting, when all common superfluities are disposed of, with some exercise preceding, with no extraneous flavor appearing in

[371]Ibid., 7. 701.

the mouth. After drinking milk they impose rest lest it spoil or turn sour in the stomach. They also forbid sleep or the taking of other foods until the milk that has been drunk has descended.

MILK FROM QUADRUPEDS

On account of its difficulty of digestion all milk from animals whose flesh is eaten except that from cows is constipating, says Theodorus Priscianus [iii]. Milk embraces a diversity of features according to the species of animal from which it is derived, its age and size, whether small, large, or middle-sized, and according to form, whether its flesh is smooth, soft, or hard, fat or thin, and according to color, whether a white animal or of another color. After human milk the milk of an animal whose time of pregnancy is closest to that of the pregnant woman is recommended, such as the cow. Cow's milk is particularly preferred in special remedies in the resumptive regimen for its nature is closest to that of the human, corresponding proportionately. The odor of the animal flesh is a sign of the goodness of the milk and its blood, sustained health, and closeness to human nature as well. Hence they think that the milk of that animal whose flesh men eat, whether wild or tame, is more praiseworthy, such as the she-goat and the deer, although sheep are the most nourishing; then follows the goat, fat and snowy. M. Varro[372] recommends both the latter as light and good for the stomach. Ass's milk is more nourishing than other milk, has a purgative effect, and provides much strength, as Theodorus says [iii], being thinner and more watery than the rest. The cause of this is the thickness of substance in ass's milk, which has an earthier and thicker part; in respect to nourishment it is similar in nature to thick or heavy food. Galen[373] thought ass's milk especially safe as food even if anyone drank it continuously. It is less unreliable than other milk and swiftly purges the stomach even if eaten without bread. It is least flatulent nor does it turn to cheese in the stomach especially if it is drunk with salt and honey. They recommend the use of goat's milk because of its medium heaviness; it should be added that it is more nourishing and less

[372]M. Varro, *R. R.* 10. 11.
[373]Galen, 6. 346, 682.

softening to the bowels. Although human milk contains the most nourishment goat milk is praised next to it as most useful for the stomach since the goat eats largely leaves and grass although Celsus[374] lists milk as among foods alien to the stomach. Of all kinds of milk that is more helpful which comes from a young animal and especially in the spring because the milk is more watery than in the summer and more temperate than milk at any other season of the year so that milk in the spring is regarded as most healthful although Avicenna[375] says milk in midsummer is better. It is feared, however, that heat will turn the milk sour after it is drunk, which is not feared in the spring. Milk very close to the time of birth is not recommended for it is hard to digest and watery because of the humors collected in the veins of the udders and uterus from the beginning of conception. But at a space of forty or fifty days from the time of the animal's birth that surplus previously collected is now used up and the natural humidity of the substance remains temperate, praiseworthy, easy to digest, inconvertible into bad humors with putrescence, especially if the old man drinks it in good health without blemish. Nor should the recognition of pasturage be overlooked, for its virtue or quality is of great importance in creating good milk. Galen[376] says that animals who feed upon scammony and spurge have a purgative quality in their milk because of which it has a heavy odor, acidity, and bitterness. Bad pasturage has a similar effect upon the milk of the animal who feeds on it continually. The milk of an animal who feeds on fresh grass purges the bowels more than the milk of one that feeds on dry grass or hay. For this reason its pasturage on lentiscus makes goat's milk preferable. Hence Democrates the physician (as Pliny tells us[377]) in caring for the health of Considia, the daughter of the consular M. Servilius, who was not responding to strict treatment, made efficient use of the milk of she-goats pastured on lentiscus. Therefore it is important that the food of animals whose milk is to be the best should not be of heavy odor, acid, nor bitter if old people are to drink it. Galen[378] therefore in consideration of

[374]Celsus, *De Medicina* 2. 25.
[375]Avicenna, II, cap. 444, f. 129v.
[376]Galen, 6. 345; Varro, *R. R.* 2. 10. 11.
[377]Pliny, *N. H.* 24. 43.
[378]Galen, 10. 363, 365.

the environment of Gabii near Rome praises its milk highly. It excels all milk in perfection because of the elevation and dry air of the place and because its pasturage is praised as nourishing. The old man who drinks milk as food does not have fever nor a flux of the bowels, a weak or aching head nor rheumatism. In its use as medicine milk is sometimes useful for catarrhs and removes them. Nor does his stomach rumble or hang down or become prone to flatulence. Milk is listed among those substances which produce flatulence and there are few who drink it who do not suffer from flatulence. Those old men whose nature is frigid and who have narrow veins and who cannot tolerate any noxious and abominable substance are advised to avoid milk. For if old men who suffer from these ills are given milk it would be harmful to their head and nerves, producing nervous disorders both chilling and phlegmatic together with dim vision and blindness. In fact, much use of milk creates body lice. Galen[379] says an old man sometimes who has used milk for a long time has lost all his teeth, for the teeth are easily rotted through the use of milk and the gums softened. To counteract this condition some honey[380] should be mixed with the milk. This makes the milk more detergent and cleans away the cheesy part of the milk which adheres to the teeth. It is not unknown for the rather frequent use of milk to stop up the meseraic or mesenteric veins. Such prolonged use of milk creates kidney stones. All in all, milk and milk products quickly spoil inside the stomach; Galen[381] calls it one of the most quickly changeable of foods. If it is exposed to more heat than is necessary it is quickly turned into smokiness; if to less heat than necessary it becomes sour. Thus it is not enough for its users that the milk be of good chyme for even good chyme can be made into bad.

CHEESE

Cheese *(caseum)* is so called from coming-together *(co-eundo)*. It is not forbidden in the resumptive regimen whether made from milk (which is the source of real cheese) or from the thin watery portion recooked,[382] or laur, as Abulkasim calls it, or the cream.

[379]Ibid., 6. 344.
[380]Ibid., 6. 683.
[381]Galen, 6. 682–83; 12. 263; see 6. 345 on pasturage.
[382]Ricotta, or cottage cheese.

However, cheese is pronounced to be very bad, heavy, and alien to the stomach, producing flatulence and easily corrupted within the stomach, difficult to digest, and lying in the passages of the liver it stops them up. It is of bad juice, especially old cheese. Fresh cheese is soft, especially without salt. They say it is close to frigidity and humidity to the first degree; others extend its nature to the second or third degree. For other people than old persons it is more nourishing. Since it humidifies the stomach, does not harm it, and is of good juice it is allowed to old men of warm, dry nature in warm regions and in the summer time. The cheese which they call green here, that is, fresh, soft, and unsalted, is good for the stomach. It contributes to fattening, provides good blood, gives good nourishment which does not remain within the body especially if the milk from which it is made is such that little or no butter has been extracted from it [as for skim milk]. However, on the contrary, old dry cheese softens the bowels although boiled or roasted it constricts the intestines. Galen[383] praises highly that cheese which the Greeks call *oxygalacticum,* that is, of acid milk, at Pergamum, where Galen was born, and which he says is regarded as most delectable by the people of the surrounding regions; it is innocuous to the stomach. With other cheeses it is less difficult to digest and easy to pass through the alimentary system without bad or heavy chyme, which is the common accusation brought against all cheeses. Perhaps it is this cheese which when fresh contributes greatly to extending life and retarding old age. They say that Zoroaster lived in the desert on cheese for thirty years so moderately prepared that he did not notice old age.[384] The best cheese according to Galen[385] greatly esteemed by the rich men at Rome is named *vatusicus* [βαδμ́σικος]. It is no wonder that cheese is praised at Rome, where the good things of the whole world are judged. Some people call cheese made of cow's milk that which, pressed by hand, Caesar Augustus frequently ate, as Suetonius[386] relates. Salted and dry cheese are bad for the stomach since they are hot and dry in nature to the third degree, inducing

[383]Galen, 6. 697, 339; 12. 272 on sour milk; also Pliny, *N. H.* 28. 134; Columella, *R. R.* 12. 8.
[384]Pliny, *N. H.* 11. 242.
[385]Galen, 6. 697; Pliny, *N. H.* 11. 240.
[386]Suetonius, *Divus Augustus* 75.

fever, or possibly the cheese called bitinus [Bithynian] with one vowel changed from batyncitus *[vatusicus]*, which is much prized among overseas cheeses, Pliny reports.[387] Daily experience teaches us that cow-milk cheese does not have such a great quality of remaining unspoiled since it is of a substance viscous and hard to digest although savory to the taste. Fresh cheese is judged more ideal for the regimen of old age since it is made of milk more adapted for the elderly without any other adverse properties. M. Varro[388] judged the best cheese for nourishment was cow's milk cheese, but it was discharged with the greatest difficulty after being eaten; next, sheep-milk cheese; of least nutrition and the most easily voided is goat's milk cheese.

BUTTER[389]

Butter is not banned in the resumptive regimen. Abulkasim allows it for old men of a dry nature in the winter and in the southern region, for butter itself is of warm and humid nature, very much praised for its nourishment and its conversion into excellent blood especially in old people if it is eaten with sugar or honey. With the addition of almonds as well they say butter can terminate a cold or catarrh. Sheep butter in winter especially is praised when it is not rancid nor salty and used moderately, for it has a superfluous humidity which when excessive can bring on phlegmatic ills, soften the nerves, stop up the head by evaporation and make the stomach rather sluggish. It also damages the villi of the stomach and softens their roughness. It discourages appetite as olive oil does and other oily substances do, for they tend to soften. It hinders the function of the orifices of the veins and stops their passages so that the veins are unable to suck. Butter should be eaten with substances which are astringent. Drinking butter is heralded as is theriac as a remedy for poisons.

[387]Pliny, *N. H.* 11. 241: *caseum bibulum manu pressum (bibulum-bubulum),* moist cheese.
[388]M. Varro, *R. R.* 2. 10. 11.
[389]Galen, 6. 683; 12. 270, 272.

CREAM OF MILK

That part of milk which the shepherds call the head of the milk and the Arabs call adog, the famous Latin physicians call cream. It is most praised as food in the resumptive regimen. It is more savory and healthful than other parts of the milk and especially nourishing when prepared with sugar and spiced with pine nuts. An especially favorite recipe is the mixture of three parts cream with two drams of fresh sweet almond oil; pine nuts prepared three days in myrrh (three drams), all ground up in a mortar for a long time until it is thick. Of all parts of milk colastra has been condemned in the resumptive diet. It is the first spongy thick part of the milk and induces jaundice and generates stone. If it is eaten it should be taken with ginger, fennel, parsley, and anise with much sugar scattered over it.

Chapter XXVIII

Birds' Eggs

The most preferred of all eggs in the resumptive regimen are fresh hen's eggs. After them come the eggs of birds which run about more than chickens, such as pheasants; these are preferred in the diet of old men. Then some people list the eggs of the calandra [a kind of lark] as Abulkasim says, and of partridge, especially for old people in spring and in a temperate region. They are thinner than chicken eggs and of less nourishment. Isaac [f. cxlv] and Rhazes [236] state that partridge and chicken eggs are better than others especially if laid by birds that are young, fleshy, and offering themselves to the males, for the natural heat of the male provides the egg with better nourishment and substance and makes it easier to cook, especially if the hens who lay the eggs feed in approved feeding grounds are nourished with convenient food such as wheat, barley, millet and such like for they have a strong heat and lack any bitter odor. Thus their eggs are easier to digest. Other eggs of both small and large birds are not to be eaten except as medicine, Rhazes says [536]. With the exception of turtle eggs, these are similar to hens' eggs and strengthen the brain; they are helpful in cases of the falling sickness.[390] Those who have examined their multifarious nature say that either because they have a cold body which is very little temperate they refrigerate their eggs evenly so that this dries them without making them pungent or because their tendency is toward evenness of temperature, as is more truly believed, the white liquid they call albumen tends toward frigidity and the yolk of the egg toward heat. Both parts of the egg are humid, especially the albumen, for the yolk is in the middle between humid and dry just as in heat and cold it tends to move more toward heat, as they say. It readily attains to inflam-

[390]Pliny, *N. H.* 32. 112, 116; Galen, 15. 898 on birds' eggs.

mation with its oiliness. The yolk is particularly in conformity with human nature. It is quickly transformed into thin clear blood by which the heart in the conversion of the blood is nourished and strengthened. It has few superfluities. It nourishes abundantly and well in the resumptive regimen and is especially good if boiled in water without the shell, [i.e., poached]. Thus the superfluities are purged away better as these appear in the foam created in the boiling. Its vapors are resolved and dissipated without the shell to impede their exit. Thus the yolk is more nourishing than in any other manner of cooking although Celsus[391] says a hard-boiled egg is a very substantial material, a soft-boiled or raw egg of very soft material. It is ideal, however, for the stomach, producing very little flatulence. The albumen is difficult to digest, as Galen[392] affirms. The yolk is propelled quickly to the heart, says Avicenna,[393] bringing relief in case of the dissolution and diminution of the heart's blood; therefore, they say, the yolk brings strength to the vital spirit for it provides temperate blood at times which functions as flesh would in supplying much energy. For this reason it is not recommended in the regimen of more fleshy and fat men. Eggs are useful in cases of congestion of the chest and throat and hoarseness of voice because of their heat. In stricture of breath, spitting of blood, roughness of the gullet (meri), cough and hectic or phthisic pleurisy, griping of the intestines and stomach,[394] burning urine and ulcers of the bladder they are helpful. Avicenna[395] writes that the yolk is of medicinal value especially if swallowed raw. Potions made of egg yolks which are soft and thin are called abula, for, as Serapio says, the egg adheres to those parts and remains there as a poultice. All in all, there is no other food which nourishes in illness, does not burden the patient, and at the same time has the power of food and drink, as Pliny tells us.[396] As to the shape of eggs, the preferable ones they say are small, long, and fresh.

[391]Celsus, *De Medicina* 2. 18. 10.
[392]Galen, 11. 35.
[393]Avicenna, II, cap. 530.
[394]Cael. Aur., *Acut.* 3. 20, 161; 2. 18, 105.
[395]Avicenna, II, cap. 530.
[396]Pliny, *N. H.* 29. 48.

Chapter XXIX

Oil

Oil is the juice of the olive whose effect they say is similar to that of butter if it were excellent oil. Therefore oil and butter are both recommended in the resumptive regimen. The preferable oil is fresh, for age makes olive oil unpleasant to the taste. Most oil is a year old and is the first juice or squeezing of the raw olive not yet completely ripe. That oil which is made of unripe olives they call *omphacium* because it has a superlative flavor. In fact, the first issuance of oil from the press which makes *omphacium*[397] is the most praised. In the whole world Italy has reached the highest estimation among the common people for the quality of its olive oil, especially for the oil from the Venafran area and that known as Licinian.[398] M. Varro in his book on human affairs[399] says the region of Casinum has the best oil for human use. In our time the oil produced at Tibur is in frequent use at Rome, but at Verona the oil from the olive groves on Mount St. Leonardo is considered the best. The best oil is the sweetest, free from all bitterness. Its nature is mild, tending toward hot and humid, ideal according to this feature for human nature, especially for the liver since it increases flesh and weight, particularly if the oil is made from the pulp of the ripe olive with the olive stones removed. For healthy bodies it is most suitable. The oil known as *omphacium* is more recommended for strengthening the stomach and is more fragrant. Oil is of bad juice, as Celsus[400] reports. It is alien to the stomach and softens and relaxes it; it checks the appetite as do all oily substances. It should be eaten with astringent foods. A sharpness or acridity of odor and taste arising from some dominant parts of it with a notable tendency toward heat can be corrected with frequent applications of water.

[397]Pliny, *N. H.* 15. 9; 12. 130; 14. 98.

[398]Ibid., 15. 7; 37. 202; Cato, *R. R.* 62.2: produced by a certain Licinius.

[399]*Antiquitates,* written around 47 B. C., twenty-five books of which were devoted to *res humanae.*

[400]Celsus, *De Medicina* 2. 21.

Chapter XXX

Salt

Salt is recommended in the resumptive diet, white, clear, even in consistency. It should be selected when spread out in the sun's rays. Its nature is warm and dry to the third degree. Abulkasim allows its use for old people of cold and humid nature in the winter in the northern region. It is useful for digestion and facilitates the descent of food to the bottom of the stomach with the evacuation of superfluities. Salt cleanses, breaks up, causes coherence, dries out, banishes flatulence, and restores appetite and digestion. Since salt is listed among the substances which depart from the body little of it is eaten and because it is also harmful to the brain and the vision it should be used after it is washed and roasted.

SALT WATER

Some people affirm that this is of warm and humid nature, which it is formally and in actuality or because it is felt to be so when it touches the human body. Others have graded it as of warm and dry nature to the second degree according to its force and effect. If it is not bitter as it flows it loosens the bowels, which Abulkasim concedes to be helpful to old people of frigid and humid nature especially in winter in cold regions, for then it loosens the bowels. But used at length it constipates and dries out; hence it is forbidden, not according to its use as food but as medicine. Avicenna[401] says it dries out and thins the body, corrupts the blood, and creates itching and scabies. In fact, it acts like an external bath by drying out and heating the body like a salt seawater bath or one of alum or sulphur,[402] as Theodorus Priscianus [xiiii] states.

[401]Avicenna, II, cap. 624.
[402]Vitruvius, 8. 3; Pliny, *N. H.* 31. 48.

Chapter XXXI

Plants Grown in the Earth, Except for Oil, Which Has Been Discussed in Its Place, and, First of All, Honey

Honey is not truly one of the kinds of food taken from plants alone nor from animals alone but is derived from both separately; so Avicenna.[403] It is made from the leaves of plants, although it is not their juice, nor fruit, nor part of them. It is formed from dew fallen from above and hidden on the flowers and upon the rest of the surroundings which the bees collect. It is really vapor which when it arises is converted and matures in the air. When it is last condensed in the nighttime, being made into honey, it falls. Its nature is warm and dry to the second degree but not greatly beyond that. Of this kind of food are many forms of manna in use by physicians whose dew is thick and dense and when apparent is collected by men. That honey which is hidden is rare or thin and is collected by the bees.[404] This part through the labor and the faculty of the bees is more elaborate and is warmer and drier in the second degree. This thinner part of it acquires some pungency from the nature of the bees from whom they say honey derives its name: *melissa* in Greek, *apis* in Latin. People teach that pungency can be removed by frequent washing, mixing the honey with much water and boiling the combination thoroughly until the foam which continually arises from it has ceased. Thus Galen[405] says the flatulence and stickiness of honey are removed and it becomes more thin and humid nor can further constrict the bowels. Its sweetness is diminished and thus honey passes more quickly through the bodies of those who eat it. It nourishes swiftly, softens the roughness of the chest, and provokes the urine, and is in every

[403]Avicenna, II, cap. 500.
[404]Avicenna, II, cap. 500.
[405]Galen, 6. 266, 739; 10. 475; Pliny, *N. H.* 11. 11–70 on bees.

way made more suitable for the distribution of nourishment. Endowed with these properties it is recommended as most useful in the diet of old age in winter especially and in mountainous regions no less than for all whose nature is cold in their illness so that the old men can use it handily both cooked and before it is boiled with bread, as Galen affirms.[406] It is excellent for an old man since it is more nourishing. It is more quickly converted into energy, easily furnishes good blood of a temperate nature, opens the orifices of the veins, dissolves humidities and expels them from the body, breaks up bad chyme and purges it through the pores of the skin, excellently cleanses the refuse in the veins, prevents the putrefaction and corruption of the flesh, and counteracts dimness of vision, although Celsus[407] has seen fit to say that it must be listed among foods alien to the stomach. Honey made in the spring is held to be the best, tending toward a reddish color when taken from the honeycomb and elaborated by the bees feeding on almond blossoms. The honey of Sardinia[408] they say is bitter because of the abundance of wormwood upon which the bees feed. The features of good honey are as follows: delectable taste, good odor, straw color, very clear, transparent, non-viscous, and when distilled it drips down without separating. When boiled in water it becomes less hot, loses its sharpness, is more temperate, savory, and humid. Attic honey from Sicily is especially praised by the Greek authors. M. Varro[409] affirms that the honey of Tarentum is the best to eat. If this honey cannot be obtained one must use some which does not have a heavy odor nor with any wax perceptible in it and especially without apparent extraneous material. It should be rejected if of sharp odor which they call viscid, that is, pungent and biting to the tongue so as to make one sneeze. It is poisonous when its odor alone takes away the faculty of reason, bringing on alienation of the mind and a cold sweat the more of it one has eaten. The cure they say is salted fish and honey-water drunk until vomiting is brought on. Honey is usually boiled with water until its foam is boiled off and it is thus rendered less sharp in taste.

[406]Galen, 7. 702; 10. 475.
[407]Celsus, *De Medicina* 2. 25.
[408]Horace, *Schol.* to *A. P.* 375.
[409]Varro, *R. R.* 3. 16. 14: he does not mention Tarentum, however.

When it is boiled with water it does not provoke the urine or remove it. Thus the old Greek physician Antiochus took care of himself eating bread with Attic honey very often boiled but rarely raw, as Galen writes.[410] The quality of honey can be judged more or less by its use as a condiment.

[410]Galen, 6. 332; Pliny, *N. H.* 20. 112.

Chapter XXXII

Sugar

Sugar cane is held in high esteem in the resumptive diet since it is very pleasant to human nature in all its forms. Pliny[411] calls it *saccharon*. Its heat is less than that of honey; it is less dry and sharp. Its nature is warm approaching the first degree of warmth and is of the first degree of humidity. It is best when very white in the resumptive regimen in every season and every inhabited region especially when made from the decoction of the sugar cane in which the inner part is squeezed out to form the essential part of the cane. The sugar is collected after the juice has cooled. It is called *taberzet* or *caphiti* by the Arabs. Its use is to provide good blood, cleanse the body's system, assist the kidneys and bladder, serve as very close to food in its drying and opening of stoppages, as Avicenna says.[412] In its functions it is quite similar to bee honey, although it creates thirst and stirs the bile just as honey does. Its food value is less, however; its recognition and frequent use were lacking among the ancient Greek physicians, who used honey more often. Abulkasim urges that sugar be eaten with pomegranates to prevent thirst and the rousing of the bile. But if it is boiled and its foam removed it combats thirst and cough and pacifies disturbances of the stomach, kidneys, and bladder, as he affirms.

CANE HONEY

This is a cane or reed whose knots are very close to each other. The juice of its inner pith while it remains in a container drips out very sweet and thin. This is called cane honey in the way in which the juice that flows from grapes not yet trodden is called.

[411]Ibid., 12. 32.
[412]Avicenna, II, cap. 757.

Then from the juice of the canes when boiled and cooled the very white sugar is collected. After it is boiled a second time and further squeezed out something called sugar loaf is made. At the third decoction a yellow sugar results which derives its color from the final step in the process of refinement. This is the cane honey from which so much strength and food value are adapted to human nature. It serves also as medicine and is of great juiciness and sweetness as a temperate liquid, very useful in the resumptive diet especially for old people of frigid nature in every season at which the honey cane is available and in every region. Since it produces flatulence this condition can be corrected by a decoction of some substances which are adapted for this purpose.

CLARIFIED SUGAR IN ROLLS

These are sometimes prescribed for old age.[413] Their nature is warm and humid, they provide temperate blood, and are helpful for those who suffer from a cough in the chest. They lubricate the bowels and are more effective if made of a purified sugar. Portugal produces the best sugar in rolls.

CANDIES

These are of temperate warmth but humid to the second degree. The purer candies are transparent and lighter. They are recommended for old men in every season and region. They are most ideal for ills of the throat since they counteract a bilious stomach when eaten with ripe fruits, as Abulkasim prescribes.

[413] Ibid., II, cap. 557.

Chapter XXXIII

Garden Vegetables or Growing Plants

The Arabs understood by the name of vegetables both herbs and fruits which do not grow from wood shoots. The usage of the Latins embraces herbs alone, whose material or substance is the weakest of all. Some of them have a cooling effect, such as especially the raw cabbage, endive, and lettuce. The charge brought against almost all vegetables is that they produce little blood; it is acknowledged that less than ten drams of blood are made from ten drams of vegetables. This particular property can be seen in the blood that results from the eating of flesh. Therefore the eating of vegetables in the resumptive regimen is not admitted without reservation. Whatever powers they have for thinning the blood of old men so as to consume or inflame it are created by their frequent use. They cause flatulence and that disease which crept in during the principate of Tiberius Caesar which they call colum or colic.[414] They impede the digestion unless something sharp among vegetables such as fresh oregano is used to heat and provoke the urine, or nasturtium, which heats and dries like mustard. It cuts and burns vigorously. When drunk with cold water it dissipates the flatulence of the intestines, says Avicenna.[415] These and similar afflictions are relieved by this process; their course is interrupted and diminished by these vegetables. Thick vegetables produce phlegmatic blood and likewise oppress the strength of the body. Nevertheless, some of them are used medicinally to assist old age or as a preservative from illness such as figs, which are lenitive, and celery, whose seeds and leaves do not loosen the bowels. The root, however, does so, as Avicenna says,[416] as do leeks, of which a little

[414]Pliny, *N. H.* 26. 9.
[415]Avicenna, II, cap. 683.
[416]Ibid., II, 549.

at the first course controls the bowels. Hence we must treat vegetables in this *Gerontocomia.* Of garden vegetables those which grow in the fields through cultivation are sometimes preferable to others of the same species for the protection of old age as being moister and colder; others are wild: their origin and use are quite the contrary to the cultivated variety. Some of these have a great deal of nourishment in their leaves, such as lettuce; others have it in their roots, such as turnips; some are sharp, some provocative, some have none of these powers. Those which have a sharp or pungent taste are used in the regimen of old age somewhat in the way of medicine rather than food. The roots of some vegetables are suitable for eating while their seeds and leaves are sometimes not in use for nourishment. Vegetables have a more vigorous effect and greater powers in cold places in the north, they say. Since it is not difficult to recognize them it behooves the gerontocomos to know them by sight according to the example of Antonius Castor,[417] whose authority in the matter of plants and vegetables was once very high at Rome in the art of medicine, as Pliny writes. He grew many herbs in his garden and lived more than one hundred years without any illness of body and without loss of memory or of vigor. Let us list the vegetables therefore so that we may profit for the resumptive regimen from the long experience of those who are experts in this area, beginning with the root vegetables primarily.

ROOT VEGETABLES IN GENERAL

Almost all roots, especially of vegetables, are listed as alien to the stomach, producing flatulence, and are indigestible and disturbing in comparison to the other parts of the plant, according to Galen.[418] They collect in themselves a great deal of indigestible humor which awaits the end of the first digestion. Thus the great amount of humor worked up in them leaves in the body a humid and disturbing nourishment. But since they are in common use some roots in the resumptive diet should be cooked and seasoned or prepared in some other manner.

[417]Pliny, *N. H.* 25. 9.
[418]Galen, 6. 645; 794.

TURNIPS

Turnip *(rapa)* is so called from *rapiendo,* that is seizing.[419] Of this species are also *napus* (navew) and *rapuncilium,* as the Conciliator [56] writes. It is somewhere between good and bad, hot to the first degree, humid to the second degree, and of bad juice because it is raw, hard, and difficult to eat. It should be cooked twice in two different waters; at last when its flesh is very soft it should be boiled. Thus it will be no less edible than similar vegetables, Galen says.[420] Its hard substance when softened provides a praiseworthy and rather powerful nourishment for the resumptive regimen. It is not at all harmful and has a marvellous property for comforting the eyesight and increasing the illumination of the eyes. They recommend the use of turnips in our diet in many ways. They are better roasted than boiled, for whatever is rather humid resists further humidification, just as a body which has fallen in one direction needs to be propped in the opposite direction. Foods should be prepared in the same way, warm foods with cold and cold foods with warm condiments and preparations. It is better to roast turnips just as with pears and pork, but vegetables and rabbit meat should be boiled. The inner part of turnip leaves when thoroughly cooked and eaten can provoke the urine, as the son of Serapion [f. clxxvv] writes. Theodorus Priscianus [x] writes that the turnip removes vapor from the body, assists the bowels, facilitates childbirth, and prohibits nausea.

HOMEGROWN RADISHES OR SMALL RADISHES AND HORSE RADISH

Since roots are of bad juice they are allowed for medical purposes but not as food for nourishment in the regimen of old age. For old men they are warm and humid in nature and especially used for inducing vomiting in winter and in the northern region. When they remain in the stomach for a long time they produce belching and cause flatulence and vomiting. They cut the viscous phlegm and move it up to the opening of the stomach. Thus they are harmful to it and are of warm complexion to the third degree, dry to the second degree. From them the large fresh garden vari-

[419]Isidore of Seville, *Etymologies* 17. 10. 7.
[420]Galen, 6. 648; 11. 368.

ety should be chosen for the last course at dinner. It is useful for old men sometimes to eat radish for it softens the bowels. Hence Celsus[421] enumerates it among foods which move the bowels. It promotes the descent of food, makes the senses keen, provokes the urine, and breaks up and expels stones, especially as they say with its leaves.

PUNGENT ROOTS

Pungent roots fall into three classes:[422] leeks, onions, and scallions or bullum [shallot] named from the city of Judaea so-named and thought to be of the Philistines (Ascalon), from which Herodes Ascalonius derived his name,[423] and garlic. All are of bad juice. The nature of the leek *(porrum)* is said to be from *porrigendo.*[424] It is warm to the third degree, dry to the second or third degree. They write that it is good for bringing on sleep and its nourishment is more solid than that of lettuce, gourd, and asparagus, as Celsus writes.[425] It is praised as food for old men, and especially because it is of bad juice it creates head, tooth, and gum ache, disturbs the sleep, and dims the vision. It is eaten rarely and in small quantity, flavored with the lees of crushed olives *(amurca)* and oil at the first course. It stimulates the stomach, softens the bowels, brings sonority to the voice, purges the thorax and lungs, and heals hemorrhoids. Since however it is pungent and creates a puffing up of ulcerated kidneys and bladder it should be boiled twice before eating and taken out of those boiling waters into cold water. Thus its harm and its tendency to cause inflation are removed. The onion similarly is of a warm nature from the end of the third to the fourth degree and humid in the second degree, especially the white onion when it is old and juicy. When boiled in two changes of water and served with vinegar and milk Abulkasim allows it for old men of frigid nature in the winter in the northern region, especially when cooked. It is called *cepa*[426] because it does

[421]Celsus, *De Medicina* 2. 29.
[422]Galen, 6. 646.
[423]Pliny, *N. H.* 19. 101.
[424]Isidore of Seville, *Etymologies* 17. 10. 13.
[425]Celsus, *De Medicina* 2. 32.
[426]Pliny, *N. H.* 19. 102; Galen, 6. 646, 632, 794; 15. 365; 18 A. 14.

nothing else than to disturb the head *(caput)*. It opens the passages of the veins, provokes the urine, quiets acid eructation, excites the appetite, rarefies the surface of the body, stimulates perspiration, constricts the bowels, and stirs up sexual desire. Yet it is not without nourishment although the onions boiled in two waters are more recommended if served with very fat meat seasoned with spices. However, the onion induces disturbed dreams and is harmful to the intellect, causing vitiated humors in the stomach, and increased saliva. In many ways it is unsuitable for old age although it is of some value for a few people. They say it should be rejected from the resumptive diet. Theodorus Priscianus says that onions *(bulbos)* heat the body and dispose of phlegm through the stomach. They are of bad juice. Garlic is so called because it smells, as they say.[427] It has a small amount of acidity; when seasoned with vinegar and oil it may be given to the elderly, Abulkasim says, of cold complexion in the winter and in mountainous regions. It is warm and dry in the third to fourth degree. When cooked it may be used as medicine rather than food just like a theriac for those of frigid nature. It induces an ulcerative and burning heat, thins out thick, humid and especially cold humors and dispels them. It also drives away flatulence even if it is itself flatulent. It stirs the bowels as onions do and thereby worms are killed straightaway. It cleanses the throat but is harmful to the eyes and brings resonance to the voice. Its odor is prophylactic if suspended from the neck, as Theodorus Priscianus [x] writes. It is prophylactic and preservative, as Alexander says in writing about epilepsy.[428] Too much use of it is burdensome to the head. It brings relief to old people especially of warm nature and to the chest afflicted with a cough. It is very effective for poisonous bites, especially that of a mad dog. It cleanses polluted water. It is recommended that one abstain from continuous eating of these foods, which are rather viscid and pungent. They are judged ideal only for those who have collected in their bodies a phlegmatic or raw or viscous humor, as Galen says.[429]

[427]Isidore of Seville, *Etymologies* 17. 10. 14.
[428]Alexander of Tralles, 6th cent. A. D., who wrote on fever and worms; ed. T. Puschmann, Vienna, 1872–79.
[429]Galen, 6. 648, 652–54.

DOMESTIC AND WILD PARSNIPS AND CARROTS

Parsnips are so called because they are food *(pastus, pastinacha)* for old people,[430] especially those of frigid nature in winter and in whatever region. They are warm to the second and humid to the first degree. They clearly warm an old man and thin the body; they are somewhat aromatic. They provoke the urine and soften the bowels. The more preferred of these vegetables are reddish carrots, especially sweet and in winter, although their nourishment is less than that of turnips. They retard the digestion; they must be cooked a long time in order to avoid their ill effects. Wild parsnips provoke the urine, require much cooking, and are used more for medicine than as food. Lesser hemlock is very similar to parsnips in form; the common people call it *maiuscula.* It is quite dissimilar in powers since as a narcotic it must be rejected not only in the resumptive diet but in any other diet for healthy people.

ELECAMPANE OR INULA

Garden inula[431] root fresh and brittle is recommended for old men of a cold nature in winter and in a cold region. It assists the digestion, opens the stoppages of liver and spleen, gives strength to the mouth of the stomach especially when it is full of humors. It aids the descent of food through the intestines, drives away flatulence, banishes anger and sadness, cleanses the chest, heals ills of the lung and breathing difficulties such as asthma which are very familiar to old men in winter, as Theodorus [x] says. It draws out the superfluities of the veins through the urinary passage. They say that wine carefully combined with it is among the salutary remedies for the ills mentioned above as a very good additional remedy.[432] Inula root is listed as of warm and dry complexion to the second degree. Its immoderate use corrupts the blood and lessens the sperm although when seasoned with rob or mixed with other foods it is praised in the resumptive diet.

[430]Isidore, 17. 10. 6; Pliny, *N. H.* 19. 89; Galen, 6. 654.
[431]Pliny, *N. H.* 19. 91.
[432]Ibid., 20. 38.

WANDERING ENDIVE OR CHICORY

Wandering endive[433] is called chicory in Egypt. Its root and leaves are both edible and the wild species is recommended for liver troubles and for every kind of illness due to kidney stones. It removes the stoppage of these organs and creates a healthy color. It is ideal for the stomach although it is listed among bitter plants in the resumptive regimen of old men of warm and dry nature in summer and in warm regions especially when cooked. Although it has a cooling effect due to its frigid nature nonetheless it tends toward warmth. This is proved by its bitter taste and by the fact that it warms less than the artichoke. It is helpful to the liver, as Theodorus Priscianus [x] says, in its leaves, roots, shoots, and tender stalks when they grow to the emission of seeds. Its flowers are eaten in great quantity at Rome, which at once the nursling and the mother of all other lands became the fatherland of all races.

BUGLOSS *[ANCHUSA OFFICINALIS]* IN GREEK, THAT IS, OX TONGUE, CALLED ALSO BORAGE OR *EUPHROSYNUM,* THAT IS, OF GREAT JOY[434]

These vegetables are praised for use by old people no less in their flowers than in their leaves and sap; they are even better in their root. Bugloss has warming powers to the middle of the first degree and drying power to the end of the first degree. Borage is more humid than bugloss but not different otherwise except between garden-grown and wild borage, whose juice when purified and mixed with wine makes a potion which retards gray hairs and cleanses the face. It has been discovered that borage gives rise to much flatulence and frequent belching when very much of it is eaten. They write that bugloss is more suitable for old age since it brings gladness[435] to the heart and repairs the vital powers by a simultaneous effect of its special property and complexion, as Avicenna says. In every illness of the heart, in every manner of use, it separates the turbid and melancholic vapors from the vital spirit with a marvellous efficacy, as all the authors agree. Its root with unwashed cortex is more helpful than other parts of it, as Judeus

[433]Ibid., 19. 129; 21. 88.
[434]Pliny, *N. H.* 17. 112; 25. 81; 26. 116.
[435]Galen, 11. 852; Pliny, 17. 112; 25. 81; 26. 116.

[f. cxiii] sets forth, since by its peculiar quality it dilates the soul, as they say, destroys the melancholic humor, and removes the suffering which proceeds from it. Mixed with wine it promotes jollity at meals. Pliny's words[436] on it are these: Bugloss when mixed with wine increases the pleasures of the spirit.

BALM MELISSA

This type of vegetable is also included in the resumptive regimen, for although it warms and dries to the second degree it has a marvellous property of increasing the pleasures of the spirit and the liver. It purifies both spirit and the blood in the heart of the melancholic vapors, clears the stoppages of the brain, assists digestion, and replaces the melancholic frame of mind with happiness.

MINT

A moderate amount of garden mint, which they also call *sisymbrium,*[437] is allowed in the resumptive regimen for they say its property of warming and drying is of the second degree and with its odor and flavor it promotes appetite and digestion. It dispels the hiccups, checks vomiting which arises from cold humors, and is generally helpful to the stomach so that with its pleasant smell it is passed abroad at table in country banquets, as Pliny says.[438] It excites the sexual passion. When a great deal of it is given to be eaten it causes thickening of the humors with its excessive humidity. They say it should not be eaten by itself for the experts say it induces itching.

SALVIA WHICH THE BOTANISTS CALL *ELELISPHACOS* IN GREEK [SAGE]

Garden salvia[439] is accommodated to the resumptive regimen because it drives away old mens' flatulence, opens stoppages in

[436]Pliny, *N. H.* 25. 81.
[437]Galen, 12. 124; 19. 172, 176; Pliny, *N. H.* 20. 247; 25. 93.
[438]Ibid., 19. 160.
[439]Ibid., 22. 147; 24. 146; Avicenna, II, cap. 607, 621.

the inner organs arising especially from the phlegmatic humors and strengthens the brain, nerves, stomach, and intestines. It is warm and dry by nature to the second degree and with its astringency dries out the superfluity of humors in these organs. It should not be mixed with wine, we are warned, since wine when so mixed brings on drunkenness more swiftly, according to Avicenna.

ROSEMARY, MARJORAM OR SAMPSUCHI, RUE, CELERY, AND PARSLEY

These vegetables are eaten by old people more as medicine than as food. They are hot and dry to the end of the second degree up to the third. They warm, dry, remove, and thin out the phlegmatic humidity with which old age abounds. Rosemary, which the Latins call salutary from the effect of the herb and others call tree of Lebanon or libanotis, is redolent of the scent of olibanus[440] with which the ancients were used to placate the gods before they used incense, as they write, is a special remedy for colds issuing from the brain [head colds]. It sucks away flatulence, provokes urine, opens the stoppages of spleen, liver, and intestines. Mingled with foods at dinner it exhilarates human nature and protects against the harm of poisons. Marjoram also is of hot and dry nature to the third degree. It is sharp and strong, opens stoppages of the brain and liver. It has the power to thin the body and to cure the pains of flatulence and of the humidities of the brain. Rue grown in a garden near a fig tree is of a warm, dry nature to the second degree, dries to the third degree and although of bad, bitter juice is allowed older people by way of medicine. It has the power of cutting, dissolving, and banishing pain *(carminandi),* of purifying the veins, assisting digestion, increasing appetite and thus of strengthening the stomach. It is ideal for the spleen, relieves constriction of the chest, paralysis, and chilled nerves. It sharpens the vision. From rue, roses, fennel, verbena, and ceridonia, a water is made which makes the eyesight keen. Parsley, which is called as it were rock celery from *petra* and *selinum, -on,*[441] which is celery *(apium),* is hot and dry in nature to the second degree and is a diuretic. It

[440]Avicenna, II, 535.
[441]Isidore of Seville, *Etymologies* 17. 11. 2.

dispels flatulence and aids the digestion. Its leaves and especially the root are hard to digest when uncooked. Old people are allowed to eat parsley with lettuce if they are of cold nature in winter and in a frigid climate no less than garden celery. Both vegetables open stoppages, provoke urine, and constrict the stomach. Too much of them is harmful to the stomach because they attract sharp matter from elsewhere to the stomach, as Rufus[442] says, and because they bring on headache. They should be eaten with lettuce, as Abulkasim says. Parsley should not be eaten at the time when poisonous animals are stirring about for by opening passages it assists poisons to penetrate to the inner regions of the body.

BASIL

Basil[443] especially when steeped in citron oil no less than caryophyllum [clove] whose leaves are small although severely criticized by Chrysippus as unhelpful to stomach, urine, and clear vision as well as causing insanity (so he says) are allowed to old men of cold nature in the northern region according to their age in the way of medicine rather than food. Basil is warm in nature in the first degree, dry in the same or rather to the second degree. As a property of its leaves and seeds it brings happiness to the heart and is assisted in this function by a certain aromatic quality and an astringency associated with thinness, as Avicenna writes.[444] The very great use of basil as food is not recommended because it is enumerated among foods of bitter taste and those which stir the bowels to action and cause superfluities of the humor which give rise to turbid blood and a melancholic flatulence of the veins. It creates headache although the odor from eating it they say provides a remedy for stoppages of the brain and nostrils as well as for hemorrhoids and heart trouble.

THYME *[SERPILLUM]* SO-CALLED BECAUSE ITS ROOTS CREEP AFAR[445]

Thyme is ideal for use in a country dish made of rue, vinegar, oil, etc. *[moretum]* and for pickling as well as for the resumptive

[442]See note 240.
[443]Pliny, *N. H.* 13. 86; 19. 176; 23. 88; 26. 93; 20.17 (Chrysippus).
[444]Avicenna, II, 318.
[445]Pliny, *N. H.* 20. 185; Isidore of Seville, *Etymologies* 3. 3. 3; 17. 9. 51.

diet. Its nature is warm and dry to the second degree. It excites the appetite, provokes urine, and is very useful to stomach and brain with its warmth, astringency, and aromatic quality.

BLITUM OR BLITIS

Blitis, known also as beta and bleta,[446] is so called because of its marvellous flavor. This is understood of the garden, not the wild, variety and is recommended especially in winter in dry regions for old men of dry intestines. Although it is of warm, dry nature to the first degree that which is white in color which they call candid is rather more cool. Thus it is listed among cool foods. It has a capacity for soothing. It is astringent to the bowels by reason of its pungency *(baurachia).*[447] It thins and dissolves; its juice more than its substance is helpful to the stomach; hence it is listed among laxatives. Although of bad juice and less nourishing than other vegetables it is more firm than lettuce, gourd, or asparagus, as Celsus writes.[448] It should be eaten without much cooking in order to relax the bowels. When cooked thoroughly it is astringent to the bowels. Blitum burns the blood, they say, and should be eaten with vinegar and mustard, according to Abulkasim; so that it does not bring lassitude to the stomach or a feeling of sharp biting it should be eaten with sweet spices and almond milk.

ANETHUM OR DILL

Sweet green dill is ideal because its juice is good for the stomach although its substance is of bad juice. It has an adverse effect upon the kidneys. It relieves flatulence and is listed among laxatives. It quickens the cold humors by warming them, purges the bowels of inner defects, and soothes their acute colicky pains. It brings on sleep, restrains hiccups due to overeating. Too frequent use of it brings on dimness of vision, nausea, and vomiting, especially because of its seeds. Therefore if it is eaten with small lemons by old people of cold nature in winter in a cold region it is

[446]Isidore of Seville, *Etymologies* 17. 10. 15.
[447]Avicenna, II, 88.
[448]Celsus, *De Medicina* 2. 21. 22. Arabic *baurachia* = borax.

useful. Its nature is warm and dry to the second degree; others place its warmth at the end of the second degree but its dryness at the end of the first degree.

FENNEL, ANISE, ASAFOETIDA, ARTICHOKE

Fennel is used in the regimen of health, no less its seeds than its root and leaves, especially the sweet garden variety, which is praised in the resumptive regimen. It is classified as of warm and dry nature to the second degree although it is more warm than dry. It is of bad juice like dill, as Celsus says,[449] but it soothes flatulence, opens stoppages, sharpens the vision by clearing away mist from the eyes, especially through its seeds. Pliny[450] writes that by tasting fennel serpents have been known to shed their old age and to sharpen their eyesight with its juice. Hence it is understood that the dimness of human eyes especially can be relieved by its use. It relieves a stomach suffering from nausea, provokes urine, and breaks up kidney stone. There is also a kind of wild fennel which they call *hippomarathum* or *myrsineum* which is more powerful in every way than garden fennel. Anise is endowed with these same properties in strength and sharpness. Its nature is hot to the first degree, dry to the third. Fennel makes the breath more pleasant; in fact, when mixed with wine it makes the face look younger. It is regarded in particular as inhibiting hiccups. If drunk, it can bring on sleep, delay the formation of stones, cure flatulence, colic pains, and diseases of the digestive organs, stop vomiting and tumors of the diaphragm, and heal troubles of the chest. It is most useful for the nerves and promises aid for travel fatigue, Pliny[451] declares. Asafoetida is also eaten; many write that its stalks when cooked are excellent for the stomach although others say that it causes headache. They say it is good for colic pains. Garden thistles are frequently eaten; they are commonly called artichokes. Their leaves with a spiny point when cooked strengthen the stomach, give a good odor to the mouth, and break up stones, says Avicenna. If we are to believe it, the artichoke contributes some-

[449]Celsus, *De Medicina* 2. 21.
[450]Pliny, *N. H.* 8. 98; 19. 173; 20. 254.
[451]Ibid., 20. 255.

thing to the female vulva which causes it to produce male offspring, as Chaereas the Athenian and Glaucias write; the latter was a most diligent student of artichokes.[452] Artichokes heat one up and provoke urine, Theodorus Priscianus [x] writes.

COLE WORT *(ERUCA SATIVA)*, ROCKET

Eruca,[453] or *uruca,* is so called because it has the power of sexual ignition. It is by no means acceptable in the resumptive regimen, whether garden-grown or wild, and is used rather as medicine than as food. Its nature is considered warm to the second degree, dry to the first. It is aperitive and lenitive; it is very helpful to the digestion. It should not be eaten alone beause it is of bad, acrid juice. It brings on headache. Lettuce, however, endive, and purslain remove this ill. Eruca is so smooth in its use as a condiment that the Greeks call it *euzomon* ("making good broth"). Nasturtium is quite similar to eruca in its properties.[454]

SINAPIS[455] [MUSTARD] SO-CALLED THEY SAY BECAUSE ITS LEAVES RESEMBLE NAPUS OR NAPY [WHITE MUSTARD]

Abulkasim says that mustard seed is ideal for old people of cold and humid nature in mountainous regions especially in winter, for although it is of bad, bitter juice nevertheless its nature is warm and dry to the fourth degree. It cuts and thins out phlegm, purifies the brain from humidities, and opens stoppages of the colatorium [between the basilar bone and the dura mater in the brain] so that nothing more can penetrate into the nostrils and brain; this is asserted positively. When eaten during a fast, they say, it sharpens the intelligence and when mixed with old honey it removes the hoarseness of the throat or cane of the lung. It thins the spleen and is very useful against all stomach troubles. It facilitates the excretions of the lungs. Taken with food it is given to those who suffer from asthma or shortness of breath. It softens the stool and provokes urine. Since it creates bad humors when used as food it is

452 Ibid., 20. 263; cf. 261.
453 Isidore of Seville, *Etymologies* 17. 10. 21; Pliny, *N. H.* 19. 71, 123; 20. 19.
454 Theophrastus, *H. P.* 1. 6. 6.
455 Pliny, *N. H.* 19. 171; 27. 140.

used rather as medicine than as food and hence very little in the resumptive diet. As with all vegetables that have some acrimony in them rob or defrutum [a juice thickened by evaporation to the consistency of honey] very handily breaks down the acrimony of mustard.

PEPPERGRASS, PEPPERWORT, OR CRESS *(LEPIDIUM SATIVUM)*, CARDAMINE, NASTURTIUM

The Arabs call this herb the pupil of the eye, others call it *eruca* of the water, or celery of the water. It is hot and dry by nature; hence it heats and dissolves, stirs the urine, and breaks up stones in kidneys and bladder. It is not to be rejected in the resumptive regimen. It should be eaten boiled or raw, Avicenna advises. It is a remedy for ulcers of the intestines.

LETTUCE

They write[456] that broad-leaf garden lettuce without milk is proper food for the young because it is cold and humid to the second degree. It cools off the human being without harm. It is listed among vegetables which provide little blood and bad chyme. Galen[457] says lettuce furnishes much blood but no chyme, good or bad. Thus they say that lettuce *(lactuca)* is so called because it gives much milk *(lac)* to women or because it abounds in milk.[458] It is not rejected in the resumptive regimen although it is listed among acrid foods just as is the greatest share of vegetables. It is however ideal for the stomach and brings on sleep. It is also used for cooling off the upper abdomen in young people when they are choleric. It is excellent when boiled for combatting insomnia in old age. The frigidity of lettuce has been likened to that of a lake or pool for the frigidity of a pool is less than that of river water both because the sun's heat penetrates to the depths of a pool as well as because of its closeness to land and its mixture with mud. Rightly therefore Averroes [5. 85v] declares that the coolness of lettuce is similar to that of brooks. It is preferred for the creation of good blood both in

[456]Galen, 1. 677.
[457]Ibid., 6. 624–81, 794.
[458]Isidore of Seville, *Etymologies* 17. 10. 11.

quantity and quality to all other vegetables. Since its nature is chilly the Greeks call it eumechion because it is especially resistant to love-making. In the summer it pleasantly relieves nausea, stimulates appetite, neither relaxes nor constricts the bowels but provokes urine, as the Israelite writes [f. cxxv]. Celsus,[459] however, lists it among the laxatives. Pliny[460] relates that the divine Augustus was preserved in his illness by lettuce prescribed through the prudence of the physician Antonius Musa. It is best eaten unwashed. Celsus[461] bids us select that lettuce whose stalk is full of milk for eating with *eruca,* the aphrodisiac with a tempering and cooling agent of diverse nature, since lettuce is too cool and needs to be mixed with a counterbalance of heat. Some people say that frequent lettuce in one's food brings clarity to the vision.

SPINACH

For old people of especially hot and dry nature in the spring or summer in warm regions spinach is useful since it is close to temperate and suitable for the throat, lungs, stomach, and liver. It relaxes the bowels by humidifying them. It provides better nourishment if served with spices and fried in brine; thus its ill effects are removed, for it is hard to digest.

ASPARAGUS

Asparagus[462] is so called because it grows in rough thickets. The appellation applies to the entire tender stalk when it has matured to full fruit or to the emission of seed. The Greek experts took the word *sparago* to be not from *sparto* or *sparo,* which is broom. Old men especially of cold and dry nature in regions in which the garden or fresh variety is found may eat it, especially the tips bending to the earth, boiled and seasoned with salt, vinegar, and oil. The nature of asparagus is dry with a balance between hot and cold although not far from hot, as Avicenna writes.[463] How-

[459]Celsus, *De Medicina* 2. 29.
[460]Pliny, *N. H.* 19. 28; 29. 6. See also *Tacuinum Sanitatis* XVIII on lettuce.
[461]Celsus, *De Medicina* 2. 29; Pliny, *N. H.* 19. 28.
[462]Isidore, 17. 10. 19; Pliny, 19. 145–51.
[463]Avicenna, II, 611.

ever, Isaac Israeli [f. cxxviii] classed it as hot and humid in the first degree although he states that the garden variety is more temperate. Wild asparagus is called by some *corruda,* by others *libycum.*[464] The Attic Greeks write that the wild variety is more effective than the domestic and hotter or whiter and hence of greater strength. Asparagus opens up stoppages in all the viscera, especially of the liver and kidneys, and is capable of dissolving, particularly the wild variety which is more powerful than all vegetables, while the domestic is more nourishing. Asparagus growing among rocks (which they call saxatile) they declare is cleansing and regulates the bowels without excessive heating or cooling. Therefore it is listed among laxatives. It provides a seething urine very usefully although it ulcerates the bladder itself. It stimulates sexual desire, soothes pains in the lower back and kidneys and although useful for the stomach it is considered noxious and listed among acrid substances of bad juice. It should be eaten boiled in brine. Theodorus Priscianus [x] writes that asparagus assists the bowels and urine as nettles do, but with its excessive heat it dissolves phlegm. Hence nettles are listed among laxatives.

HOPS

For old men of hot dry nature and with thin blood and inflammable spirits hops are ideal, they say, in all seasons where it is found. It is of temperate quality tending toward cooling and extinguishing all inflammations. It soothes the bowels, drawing something from the yellow bile, Mesue [f. 31] says, purifying it from the blood and clarifying it, thus cooling its inflammation. They write that it is most useful to the overheated stomach and liver. Its condiments should be carefully observed for Galen in the third book of *De Locis Affectis*[465] says that hops prepared with vinegar and salt produce melancholy blood, which is quite true if too much of them is eaten.

[464]Pliny, 16. 173; 20. 110. See also *Tacuinum Sanitatis* XXXVIII.
[465]Galen, 8. 183–84.

CAPERS

The nature of capers is so called in Greek[466] because in its round stem it has little heads of its seeds, as they say. It is hot and dry to the second degree, with extension. It can be easily recognized by its bitterness, acidity, and sharpness of taste. Its use in the resumptive regimen is acceptable for its not inconsiderable qualities as a medicine rather than food. It furnishes very little nourishment just as do other vegetables of thin parts.[467] When fresh and before it is salted it is judged to be stronger in quality. Salting causes it to lose its food value. We use capers for dissolving, opening, and cleansing passages. Overseas capers are not eaten for the Arabic variety is considered to be pestilential, the African harmful to the gums, the Marmaric to the vulva, and the Apulian causes vomiting, as Pliny[468] writes. The Italian variety is less harmful. The Alexandrian is much praised, second to that of our own time. Those who eat capers daily are not threatened with paralysis nor splenetic ills. The stomach and bowels when loaded with phlegm are purged by capers, and congestion of the chest is relieved by it, as many authors agree. Salted capers brings on appetite before meals, exciting it if it is lost, deadened, or dejected in any way. It thins out black bile and is a laxative. It is regarded as excellent for the spleen, for by evacuating the thick humors through the urine it purges the spleen just as the liver is purged with wormwood; obstructions and hardnesses of the liver are banished by capers prepared with vinegar. It is not recommended as food for although it dissolves melancholy by its peculiar virtue by means of its substance nonetheless it provides melancholic nourishment and is convertible to bile and black blood. They write that its frequent use is damaging to the nerves; authors agree that it is useless for the stomach. Old men may eat it even in time of pestilence when it is placed in boiling water, then seasoned with oil and vinegar as well as coriander. They say that capers is very effective against the harm created by the temperature.

[466]Isidore of Seville, *Etymologies* 17. 10. 20.
[467]Galen, 6. 615–66.
[468]Pliny, *N. H.* 13. 127; 19. 163; 20. 165.

OLIVES

Although their substance is of the weakest just as with capers, as Celsus[469] says, olives are difficult to digest, provide little nourishment, and produce thick astringent humors. Served with salt and lemon juice they stir the appetite and make the breath more pleasant as well as strengthening the stomach. For old men of frigid nature in winter in cold regions it is acceptable at the second course although when eaten at the last course the ascending vapors it produces compress the head. The olive which is in the middle of its completion or maturity is to be selected. Overseas olives are preferred to the Italian olives, and in Italy itself the olives of Picenum are preferable, according to Pliny.[470] No less praised, however, in our time is the olive which Bologna, mother of studies, produces nor does Tibur lack good olives for although in comparison to others they are small nonetheless in flavor, sweetness, and smooth quality they excel others. The white olive is more useful for the stomach but less so to the bowels. Pliny reports that it has an excellent use before it is pickled;[471] it is eaten fresh by itself. It cures sandy urine and worn or pulled teeth from aching. The black olive they call hyacinthine is less useful for the stomach, head, and eyes but easy for the bowels, writes Galen[472] in the sixth book of his *Sanative Method (De Sanitate Tuenda).* The olive from Spain is useful for softening the bowels and is therefore especially praised in the regimen of old age.

[469]Celsus, *De Medicina* 2. 21.
[470]Pliny, *N. H.* 15. 16.
[471]Ibid., 15. 18, 21; 23. 73; Cato, *R. R.* 117.
[472]Galen, 6. 608–609; 11. 648, 869, 871.

Chapter XXXIV

Legumes and First Chickpeas

The experts properly call legumes those grains which are eaten but are not used in bread baking. They are so called because they are picked up *(leguntur),* as Pliny says.[473] They are pulled from the earth, not cut away. Almost all except wheat from which bread is made or not are of bad juice, alien to the stomach, especially all those which produce flatulence, for almost all of them do so and produce harm very quickly, with the exception of bread, they say, and *candarusium,* that is, broth made of wheat. To these two they add chickpeas for the regimen of old age with a few others. These may be eaten by old men of a particularly frigid and dry nature in autumn and in the northern region, as Abulkasim says. The white chickpea is hot and humid to the first degree. Others say it is dry. The red variety is hotter and stronger than the white, much more nourishing and more capable of opening the bowels. It makes the voice more resonant and is of more food value to the lung and any other part. Rufus[474] says the chickpea operates on the flesh as yeast works in dough and vinegar on earth. The thicker non-corrosive variety should be chosen. The black chickpea breaks up stone, the white is astringent and purges the kidneys, liver, and spleen. In each two substances are found, salty, which controls the bowels, and sweet, which provokes the urine. Because they also induce abscess of the kidneys and bladder they urge that chickpeas be eaten with poppy seeds. Since they produce flatulence at the second course of a meal they should be eaten between two courses. Old people are urged by no means to eat fresh green chickpeas for almost like the fresh bean they produce thick phlegmatic humors

[473]Ibid., 18. 60, 165; Isidore of Seville, *Etymologies* 17. 4; Varro, *R. R.* 1. 23. 3; Celsus, *De Medicina* 2. 25. 26.
[474]See note 240.

from which sometimes arise dysentery, colic pains, and a fetid breath.

RICE

Rice is warm and dry to the second degree. It is of good food value in the regimen not only of old age but also of whatever age in every region especially in winter. It furnishes a uniform nourishment if it is properly prepared and is more acceptable when thoroughly cooked so that its grains swell. It is ideal for stomach and intestinal gripes, they say, and is listed among substances very suitable for the stomach, says Theodorus Priscianus [*Eup.* 200]. When rice is washed a little of its juice can constrict the bowels and repair and nourish strength. However, it is harmful to those who suffer from colic because it tightens the intestines and thus removes their ill if it is seasoned with milk or almond oil or sesame. Although with fresh milk it brings on obstructions its dryness is removed and it promotes fattening. They say that rice adds to the sperm and diminishes the bad odors of perspiration and urine.[475]

KIDNEY BEANS

Abulkasim says that kidney beans ought not to be absent from the diet of old men of particularly cold and dry nature in winter and in frigid regions. They promote fattening and provoke urine, especially the red bean, which is not corrosive or hotter than others of dry substance. Avicenna[476] writes that they are helpful to chest and lungs. They provide a thick humid sustenance with phlegm. They induce vomiting and troubled dreams. Therefore they should be eaten with oil, brine, and mustard; others say with vinegar, honey, pepper, oregano, and a drink of pure raisin wine to counteract their ill effects.

LUPINE

Abulkasim suggests that old people should eat heavy white lupine, especially those old people of phlegmatic nature in winter

[475]Galen, 6. 525; 12. 92.
[476]Avicenna, II, 253. See Chap. XXXIV for *candarusio,* broth made of wheat (see under *spelt*).

and in the northern region. It is warm and dry to the second degree; it is nourishing and digestible. It loosens the bowels, as Theodorus [x] writes, functioning rather as medicine than as food. When well seasoned it provides good nourishment. Not all of its bitterness should be removed by infusion or dilution since thus its penetration is more rapid. They say it should be eaten with vinegar so as to remove obstructions of the liver and spleen and when properly cooked with rue, honey, and pepper. If by means of infusion its bitterness is removed it is called nutritive medicine. Lupine when washed and salted provides a special means called *corre bezare* of improving the eyesight, Judeus declares [f. cxii].

SPELT

The nourishment provided by spelt is midway between that of wheat and barley. Its nature is similar to *candarusium* as it is called among many writers. It is not entirely rejected in the resumptive regimen. Its nourishment is viscous and is said to bring on obstructions. When eaten with sugar which provides both aperience and astringency its harmful effects are removed.

SESAME

This seed produces more flatulence than other seeds. If it is not rough and is somewhat heated and stripped of its skin it does not constrict the bowels very much but inflates them and produces fat for the body, Theodorus [iiii] says. It is warm to one-half of the first degree, humid to the full degree. Avicenna[477] writes that it relieves constriction of the breath, asthma, and of the colon intestine. It is harmful to the stomach, brings on nausea, and quickly reduces appetite. Thus it should be eaten with honey so as to remove its ill effects and to retard its digestion. It softens the viscera and with its virtues is believed to be by no means adverse to old age.

[477]Avicenna, II, 650.

Chapter XXXV

Condiments for Table Use and Preserves As Well As Relishes and More Truly Relishes Eaten With Bread

There is a great deal of use and pleasure for an old man in both the vegetables and legumes thus far described which provide him with food from which preserves are made suitable for the resumptive regimen. Not only vegetables and grains but also meats, oil, butter, honey, and fish cooked together and every kind of relish have a remarkably subtle effect on his taste, together with any new recipe discovered for use in the resumptive regimen and garnished with an unsurpassed elegance, should be indulged in by old age as long as it brings pleasure and assistance. In general at the beginning are those condiments and preserves made from soft substances such as broth, gruel, cakes, starch, tisane (a decoction of barley), and the like.

WHITE RELISH MADE FROM MEAT

This is called contusion (from *contundere,* to pound up) because it is made from the solid flesh especially of birds and fowl such as chickens, castrated roosters, pheasants, and partridges which has been decocted or boiled down to which almond milk, sweet and fresh, has been added as exceedingly appropriate. The solid flesh should be cut transversely into little pieces and then pounded to a pulp so that it will serve best in the regimen of old age. A modest amount will nourish a great deal, and thus it is used for the best recovery of convalescents, which involves the same art used in caring for the aged. This juice is temperate with a tendency toward warm and humid. It is well known that the nature of those who use this relish is in harmony with it, that is, of the flesh from which the decoction is made, especially of the pullets and birds already mentioned whose nature it is to make all humors equal. Indeed, the juice of pullets rather than hens is used therein as more nourishing, as Judeus [f. cxxxv] says, and more adapted to fattening the body. Almond milk, which they call *sauich* or juice of the almonds, is heavy and with its sweetness stirs the bile, as Avicenna says,[478] in an adult warm in age and nature. In old men this is not the case. Their frigid nature in relation to that of youth requires a lighter almond juice for a better nourishment; although modest in amount they say its equable nature tends toward little humidity.

BAKED BREAD

Some nutritious liquid should be baked with or poured into bread intended for old people, especially decoction or purée of meat from preferred animals. In this way old people of especially cold and dry nature in autumn in the northern region should be nourished. If this condiment should be used in bread which is thoroughly permeated with yeast the quality of the yeast will be removed along with its dryness and viscosity. It will give good, humid, strong blood and fat to the thin or slender or skinny bodies. It is agreed among authors that it will nourish and quickly descend from the stomach, constrain the bowels, and heal coughing and hoarseness of the throat. Spices should be scattered on the bread; I shall describe these shortly. This is the bread which Averroes [5.80v] describes. In addition to bread a good food is *panata* [a recipe of bread, water, milk, and sugar boiled into a pap] which is of the first degree in agreeableness. It is among the chief types of bread which are listed as very good for the weakest constitutions. The grains from which they are made are farina [spelt], rice, pearl barley, and gruels made from them[479] or moistened bread. This kind of potion made from wheat is stronger although water makes it very weak.

A LIST OF DIFFERENT CONDIMENTS, PRESERVES, SEASONINGS, OR SPICES

There are in addition to preserves made with meat many praiseworthy foods of the same kind such as Abulkasim lists made

[478]Avicenna, II, 58.

[479]Celsus, *De Medicina* 2. 28, 29, 30. Zerbi, *Libellus* etc. f. 62, also describes the concoction of chickpeas below in detail. See also Avicenna, II, 132.

from fried meat prepared with vinegar, salt, spices, and warm seeds which are helpful to the digestion of old people of cold and humid nature in winter and spring. Such a condiment stirs the appetite, checks belching, thins out the humors, and cuts phlegm. A preserve made of meat and eggs and one made of meat, rice, milk, sugar, and chicken fat with spices is beneficial. It provides a temperate nourishment suitable for every age, especially for those who have a similar temperate nature in winter and in a temperate climate. Condiments sharpen the intellect and induce pleasant dreams, according to Abulkasim. Rice and millet prepared with milk, especially pure goat milk, has a similar benefit. Condiments provide a very helpful nourishment for every temperate nature and age, especially in spring and in temperate regions for although rice and millet are dry milk counteracts their dryness so that from them there results a mixture which, eaten with sugar, is readily digested and prevents obstructions. There is also a recipe (as Abulkasim writes) of meat with vinegar cooked in a pot whose opening is covered with clay or dough which he affirms is useful for old age in summer and in warm regions for it aids a phlegmatic stomach. A decoction of chickpeas is good for old age of a cold nature in spring in the northern region for it opens and cleanses the veins, capillaries, and passages of the liver and urine, preserving the person from sand and stones with which morbid old age is frequently afflicted. The recipe follows: Soak a pound of chickpeas in twenty pounds of sweet river water overnight to soften them. Boil them in the water in which they were placed for the following day with a slow and gentle heat. Then drain them, cool them off from their long boiling, and serve them with a bit of salt and spices. This dish has great medicinal value for old age. With the humidity of the chickpeas the nitre or salt (*baurachia,* borax) is expended by the low heat in the shells of the peas and is left behind in the boiling water. The water is thus rendered astringent, useful as a lotion, capable of opening obstructions of the epigastric region and the alimentary passages as well as of the urine. It can break up stone and cleanse the inner organs, as Johannes Nazarenus says. Since it does not quench thirst this defect must be corrected with poppy seeds. If that water mentioned above receives a final boiling so that it acquires a consistency between thin and thick, it provides a good food against phlegmatic ills, but it should be taken after it is strained. From chickpeas which have had their natron removed they make a juice which stimulates sexual desire. It also increases fat and creates a vivid color in the flesh. Another recipe requires animal flesh cut up into little pieces and boiled thoroughly so as to produce a good chyme. It increases fat and provides a temperate blood. In a marvellous manner it removes supervacuities resulting from exercise and frequent sexual activity or from other incidental causes and relieves languor and fear, for the greater part of the meat in this concoction prepared in this way is easily changed into blood by its unchanging quality and restores the body. This preparation is therefore recommended for old men of temperate nature in temperate regions and especially in the spring. A preserve made of meat which has been first fried and then seasoned with acid and sweet substances which have been partially fried is recommended also for old men of frigid nature in winter and in the northern region. It ameliorates a humid stomach and strengthens the faculty of memory. Thus it is ideal for those who happen to lose their memory. A food partly fried and roasted is very nourishing, satisfying an old man's hunger, converting humor into blood readily and restoring the vital power. Another dish made with cooked meat mixed with eggs the Arabs call *ziburbegi;* it has the same benefits. *Cocetum*[480] also sometimes restores the ability to go to sleep for it is a kind of food made from honey and poppies. There are also foods made with eggs and butter both boiled and fried in a skittle, especially from the yolks of eggs without the albumen, with white butter, spices, and sugar. It has a good nourishment, warm and humid. Nor should any foods flavored with sweet and sour be overlooked in this account of concoctions and decoctions for the old folks. There are other excellent dainties such as *mirtata* and *salviata.* Some are well known to the common people, such as *rapata* and *alleata. Intrita* is of this kind of food, that is, food made of garlic triturated in a mortar. And among the Romans of our time *caulata* is famous. Old people are urged to eat some of all these foods. As advantageous to the bowels of the elderly one must not overlook a food made of vegetables with oil or butter or whatever oily substance and salt, which old people eat as the first course of a meal. Ideal for this purpose are blitis, anethum or dill, parsley, mallow, chenopodium *(mercurialis),* and similar herbs.

[480]Paul. ex Fest. 39. 8 Müller; Tertullian, *Adv. Valentinianos* 12.

SALAD *(MORETUM)* WHOSE FLAVOR FOR PICKLING IS RECOMMENDED TO OLD PEOPLE

An inventive taste has discovered the process of dipping or immersing for pickling bread to excite an appetite or for the sake of pleasure. For we will show that pleasure can be mingled with the necessary nourishment, a practice also followed by healthy people. Celsus[481] rejected it as useless, along with all condiments both because more food is eaten on account of its sweetness and because part of it is badly digested. But in the resumptive regimen of old people whose appetite is almost dead it is quite useful and a matter not unknown, i.e., to sweeten or otherwise season food to make it more palatable. There are various dishes which are not to be rejected in the resumptive regimen which should vary according to the seasons of the year and the nature of old people materially and formally as well as according to the geographical regions involved and other differing factors, such as those made with beans and prepared with a thorough boiling down into a must. This food is stronger the more raw it is, mixed with honey, sugar, or wine and similar sweetenings or those which are mixed with the juice of unripe grapes, pomegranates, lemons, tartar, sour herbs, unripe cherries of the sour astringent sort, or vinegar itself and such like liquids of a sour, acidulous taste. One may add such astringents as *myrtatum,*[482] for it is a much-prized flavor pickled with myrtle, as Pliny says. These spices are also used with almonds, baked bread, pine nuts, garlic, or some pungency and herbs such as thyme, mint, basil, pennyroyal, oregano, salvia, sansuchi or mastic, and similar herbs separately or in combination bring pleasure to the food and are praised in the resumptive diet as are many delicacies.

[481]Celsus, *De Medicina* 2. 25.
[482]Pliny, *N. H.* 15. 118. See *myrtata,* above.

Chapter XXXVI

A Description of Aromatic Spices Useful for Old People

The experts write that the strength and innate heat of old age can be restored by the use of spices and that they can greatly increase the serous humidities which are consumed by old age as well as counteracting some accidental ills that accompany that stage of life. As Avicenna says ginger and spices are among foods which assist old people. In their use, however, one must observe their quality insofar as they heat and promote digestion but not those which dry the body for according to fixed measures old age ought to be fed on foods which humidify. Old people should not use spices except for the power of warming the body and promoting digestion. Although there are many spices which are suitable for the regimen of old age the following recipe is particularly recommended. Take some good cinnamon, that is, of good odor as an indication of its high quality, and of unmixed color, a part made up of three portions of ginger, galanga, and pepper to the total of six-eighths of a handful; an eighth finger each of cloves and nutmeg, one finger of very white sugar. Grind these up separately, then mix them, and use as condiments. In their use one must consider the nature of the old man, the region, the exercise taken, the season of the year, and other factors as to the amount of such a mixture ideal for him and the nature of each ingredient, which is easy to recognize.

CINNAMON

Cinnamon is hot from the second degree to the third. Its dryness is said to bring pleasure. Its aroma is stimulating and it combines strength with fine texture, Avicenna writes.[483] It serves the

[483]Avicenna, II, 128.

same useful function as theriac; it has strength to attract and open, to combat putrescence and to rectify corruption which has already set in. It is very helpful in the case of a cold and in dimness of vision. It loosens chest-congestion, purges superfluities, clears up a cough, opens obstructions of the liver, brings aid to the stomach by drying up the humor congested in it as it flows in from elsewhere, and in every way strengthens the stomach, aids the digestion in the liver, and inhibits kidney pains. Averroes [6.94v] writes that cinnamon is one of the medicines in which are found aroma, astringency, and a sharp quality (all of which distinguish this spice). It strengthens all the members nor is it similar to any other spice; it also has the ability to resist putrefaction and corruption especially affecting the stomach. Galen[484] in his book of *Experiments* says cinnamon is very useful against cold and heaviness in the stomach as well as purging its humors with a remarkable property which may be described in the versifier's line:

> No man who eats cinnamon frequently will die.

They say that with its special quality it is an antidote like theriac against poisons.

GINGER

They rate ginger at the end of the third degree in warmth. It improves the memory, wipes away humors in parts of the head and throat, improves the vision, and lends aid to the digestion: authors agree on these points, Avicenna[485] says ginger dries up the humors which occur in the stomach due to eating fruit such as melons. It warms the stomach, opens obstructions of the liver and constrains the bowels, Isaac [f. cxxix] affirms. In every way it aids the digestion in old age and cures snake bites.

GALANGA

Galanga is warm and dry in nature from the second to the third degree. It makes one thin and dissolves flatulence. It makes

[484]Galen, 12. 26, 56, 63, 64; 14. 257.
[485]Avicenna, II, 748.

the breath more pleasant. It is ideal in the regimen of old age for natures especially cold and humid in winter and in a cold region. It assists the digestion in a marvellous way. The thicker root should be chosen.

PEPPER

This spice is warm and dry in its three kinds to the third degree. It excites the appetite, removes heavy flatulence by dissolving it, drives away humors collected in the stomach and the parts adjacent to it and sends them downwards, Judeus [f. cxxx] reports. Hence it is of use to old age especially because its moderate use provides relief to chilled nerves, persistent cough and colic pains, stimulates the urine, and is considered useful to all who have a cold nature.

CROCUS, SO CALLED FROM CORYCUS, A TOWN IN CILICIA

The nature of crocus[486] is warm in the second degree but dry in the first degree, as they write. It is listed among items of food which strengthen the heart and vital spirit. It cheers, illumines, dilates, and hardens their substance, as Avicenna says.[487] It is assisted in all these functions by its aroma, astringency, and dissolution which dominate in it and which facilitate digestion. It is useful to the stomach, as Serapio the son [f. clxxvr] says, fortifies the liver, stimulates urine, arouses sexual desire, creates a good color in the face and destroys the acidity of the stomach, thus promoting appetite. It fills the brain so that when mixed with wine it clouds the vision and the senses. It is ideal for the resumptive regimen. It should be used in small quantity with other spices; too great use of it exhilarates to the point of insanity. Its frequent use dilates the spirit and sets it in motion to the point where it may prove fatal. Avicenna does not assign a dosage for this contingency but Johannes Serapio assigns three drams.

[486]Galen, 13. 269; 14. 68; Pliny, *N. H.* 21. 31.
[487]Avicenna, II, 130.

CLOVE

Its nature is warm and dry to the third degree. It gives the body a more pleasant odor, clears the vision, and counteracts vomiting and nausea.

NUTMEG

This spice is also dry and warm to the second degree, according to Musa.[488] It makes the breath sweeter, improves the vision, and is ideal for the mouth of the stomach, the liver, and spleen. It checks vomiting and arouses the appetite.

[488]See note 460.

Chapter XXXVII

Fruits

Since we eat fruits for the sake of the great pleasure they provide they are so called from the upper part of the gullet with which we enjoy food.[489] Therefore we shall discuss below the nature of those fruits which are in common use by humans so that the ones which are good in the resumptive regimen may be selected, beginning with fruits in season.

FRUITS IN SEASON AND ESPECIALLY MELONS AND GOURD

Galen[490] says the Greeks call fruits seasonal not only because they are found in that season which the Greeks call the dog days in which the Dog Star rises, which are the forty days by common computation from the tenth day of July to the twentieth day of August, but because seasonal fruits are those which by their nature cannot be preserved for a longer time and are thus distinguished from other fruits which are ideal for laying aside or preserving. Seasonal fruits are such as melon, watermelon, and gourd *(battheca)*. All of these are humid by the common consensus of physicians and are easily converted into that humor which they find abundant in the stomach. By their nature they change easily to phlegm although by reason of their bubbling up they change into bile as many insist. When they are not digested in the stomach they are harmful, causing vomiting, flux of the bowels, colic, flatulence, belching, and rejection of food, especially when mixed with other foods. They are entirely subject to putrescence[491] and most weak in the material of food. They easily leave the body

[489]Isidore of Seville, *Etymologies* 17. 6. 23.
[490]Galen, 6. 558–70; Avicenna, II, 93.
[491]Celsus, *De Medicina* 2. 18. 3; Galen, 6. 559.

through the bowels, especially those fruits which have some soda and a drying property, such as the melon, which provokes the urine. Since they are of bad chyme they are not all recommended for the resumptive regimen. Abulkasim allows the sweet melon to old men of phlegmatic nature in autumn and in a temperate region, especially to those fatigued by journeys or heated by some other cause for it has a putrefying, that is, refrigerating effect because its nature is frigid and humid to the second degree, with frigidity dominating over humidity. Hence it soothes lassitude, inflammation, and heat. Avicenna[492] says it is not good to drink wine after eating melon nor after eating humid fruits in general, but a later age has rejected his advice and indulges readily in unmixed wine with melon. For either wine after eating melon in order to temper its frigidity is suitable or if it is not suitable the melon is listed as of warm nature, as Abulkasim writes of a certain species of melon which is very sweet, ripe, swiftly penetrating the veins, and bringing on burning fevers in regions not known to Galen. After eating it an acid syrup or a mixture of sugar and vinegar is salutary. It is advised that melon should be eaten on an empty stomach which has been purged of vitiated humors and some time should elapse before taking other nourishment. After eating melon it is pleasant to take a walk. If it is eaten with seeds and pulp it will be more astringent and more powerful an aid to kidney sand and bladder trouble. The excessive eating of melon is condemned for Rhazes writes that it brings on colic and is admitted to be dangerous to the nerves with its humidity. Avicenna says[493] the Roman melon or gourd is not used medicinally; it neither cools nor warms and is eaten solely for pleasure. Chrysippus[494] the physician condemned it as a food. It is, however, agreed among the authors that when thoroughly cooked and seasoned it is very helpful for an overheated stomach. Celsus[495] says the cooked gourd is ideal for the stomach and cools it; he lists it among foods which are laxative. It should sometimes form part of the resumptive diet, seasoned with spices.

[492]Avicenna, II, 179.
[493]Ibid.
[494]Pliny, *N. H.* 20. 17. See also *Tacuinum Sanitatis* CXCI. On the gourd as food see J. L. Heller, "Notes on the Meaning of Κολοκύντη"; *Illinois Classical Studies* X. 1 (1985): 88–89.
[495]Celsus, *De Medicina* 2. 24.

NON-SEASONAL FRUITS: FIRST, THE FIG

The fruits discussed earlier are of humid chyme. Those which are not seasonal are of a dry and solid nature and provide an earthy nourishment. Those among them which have a humid nature are easily expelled from the body as thin, small, and moist in substance. Celsus[496] calls these fruits those which grow on twigs according to the consensus of all the experts. Grapes, figs, nuts, and dates are stronger than orchard fruit properly so called, that is, they are more nourishing because of their fertility and of these last the juicy are stronger than the ones which are mealy. Of all of these fruits the fig has first place in the resumptive regimen by antonomasia, or the use of an epithet, as food for old men, fresh and green when fully ripe, and of figs the white one, which should be peeled since its temperature tends toward warm in the middle of the first degree and in equableness between both humid and dry while it is thin in substance, swift to ripen, and penetrative to the chest and stomach, in fact, the entire body and of difficult corruption. It is greatly praised among expert physicians in the regimen of old men of cold nature in autumn and in a temperate region. Its skin is difficult to digest and its seeds are of no food value, but its flesh is nourishing and it constrains the bowels. Dioscorides[497] says the fig takes away thirst which Avicenna says is caused by salty phlegm.[498] The fig provokes perspiration and is a preservative against poison. Of all fruits it is the one which is least harmful and more nourishing especially when it is completely ripe but less so when dried. The red fig comes second to the white one in praise; the black one is next when ripe also; it has the least hard skin of all. There are regions which bear the best figs, such as the Tusculan territory, as Marcus Varro writes.[499] Abulkasim recommends for the resumptive regimen the dry fig tending toward roundness which he calls *tartarosa,* especially for old men of frigid nature in springtime and in a temperate region for the fig is of a dry nature and warm almost in the beginning of the second degree; this one is more nourishing than other fruits and produces more flatulence,

[496]Ibid., 2. 18. 6.
[497]Dioscorides, *De Materia Medica,* I, 183.
[498]Avicenna, II, 283.
[499]Varro, *De Lingua Latina,* 7. 318.

constrains the bowels when dry and green but more so when green.[500] Avicenna writes that although its food value is not great in both flesh and seeds it is yet more nourishing than all other fruits. The dried fig called *carica*[501] is so named for its abundance because as they say it grows twenty or thirty in one clump or mass. It is useful for the chest, back, emaciation of the kidneys, hoarse throat, obstructions of the liver and spleen, and sand in the kidneys. They purify and open but are not completely free of flatulence. The white fig is of lighter substance than all other figs and of better chyme, according to Isaac Israeli [f. cxiv], when eaten with nuts and almonds. It produces less flatulence in this way. The blood generated from the fig, especially the dry one, is not at all good. Therefore eating figs produces body lice for they propel the nourishment to the upper surface of the body and overheat it in addition. It is harmful to the spleen and liver, as Abulkasim says. These last two organs desire something sweet and attract it to themselves more quickly than they should from the stomach and from those foods similar in nature to sweets which are attracted by an incomplete digestion and increase the obstructions of the passages of the spleen and liver and thus their thickness. A sign of this condition, they say, is found in the livers of animals who eat figs: it is a certain thickness along with a good flavor and fatness in these animals. There are birds which are very nourishing whose flesh when eaten creates a beautiful color in the face. The fig is so called as if "suffering from piles" in Greek, that is, because it thickens the liver.[502] The first figs which appear on the trees are called *grossi;* they are the flowers of the fig and should be rejected for they are of poor nourishment and filled to superfluity of humidity.

THE GRAPE, SO-CALLED BECAUSE IT IS MOIST *(UVIDA)* AND FULL INSIDE OF HUMOR, JUICE, AND FATNESS

Among fruits the fig and the grape hold first place, are more nourishing than all the other seasonal fruits, and have the least

[500]Galen, 6. 352, 570.
[501]Pliny, *N. H.* 13. 51; 15. 83; Galen, 6. 367; Isidore of Seville, *Etymologies* 17. 7. 17.
[502]Martial, 7. 71. 1; Cato, *R. R.* 94; Celsus, *De Medicina* 5. 12; Pliny, *N. H.* 23. 125; 17. 254.

bad chyme, as Galen says.[503] Although there are many kinds of grapes, of the early ripe, purple, hard-berry, dactylis, ceraneis, Cydonian, the one Abulkasim particularly recommends for the resumptive regimen of old men of frigid nature in autumn and in the northern region is the white, completely ripe grape, large, thin-skinned, watery and especially that which after it has been picked for some days and has wrinkled and hardened so that it is flaccid, for another grape picked and eaten at the same time is held to be better for eating. It should be eaten at the first course. It is warm in nature in the first degree, humid in the second. It furnishes good nourishment, is ideal for the stomach, moves the bowels especially when fresh and fat. Its food value is similar to and no less harmless than that of the fig except that the fig as long as it remains in the stomach or intestines creates flatulence. The grape produces flatulence at all digestions, as Averroes [5.83r] writes. Although it is copious in nourishment it is less so than the fig; it increases the body more swiftly yet the nourishment it provides is not as permanent and solid and the human flesh that results from eating it is flabby and impermanent. It is harmful to the stomach especially when fresh and creates thirst. Therefore it should be eaten with acidic pomegranates. Avicenna[504] writes that the grape is harmful to the bladder, which is not true of the dried grape.

DRIED GRAPES

The relation of dried to fresh grapes is similar as Galen[505] writes to that of dried figs to fresh figs. They are of moderate heat, as Rhazes says [537], or at least of warm and humid nature and are digested swiftly; if eaten as is allowed in the resumptive regimen they are admirably suited to the aged especially those of frigid nature in winter in the cold region. They suggest that the grapes selected should be black, small, thin-skinned, abundantly pulpy, and of pure sweetness without being dry. The best of these grapes is the Corinthian dried grape [currants]. They have a great deal of nourishment, they cleanse humidities, check the bowels, and are

[503]Galen, 6. 573; Pliny, *N. H.* 14. 40.
[504]Avicenna, II, 737.
[505]Galen, 6. 581.

more suitable for the stomach than figs. They help the chest and lungs and strengthen them as well as the kidneys and bladder, as Avicenna says.[506] They are especially good for the liver. They clear up a bad complexion and give it an excellent nourishment. They do not produce the obstruction produced by dates and are a remedy for a flux with a difficult hepatic lotion. Serapio the son says they putrefy rather slowly. They are weaker in their effects upon the entire substance of the liver and its operations than other wines and can be substituted for another wine made of grapes although they heat the blood, as Abulkasim says, especially when eaten to excess, as Judeus says [f. cxiiii]. Therefore they should be eaten with fresh lemons.

DATES

When the date is sweet and nearing that complete ripeness which Galen[507] assigns to the *cariothus (caryota)* it is useful for old people of cold and humid nature in winter in northern regions. Its nature is warm and humid to the second degree, is more digestible than dried figs and provokes the urine more. The better date grows in hot regions. The sweetest and more viscous is more quickly digested and checks the bowels although its nourishment is small. Galen says the best date is raised in Syria Palaestina at Jericho. The more humid date is considered less good. Theodorus Priscianus [xv] says the date is nourishing but is astringent to the bowels and harmful to the stomach, brings obstructions to the liver and abscess to the head, is of bad chyme and inflicts hemorrhoids and headache, generates thick blood, and is hard to digest, as Judeus [f. cxiiii] declares; hence he says dates should be eaten with poppy and rose water. Afterwards lettuce with vinegar is recommended to be eaten.

SWEET APPLE

Although the material substance of the apple is very weak according to Cornelius Celsus[508] and orchard fruit when sour or bit-

[506]Avicenna, II, 737.
[507]Galen, 6. 607.
[508]Celsus, *De Medicina* 2. 18. 319. 1; 21; Galen, 6. 594–601.

ter are of bad juice the sweet apple is praised in the regimen of old people of warm nature at all seasons and in every region. Its nature is humid to the middle of the first degree with a tendency toward warmth, as the authors agree. There are various species such as the Matianus from a place in Spain, as Isidore says.[509] Its special property is to enliven the heart and to strengthen its powers; its odor and sweetness assist in this function. Since it is of both medicinal and food value it assists the spirit by nourishing, tempering, and rectifying it, as Avicenna says. Other species include the Jerusalem apple, which Abulkasim considered the most temperate of all. Then follow the Lesbius, Socanus, and Malcius. Avicenna listed the Ascanius as more temperate and especially ideal for the heart and fragrant. In our climate before our century the orbiculate [round] apple was regarded as especially ideal for the stomach, as Celsus[510] reports. The Scandian, Amerine, Appian [from Appius of the Claudian clan], as Pliny says,[511] which Paulus praises highly are other kinds. There are also the very sweet Appian apples which Rome and its environs grow in abundance, whose praise is spread abroad thus: "All apples are bad except the Appian apple." Their odor is that of the quince and their size also resembles that of the latter. Then comes the rosy apple with which Bologna and the Romagna abound. The calamana is to be rejected. They are not very sweet, but if they are boiled they become moderately sweet and with their aroma and warmth they strengthen the stomach, bring gladness and contentment to the soul, as Abulkasim says. With their odor they restore the shattered power of the brain and comfort the heart. Cassius Felix calls this apple comforting.[512] Rabi Moyses [f. 26v] says the food value of apples is less than that of other fruits because they induce flatulence in nerves and muscles which is hard to dissolve and create pain in the nerves, especially the nervalia *[ossa paris, os iugale],* as Avicenna says.[513] Abulkasim says they should be eaten with sugar and honey in rose wine. The food content of the pear[514]

[509]Isidore of Seville, *Etymologies* 17. 7. 3; Columella 5. 10. 19; 12. 47. 5.
[510]Celsus, 2. 24. 2.
[511]Pliny, *N. H.* 15. 50.
[512]*De Medicina,* ed. V. Rose; Leipzig, 1879, 101.
[513]Avicenna, II, 569.
[514]Pliny, *N. H.* 22. 153; 23. 115.

is difficult to digest even for the strong among the aged for it is too sweet, aromatic, and savory as well as fragile, similar to water coagulated and congealed with sugar, not sandy in texture or mealy. Those which are reddish, pleasant of odor, thin-skinned and very ripe are approved. Pears endowed with these features are among those in which there is no harm, as Avicenna[515] writes. Best suited for the stomach, as Celsus[516] says, are the mealy pear from Crustumeria or the Mevian, Tarentine, or Signian, and in our age the glacial pear, very ripe, of which the poet writes:

> And the icy pear commends itself everywhere.

Then there are the Musea, Sementina, and the Ricarda as they are called at Rome, very similar to the glacial pear. In ancient times the following pears were held in high esteem: Dolabelliana, Crustumerian, Royal, Venus, Volema, Veniana, Laterisiana, Decimiana, Laurea, and Mirappia. It is listed as of frigid nature[517] to the first degree, dry to the second, although the glacial pear is very full of humidity. Judeus [f. cxviii] writes that the pear strengthens the stomach; when eaten at the last course it quenches thirst nor is it harmful to the nerves. By reason of its constipating effect and its aroma it is peculiarly effective against the illness that arises from mushrooms. Because it induces colic and intestinal disorder oily foods should be eaten after it, as Abulkasim urges. The pear except for small portions and when boiled or spiced is not recommended in the resumptive diet. Ginger should be eaten with it.

QUINCE APPLE OR QUINCE

The quince is by nature frigid at the end of the first degree, dry at the beginning of the second degree. It is allowed to be eaten by choleric old men in the resumptive regimen as ripe fruit with honeyed dates in all seasons and regions. It produces a cold humor, softens the nature, and provokes the urine. By accident,

[515]Avicenna, II, 550.
[516]Celsus, *De Medicina* 2. 24. 2. et glaciale pirum sese commendat ubique: poet unknown.
[517]Galen, 11. 631, 648, 834; Pliny, *N. H.* 15. 53; Cato, *R. R.* 7. 3. 4; Varro, *R. R.* 1. 59.

however, Serapio the son says it constricts the bowels when eaten at the first course nor is it corrupted in a sick stomach any less than in a healthy one. It does not produce colic and is medically useful for asthma, the chest, gullet, and hoarse throat, especially the musty juice of its seeds. It inhibits the spitting of blood. In every way the quince is remarkable beyond other kinds of apples since it is more astringent and provides a more stable chyme or digestible juice. When not ripe[518] it nevertheless stirs the appetite and assists the digestion. It increases and nourishes the forces of the stomach, as Theodorus Priscianus [xv] says and with its juice it checks stomach upsets and nausea. In general, it is of comfort to the stomach and strengthens it, especially in keeping it from receiving bad humors from elsewhere. Avicenna[519] says cooked quince is more helpful because when eaten at the last course it constrains the bowels. Judeus [f. cxvii] says the same: the quince brings pleasure to the body. Avicenna gives the recipe for preparing quince: remove the pulp and throw away the seeds. Fill the empty shell of the fruit with honey and sugar and the yellow pulp; cover with tow or a similar material and bake in the ashes.

POMEGRANATE OR PUNIC APPLE

The pomegranate or Punic apple derives its name from Carthage.[520] The ancient physicians called it *apyrenum,* which means sweet and without pips or seeds. It was recommended in the resumptive regimen for old people of equable nature in autumn in temperate regions. Its nature is said to be warm and humid with temperament although Avicenna lists it as cold and humid in the first degree. Its nourishment is good although modest and it is helpful to the liver which has lost its natural spirit. By means of its goodness and sweetness and a certain wonderful property if it is eaten with bread it checks the corruption of bread in the stomach, soothes hoarse throat and cough, and strengthens and soothes the chest, as Abulkasim reports. It is believed that the sweet quince excites sexual passion. The Spanish quince, rather thick and easily

[518]Celsus, *De Medicina* 2. 30.
[519]Avicenna, II, 156.
[520]Pliny, 13. 112; 15. 47; 23. 106; Theophrastus, *H. P.* 4. 13. 2.

skinned, is recommended and especially from Valencia, the quince of Gaeta and the regions around Naples, Tivoli, and Florence. Theodorus Priscianus [x] says the African pomegranate constricts the bowels but benefits the eyes. The sweet pomegranate induces inflammation especially in a choleric stomach because it often brings on acute fever. Therefore the pomegranate should be eaten with vinegar.

THE CITRUS APPLE, ORANGE, AND LEMON

Insofar as these fruits pertain to our purpose in the resumptive regimen they are acceptable as food for it is well known that fragrant foods are useful for the aged since the odor in which they abound is exceedingly adapted to human nature, clearing up the corruption of the air with its pestilential pollution, as Avicenna says.[521] The citrus apple is most acceptable in the diet of old people of frigid nature in winter and in cold regions if as is proper it is eaten with seasoning. Its nature is equable or temperate as a whole, but its skin is warm in the first degree, dry in the second, although Avicenna in his little book on the powers of the heart says it is warm and dry in the third degree to which both its leaf and flower approach although these are more delicate. Its flesh or pulp is warm and humid in the first degree. The acidity of its juice is of a frigid and dry nature to the second degree, its seeds warm and dry to the second. That which is to be eaten in the resumptive regimen are the skin and flesh flavored with sugar or honey, for the skin alone is not digestible because of its hardness. The flesh is not good for the stomach; they say that produces slow digestion and colic. Therefore Avicenna bids us to eat it with pickling brine. It is more salubrious when flavored with honey for its aromatic property assists the stomach, lends force to the digestive power, and is salutary to the throat and lungs. They say the citrus skin makes the breath more pleasant, strengthens the heart, exhilarates the soul, and performs the function of theriac with a peculiar quality it possesses to preserve with its warmth against putrefaction. Citrus seed counteracts poison. The leaves fortify the stomach and

[521]Avicenna, II, 120, 156.

viscera as do the flowers. Citrus should be eaten alone and not mixed with food either before or after at table, as Avicenna warns. Citromilus or citrangulus (which I think is the orange apple) whose acidity among the rest of its parts almost alone is used in the regimen of the aged is of warm and dry nature in summer and in warm regions is especially praised because of its sweetness together with what is believed to be a more moderate frigidity than that of citrus and lemon. Its skin is almost similar in nature in its warmth to the citrus skin or perhaps a little warmer and with less humidity. Its flesh is warmer than citrus flesh; this is shown by the bitterness perceived in it which is not found in the citrus. It is as ideal for the aged as the citrus when eaten with sugar and honey. The experts rarely mention the orange. It is not the Median or Persian apple which Vergil[522] mentions in the *Georgics:*

> The lingering taste
> Of the blessed apple than which there is none more
> Quick to bring relief

nor is it the Assyrian apple of which Pliny[523] speaks, for Macrobius[524] is authority for the statement that they [Vergil and Pliny] understood it to be that, but it is the citrangulus of which Avicenna[525] writes in *Canon* IV, the chapter on the cure of variolae, in his description of a certain syrup. The appraisal of the lemon in its nature and property for aiding and harming as almost similar to citrus is given in addition by Abulkasim in *baldach* and Avicenna, *Canon* I, fen 4, on acute fevers. Beyond these I have read no other of the experts on the subject. [Zerbi evidently confuses Abulkasim, author of the *Liber Theoricae,* with Ibn Botlan, also known as Ellbochasim, Albulkasem, Ububchasym, and Albullasem de Baldach, Baldac, or Baldak in four MSS of his *Tacuinum Sanitatis;* see the bibliography.]

COCCYMALUM OR PLUM[526]

As a laxative for old people Galen[527] vouches for the plum although it may also be eaten to counteract the ill of choler with its

[522]Vergil, *Georgics* 2. 126.
[523]Pliny, *N. H.* 14. 7; 16. 135.
[524]Macrobius, *Sat.* 3. 19. 3.
[525]Avicenna, *Canon* IV, cap. x, p. 418.
[526]Macrobius, *Sat.* 5. 3. 19; Isidore of Seville, *Etymologies* 17. 7. 10.
[527]Galen, 6. 353, 613; 12. 32; Pliny, *N. H.* 15. 41.

coolness, for its nature is frigid in the second degree, humid in the third; it easily corrupts in the stomach. From a huge number of kinds of plums the experts suggest that the following be chosen: the parti-colored, black, white, the one called hordearia [because it is ripe at barley harvest] and the one called asinine [held in little esteem]. The black is preferable; even better is the cerine or purple and the Damascene from Damascus in Syria; each of these should be completely ripe. They should be eaten before the meal; when eaten after it honey water should be drunk or wine from dried grapes, or sweet wine, as Avicenna says.[528]

CHERRY

The nature of the sweet cherry as of the plum is cold and humid to the second degree. Its usefulness as a laxative is moderate in the resumptive regimen but not without praise. It descends from the stomach quite rapidly and therefore constrains the bowels. Although according to Galen[529] prunes serve as a laxative along with figs, vegetables, and other similar foods which grow in the summer and autumn sweet cherries especially of all species of foods are ideal for the stomach and are numbered among foods which relax the bowels. Although because of their pleasant flavor the hard-berried cherries as Pliny[530] says they are called in Campania hold first place nevertheless the smaller of these are more desirable as a laxative. Yet they are of bad chyme, burdensome to the stomach and intestines, ideal for the generation of putrefaction and worms, and create putrid fevers. Therefore a small amount of these cherries and only at the first course can reduce these ills. The sour cherries especially are to be eaten for the sake of drying and bursting obstructions which are created by superfluities in a replete phlegmatic stomach and sometimes for quenching thirst and checking the bile as well as for stimulating the appetite, as Serapio the son [f. clxxx] reports. Nor are they convertible to putrefaction as are the sweet cherries. The dried cherries are better preserved. The large sour cherries are to be rejected entirely.

[528]Avicenna, II, 541.
[529]Galen, 6. 353.
[530]Pliny, *N. H.* 15. 103.

PERSIAN APPLE (PEACH) AND CHRYSOMALUM[531]

When quite ripe this fruit loosens the bowels. It is especially good for a hot dry stomach and excites the appetite. In the resumptive regimen especially of old men of hot and dry nature it is allowed at the first course. It is frigid in nature to the second degree, humid in the first. They prohibit the drinking of wine mixed with the Persian apple. Isaac Israeli [f. cxv], however, permits a small amount of wine in order to counteract its frigidity and to prevent its easy corruption in the stomach. No other food is to be eaten after the peach is eaten for it is corrupted, they say, and corrupts the food eaten with it quite readily. A sign of this is the fact that nothing is more perishable than the peach; the longest delay it can sustain after being picked is two days, as Pliny[532] states, and must be sold. Of all species the hard-skinned *(duracinus)* is considered the best as being more valuable than the nut. Martial writes of them:[533]

> Of little worth should we peaches have been on the branches of our mother tree; now on adoptive boughs we peaches are prized.

The chrysomalum (golden apple) is similar in nature to the peach; it is not suitable for the elderly except sometimes at the first course, with the addition of anise, mastic, or with unmixed wine, raisins, sugar or honey.

THE ALMOND, AND FIRST THE NON-EDIBLE OR BITTER

It is prescribed that the almond is acceptable as medicine in use for the aged and therefore it is called non-edible; for old men of frigid nature in winter in the northern region it is ideal. Its nature is warm and dry to the second degree. It is astringent, cleansing, and aperitive. In these properties the edible almond is superior; it does not constrain the bowels. They write that it will destroy foxes.[534] It is chiefly used as medicine without food value since it creates a raw humor. Its special function is to open obstructions of

[531]Pliny, *N. H.* 15. 39, 44, 48, 113; Galen, 6. 592–98.
[532]Pliny, *N. H.* 15. 40, 42.
[533]Martial, *Epigrams* 13. 46, of peaches grafted on an apricot tree *(malum praecox)*.
[534]Pliny, *N. H.* 23. 145.

the liver, spleen, kidneys and bladder and those which occur in the extremities of the small veins. It provokes the urine. The more bitter it is the more effective it is in these functions, they say; because it is harmful to the intestines it should be eaten together with the edible almond, as Avicenna says.

WALNUT

The walnut *(iuglans)* is so called because it pleases *(iuuat)*[535] or because it is said to be the tree of Jove, says Macrobius, and thus is very flourishing. It is acceptable in the resumptive regimen because it is less warm than dry and because of its imperfect humidity especially for old men who live in mountainous places and whose stomach or nature is temperate or who have at least as much frigidity as warmth which can counteract the nut, as Isaac [f. cxix] says. Avicenna[536] says it is thus ideal for old men and provides a praiseworthy nourishment for them. It is more swiftly digested than the almond[537] although more quickly converted to bile and is therefore listed as harmful to the stomach. More acceptable is the fresh or green walnut eaten with sugar or honey. The dry nut should not be eaten by old men, for it is warm to the third degree, dry to the beginning of the second. It is more oily than the almond and thus causes hoarseness more quickly; it provokes vomiting and with immoderate use it causes paralysis of the tongue. Judeus [f. cxix] writes that the nourishment given by the walnut produces retention of words and therefore it is forbidden as food for children since its substance is imbibed into the muscles of the tongue. If the dry walnut is eaten they urge that the one which is more quickly shelled should be selected; it should then be steeped in hot water overnight so that with its humidity the nut may be brought back to its original freshness. It should be eaten in cold seasons because it is thought to be obnoxious in warm seasons, especially when eaten with oxymel. For those whose stomach is weak Avicenna recommends that it be eaten with brine and vinegar. I believe it is useful to mention here what Pliny[538] says of it.

[535]Pliny, *N. H.* 15. 86; 17. 89; 23.147; Varro, *L. L.* 5.102; Macrobius, *Sat.* 3. 18. 2–3.
[536]Avicenna, II, 505.
[537]Pliny, *N. H.* 15. 89.
[538]Ibid., 23. 149.

Gnaeus Pompey found in the private archives of Mithridates the Great in a set of notes written in his own hand an antidote made of two dry nuts, likewise the same number of figs and twenty leaves of rue ground together with a grain of salt added. If one takes this antidote while fasting no poison will harm the person that day. Fresh Indian nut is useful for old men of frigid and dry nature in autumn and in southern regions, according to Abulkasim. Its nature is warm in the second degree, humid in the third. It sharpens the intellect, as they say, and promotes fat and corpulence. It should be eaten with clarified sugar made into rolls because it descends slowly.

HAZEL NUT

This nut is less warm than the walnut but more nourishing although its food value is more solid and earthy and less oily than the walnut. Therefore it is digested more slowly and eliminated more slowly from the body nor does it promote vomiting as the walnut does. It produces flatulence, they say. In the resumptive regimen it is not to be rejected, especially for old men of frigid nature in the winter and in the northern regions. It is of warm nature near grade three, humid in the second. Since it is warm and dry in the beginning of grade one it is thought to add with its astringency to the brain, Avicenna says.[539] When cooked and eaten with a little pepper it is effective against colds and rheumatism. It has a good influence on the jejunum intestine in expelling its bad quality, as Judeus [f. cxix] writes. They say that the hazel nut is beneficial against scorpion stings especially if taken with fig and rue or placed in a poultice upon the sting. It removes the thicker humor. Since it is bad for the stomach it should be eaten with clarified sugar made into rolls. When the inner shell is removed the hazel nut loses its inflationary power or at least relaxes it.

PINE NUTS

It is suggested that the kernel of the pine nut be extracted from its shell and steeped in hot water so that its sharpness or

[539]Avicenna, II, 43.

burning quality may be removed so as to make it available for old men. It is warm to the end of the second degree but dry to the beginning of the same although Avicenna asserts that the degree is the same for both warmth and dryness, with little warmth. Its food value is not unimportant, in fact, it is praiseworthy. It does not cause flatulence although the common charge brought against all nuts is that they cause it. Hence the pine nut kernel is reckoned among light foods. Its property is in the final power that of nutrition so that there is little in it which does not contribute to nourishment, as they say. It is helpful in adding weight to the body, in rectifying corrupt humidities in the intestines, in drying up and easing the hawking-up of phlegm, and in curing cough, chest and kidney pains, as authors agree. It cleanses the viscous humors in both kidneys and bladder. Therefore it is listed among diuretics. It should be heated and eaten with sugar; when cool it is eaten with honey after it has been poured into hot water, as Serapio the son [f. clxxxii] says.

PISTACHIO

Syria[540] grows certain trees which provide pistachio nuts; these are included as food in the resumptive regimen. The pistachio has an effect and properties similar to those of the pine nut and in addition is helpful against snake bite, whether it is eaten or drunk. It is ideal for old men of frigid nature in winter and in a cold region, writes Abulkasim. Its warm nature is placed in the middle of the second degree with some humidity. Some people consider the pistachio warmer than the almond. Avicenna says its heat is vehement although Judeus [f. cxxiiii] insists it has an equal amount of heat and dryness. It provides good although small nourishment. It has the power to cheer and restore the heart. It is also enumerated among theriac medicines, as they say. It contains a spicy fragrance with viscosity. It purifies the liver and increases its powers throughout its substance while they say it opens up obstructions of the alimentary passage. Its fragrance and astringency are also beneficial for the reparation of the mouth of the stomach and the entirety of the latter. Its effects are good for nausea and

[540]Pliny, *N. H.* 13. 51.

upset stomach. It neither relaxes nor constrains the bowels. Judeus [f. cxxiiii] writes that *fisticus* or pistachio is more helpful than all other fruits or nuts; its property is to strengthen the stomach and the liver when the stomach is smeared with its oil. Pistachio is useful at the first and last courses eaten alone or with raisins or with sugar and is ideal for all ages. It is listed among foods which have a great deal of benefit, as Averroes [5.83v] says. The large nut should be chosen and as the ancients say eaten with dry chrysomalum, according to Abulkasim; it is thus less harmful and does not produce dizziness.

CHESTNUT

The chestnut[541] (although more suitably classified with acorns) is called a nut by Pliny. Although it is of little value it is surprising that nature has hidden it with such great care [in its prickly shell]. The Greeks call it *castanon* because its fruit grows in the shape of testicles. It is acceptable in the resumptive regimen of the elderly of warm nature in the winter in mountainous regions. It is of warm nature in the first degree which is proven by its sweetness. It is dry in the second degree and is detergent. It is very effective against flux of the stomach and bowels. It stimulates evacuation and is salubrious for those excreting blood, nourishes the flesh, and provides a praiseworthy aliment. It is better when eaten with sugar. It strengthens the jejune intestine, says Israeli [f. cxix]. Judeus writes [f. 26r] that in every fruit of the trees there is some defect except in the chestnut; if it is well digested with its density it does not produce bad chyme. It should be cooked before eaten so as to rarefy its substance. If it is placed in tepid water this modifies the dryness of the chest and body and removes difficulty in passing urine. Its complexion is tempered by such an infusion by the softness and humidity of the water because the chestnut is of good chyme although difficult and slow of digestion. Thus it is sometimes burdensome to the brain. It purges the constrained bowels but causes flatulence although it does so less when cooked, as Theodorus Priscianus [xv] reports.

[541]Ibid., 15. 92.

Chapter XXXVIII

The Advantages of Sleep in the Resumptive Regimen

Old age requires a substantial conservation of its humidity not only because it has a short supply but because it also requires a continual replacement of that humidity which is lost. It is well known that this regeneration of humor is most conveniently accomplished through sleep. Sleep rivals food and drink in the task of humidifying; hence sleep is listed among the causes of humidification. It accomplishes its purpose by moderate use and by offering aid to the powers of digestion in old men, for sleep assists digestion, removes the fatigue due to labor, warms thoroughly the inner parts of the body, promotes the increase of weight, exhilarates the mind, and lends strength to all the faculties or powers of the individual. Thus it increases and kindles the natural heat and rectifies the other humors and the thoughts of the soul if nature is not reluctant, as is agreed among authors. A sign of the beneficial effects of sleep, they say, is the fact that those who awake from it exhibit a lightness, alacrity, and greatness of spirit. Sleep does not occur except through the powerlessness brought about by staying awake, which is usually followed by a breakdown of spirit and heat in the operations of sense and motion.

LENGTH, TIME, AND MANNER OF SLEEP TO BE OBSERVED IN THIS REGIMEN

A sleep therefore rather longer and more complete but not too long with too great a lingering in bed for older people in all seasons and regions than for healthy young people is recommended as quite helpful for the restoration of their humidity. For all their animal powers of motion and sense are thus put to rest; these must be protected in old people as long as the raw or at any rate vitiated humor remains in their stomachs, resisting digestion. Through a rather long period of sleep their digestion is repeated and that which is corrupted in it from languor and inactivity is rectified and corrected, says Averroes [6. 94r]. Sleep will also be more beneficial to old men if they sleep as long as they are accustomed to sleep. Let the time at which they go to sleep be at the end of their power to keep awake which for many will be more opportune after the evening meal when the sun is setting, for then humid night falls from the heavens and the wheeling stars persuade them to sleep, especially when the old man needs it. Therefore sleep at night is preferable than during the day preceded by the descent of food to the bottom of the stomach. This can be accomplished by means of some light exercise especially with an animal and preceding sleep as well as by a conversation with which old age is accustomed to be soothed. Daytime sleep retains as they say the respiration customarily exhaled from the body which prepares the man for rheumatism. This should not be allowed except through urgent necessity or by the demands of habit, especially in the summer time. It is suggested that during daytime sleep old men should sleep with an elevated pillow, which is more conducive to a thorough digestion. Both by night and day old men should shed their clothes and shoes and the top of their heads should be covered with a cloth, as Aristotle[542] says, for cold in the extremities during sleep can bring great harm to the brain. Care should be taken that they should sleep in a dark place where the moonlight cannot enter. They should also lie with legs bent up and not extended and by no means on their back. This manner of sleeping produces nightmares and catarrhs in a healthy man. Lying supine, according to Pliny,[543] causes many dreams in autumn and spring and is helpful to the eyes; lying prone is helpful for the cough. Sleeping on both sides alternately is considered more beneficial for they say that lying on one's side counteracts distillations. In this manner sleep is somewhat more profound and not interrupted by slanting the body below the right side. Hence the food is more quickly digested on the right side in sleep, as Theophrastus affirms, for the food descends more quickly to the bottom of the stomach which is the place for digestion. Then one must make a turn to the left side. Thus the process of digestion is assisted most

[542]Aristotle: see Plutarch, *Sympos. Quaest.* VIII,10, 1, p. 734.
[543]Pliny, *N. H.* 7. 171; 28. 54.

greatly by the virtue or power of the stomach. In this way the liver within the embrace of the stomach aids the digestion. Finally let a return to the right side be made; thus a descent of the food to the intestines is brought about, as Avicenna writes.[544] All this manner of sleeping is more beneficial if the old man of weak stomach holds a girl who is close to her menstruation in his constant embrace or a feather bed. Diligent observation must be maintained that for old men who are frequently wakeful sleep should be induced with hypnotics, that is, substances which bring on sleep or drowsiness. Adapted to this purpose out of many are poppy or lettuce,[545] especially summer lettuce whose stalk is already filled with milk, Celsus says.[546] The same is true for cinnamon. Mulberry and leek promote sleep, likewise moist coriander and edible almonds, especially if eaten with some wine and conversation. These foods are especially pleasing and convenient to an old man with a nature that is willing to sleep for we learn that they induce sleep whether truly or falsely the cause of which I think it is not useless to insert at this point. The hearing receives that which is presented to itself without actual motion since the process of hearing is spiritual as they say; it receives with greater delight that which is pleasing. These perceptions it then transmits to the imagination; the latter transmits them to the reason. But the reason at least partially is astonished concerning the objects presented to it, for wonder is uncertainty as to their cause. The reason is wearied by wonder or surprise but the continuation in reason of its wonder at the perceptions toward which the auditive power is directed does not bring back the audible experiences, for the organ of hearing rests from its apprehension of sense impressions just as do the organs of the other exterior senses. When these are at rest sleep supervenes while reason nonetheless continues to make distinctions among the sense impressions presented to it. Thus they assign this as the cause why in many dreams there appear to those who are sleeping the sense impressions experienced by them when they are awake. It is also urged that the speech of conversation ought to be marked

[544]I, fen. III, cap. ix, f. 61v.

[545]Pliny, *N. H.* 19. 26; 20. 61. For the reference to Theophrastus see the edition by F. Wimmer, Leipzig, 1854–62, III, 135.

[546]Celsus, *De Medicina* 2. 32. On sense-impressions in dreams, see Cicero, *De Rep.* 6. 10. 10 as mentioned below.

by an elegance of language that is more delightful and which will cause sleep to be more prolonged and also in order to keep the sleeping man from having bad dreams. Such dreams are disturbing to the sense perception as well as to the spirits and blood and hinder the completion of the digestion. It may be added that sleep is promoted by other means such as boats or cradles and any motion such as is used in the rocking of a baby. In this way the vapors of humidity ascending seek the brain and clog its passages, thus inducing sleep.

Chapter XXXIX

The Advantages of Wakefulness

Since the state of wakefulness is the purpose of a living creature and since to perceive and to know is the purpose or end striven for by all, this is achieved by wakefulness, for wakeful *(vigil)* is said as though it were "agile for seeing" *(ad videndum agilis).* This end is sought as being the best; therefore there is more desire for wakefulness than for sleep as there is for living and being. The purpose of sleep is wakefulness, for we sleep in order that we may be wakeful in a better way. Wakefulness is said to be a kind of exercise of the senses; hence it is most acceptable in the resumptive regimen of old men in whatever season and whatever inhabited region since by its mediation heat is distributed, the pores are opened, and assistance is lent to the excretion of superfluities by which digestion is improved and the body acquires those things which are necessary to the regimen of life. That wakefulness is not however excessive by which the senses are stirred and the body's forces disposed so that they may exercise their accustomed operations. The entire body is thus purged of superfluities because motion disposes of them and diminishes them. Therefore the appetite for food is increased by wakefulness rather than by sleep not because wakefulness is more advantageous to digestion than sleep (since beyond doubt a better digestion is carried out during sleep rather than during wakefulness) but because superfluities are dissipated by wakefulness and the expulsive powers are increased. Therefore old age requires for its resumptive regimen a greater amount of sleep than it chooses in its restorative regimen. Much more wakefulness is required for the perfection of health in order to make up for the lack of it caused by the process of restoration. Hence old men do not need a more ample sleep since the restoration created by the digestion of food which had been lost is brought back by means of that heat and strength which, due to old men's lack of power had retreated inward, are now awakened and brought out to the exterior.

THE LENGTH OF WAKEFULNESS IN THE RESUMPTION OF OLD AGE

According to Hippocrates *[Aphorisms,* II,3*]* sleep and waking can cause harm in each of their ways. Sleep enervates the animal powers and breaks them down, relaxes the passages of the heart, increases phlegm, weakens the natural heat, corrupts the color, slows movement, often induces asthma, and finally extinguishes the innate heat just as a fire is extinguished when covered with many ashes. Too much wakefulness diminishes the body's strength, destroys the organs of sense, and cools off their heat as the heat of a fire is cooled by excessive motion, as Averroes [6. 94v] reports. It is urged that too much wakefulness no less than excessive sleep should be avoided by old people for superfluous wakefulness in them results in the domination of humidity although a false and nitrous humidity, as Galen[547] says, in old men causes insomnia also because of the sadness which old age brings. From whatever cause, however, it should be repelled as long as it creates superfluity. Not only does it bring weariness to old men but it dries the body, corrupts one's normal way of life, is harmful to the brain, and causes an intermixture of the senses from which arise acute illnesses. The eyes become hollow with too much wakefulness and a general weakness of the body follows, infirmity of digestion, deterioration of the innate heat, inflammation, dissolution, increase of the reddish bile especially in thin bodies. When there is too much of this care must be taken to remove it both by bringing on sleep and avoidance of everything which excites the senses. As Celsus[548] reports, these are catmint, thyme, satureia, hyssop, and especially pennyroyal, rue, and onion. Concerning air, exercise, rest, food and drink, sleep and waking, those things which conduce to the resumption of old age and which are common to every age so much has been said. Nothing has been said as to sex. Galen[549] says this is only suitable for the young. Age-

[547]Galen, 8. 162; 16. 619; 17. B. 450.
[548]Celsus, *De Medicina* 2. 32.
[549]Galen, 6. 84; 1. 372; 5. 911; 4. 179, 402.

groups anterior and posterior to adolescence either do not emit sperm or produce an infecund or poorly fecund sperm. Concerning sex something will be said in the following chapters, especially chapter XLIII.

Chapter XL

Bodily Elimination to Be Observed

The emptiness which lack of food creates and how it must be taken care of has been discussed in its place, chapter III. Now we must discuss bodily elimination, which also comes under the heading of inanition and likewise we must next discuss purges or enemas and the retention which is properly their opposite. The consideration of these needs is quite imperative in the care of the aged and should be observed so that superfluities are not retained but are evacuated from the body. If the inner members are purged of that with which they are replete the superfluities will not remain therein and the individual will be healthy and young a long time, as Galen[550] rightly declares. Blood-letting is included in this process and sometimes purging by use of solvents and diuretics which promote perspiration, loosening of sputum, and similar methods which purge through the visible passages of the body.

BLOOD-LETTING FROM THE VEINS

He who prescribes evacuation in the resumptive regimen which is properly the letting of blood or of some other humor mixed with blood when the humors are amiss only in their quantity and makes an incision in a vein which they call phlebotomy should be a very careful judge of the strength and natural complexion of the old men. It does not make any difference what the age or the powers may be of the person who is to be blood-let. Galen[551] says that a septuagenarian who has much blood and is very strong can be blood-let nor does his age alone need to be taken into account but also the general condition of his body.

[550]Galen, 6. 79; 16. 120, 752.
[551]Ibid., 11. 291.

Some sexagenarians cannot tolerate phlebotomy but some septuagenarians can tolerate it. Every letting of blood is to be feared in the elderly (insofar as it can be performed) says Avicenna[552] unless you have confidence in the old man's general nature, the solidity of his muscles, the amplitude of his veins, their repletion and the reddishness of their color. But if all these factors are not favorable to the letting of blood then the evacuation of the elderly must be performed rather by medicines than by phlebotomy for it is more helpful to loosen their bowels by using them. But if the factors mentioned as the proper conditions for the use of phlebotomy are favorable the sexagenarian also may be blood-let twice a year if he is fat and fleshy. Avicenna forbids phlebotomy for such a man from the cephalic vein for the heads of old men are weak and cold. Those approaching their seventieth year can be blood-let once a year nor can it be repeated however flourishing they may be. The median vein should not be cut for it is composed of the cephalic vein which is located in the upper part of the arm. When a person has reached the age of seventy-five he can be blood-let twice in two years from the basilica vein. There is a great possibility of error in this respect since there is less strength in an old man. Everything which has been mentioned in the curative regimen of the elderly must be adhered to if phlebotomy is necessary due to contingent illness, but in the resumptive and conservative regimens phlebotomy must simply be restrained because there is an exuberance of phlegm in old people and by the opening of a vein a removal of watery and humid matter as well as of blood and heat takes place, a very dangerous condition for the aged. In all of these matters just as in general in the administration of the six non-naturals there must be observed the difference in regions or climates for according to these complexions, ills, and natures, diets and medicines will vary daily, says Damascenus [f. 59]. Hence that which is carried out in the second climate differs from that which is carried out in the fourth. Inhabitants of the fifth and sixth climates can tolerate more the letting of blood than those who dwell in the seventh, first, second, and third.

[552]Avicenna I, 69–70. 73–75. See a long footnote on venesection and its history in my *Pre-Vesalian Anatomy,* etc., 228, listed in the bibliography.

PURGING THE BODIES OF OLD MEN AND, FIRST, BY USE OF A PRIVY ENEMA

The evacuation of the three humors different in quality from the blood which make the body sad they call a purgation or cleansing; this must be observed in the regimen of old age. This cleansing is indicated for old men of whatever nature in all seasons and regions as long as the superfluities are expelled since these are rather frequently collected in their bodies nor does exercise alone suffice for their removal. Therefore medicinal foods with a laxative effect are recommended for the old men lest their bowels remain clogged entirely. It is safer for the old men to purge themselves with medicinal food or food which acts like medicine than to use drugs for this purpose; thus their bowels should be kept as soft as possible so that no superfluities are contained in them. For an old man's bowels are in good condition if elimination takes place daily in them. Avicenna says that harm due to the looseness or weakness of the bowels is to be feared. Care should be taken that whatever you use as a laxative should be pleasant and not adverse, that is, bitter, so long as the power of expulsion is not harmed for the sake of pleasure. When the old man's dry bowel after two days does not produce anything its contents must be eliminated by various means, both by the use of certain simple medicines as well as by compound syrups *(eligmata, electos).* By the use of simple medicines indeed just as by drinking juicy broths oily and fat such as olive oil and similar unctuous foods especially when accompanied by sugar humidity and lubrication are created which cause a cleansing of the bowel, swiftly descending at the first course as well as with all sorts of herbs and vegetables seasoned with *garum,* that is, *salmuria* [pickle juice], for food and vegetables seasoned with these condiments begin the meal better. Figs and plums or prunes and raisins which, as Galen[553] says, grow in summer and autumn, should be eaten. In winter the bowels are moved by caricae, or fat dry figs, from which the outer skin should be removed, and Damascus plums either alone or mixed with honey, and olives seasoned with pickle juice. Olives from Spain loosen the bowels more than Damascus plums, according to Galen, and the roots also of polipody [fern root] or what Marcus Cato[554] calls *felicula* in a broth

[553]Galen, 6. 613.
[554]Cato, *De Agricultura* 158; Galen, 6. 354.

of boiled chicken and cabbage leaves are ideal for the same purpose, although the mercury plant[555] steeped in water checks the appetite and is a hindrance to the stomach, as the Conciliator led by experience affirms. Running water in or from the sunshine loosens the bowels. In order to give it a pleasant flavor it should be seasoned with almuria, that is, salt water and oil. The water should be running as fast as possible. The whitish leaves with emission of milk should be used of an herb whose root is called scamonea [scammony, *scammonium Syriacum*] at Antioch.[556] The inner part of saffron seed ground up with barley and turpentine to which one hazel nut or two or at most three are added forms a salutary remedy as a laxative. Turpentine has a special quality for this purpose; it softens the lining of the intestines without lesion and cleanses them as well as purging the liver, spleen, kidneys, lungs, and bladder, as Judeus [f. cxxiii] writes. Of compounds good for a laxative, as Galen[557] writes, take saffron seed with the shell removed, with figs and nuts. Another recipe that is efficacious is an ounce and a half of cinnamon, tartar, leaves of senna, six drams of each, saffron two drams, nitre one dram, anise and pepper one dram and a half, turbit, rhubarb up to two scruples with sugar or honey as an electuary or in powder with a decoction of flesh can be given to the old men. Another very useful recipe for choleric old men is ten drams of tamarind dissolved in hot water, one dram of pounded fresh rhubarb, mixed and poured together and then laid aside for a day and a half. Then strain the entire concoction and add one ounce of syrup of citron peel. Another recipe for melancholic old men: take equal parts of senna, fern, epithymum *[cuscuta Europea]* or thyme, tartar, cinnamon, gum Arabic. To the mixture add sufficient sugar or honey. It is allowable to use these laxatives of simple or compound medicines for the bowels of old men sometimes as well as eligmata, electuaries, pills or any other method nor to persist in any one approach for the individual's nature becomes accustomed to them in time and rejects the drug. It is advisable therefore to vary the kinds of laxatives, as Galen[558] prescribes, and to suit them to the natures of

[555]Galen, 12. 63; see note 160.
[556]Ibid., 19. 732; see also 4. 760; 17 B. 306.
[557]Ibid., 13. 879; 6. 353, 355.
[558]Ibid., 6. 353–54.

each individual. Thus the dry nature should not use astringent laxatives which some reprehensibly do employ, according to Galen,[559] with cabbage juice or spices and make pills from these. Others mix humid ingredients only such as water or honey. Other rich men make a bitter brew of aloes which they call holy, hence *hieron,* which they sprinkle into a potion or they use this with a moderate amount of unboiled honey. But none of the remedies should be used except under great necessity for although their use may perhaps be helpful in the conservative regimen yet they are not a protection to old age; a liberal use of drugs is not recommended for old men. One must always remember that while most of them have pleasant evacuations yet the more they evacuate the bowels will still contain feces in the days that follow so that purgations will sometimes be necessary. When they are frequent they become dangerous for the body becomes accustomed to not being nourished and will thus become infirm. For this reason Avicenna[560] advises that old men be cleansed by massage and sweating and that they should be given figs now and then and softening foods; attacking the situation with drugs is strictly forbidden. I approve of figs used at intervals but their excessive use is to be avoided for as Averroes [6. 94r] says figs create obstructions in old men. Galen advises their occasional use with seeds of nettle, crocus, and the like.

CLYSTER

The enema which Avicenna[561] calls a noble medicament should be made of oil or anything else that is pleasant and unctuous; it is helpful to old men. Its effect is to soften the intestines for evacuation, especially if made with sweet olives or with the oily juice of almonds and something fatty added with some sugar or honey or salt and the yolk of eggs. Averroes [6.94r] writes that the clyster is the last lenitive method that should be used in the regimen of old age and that softening suppositories are similar in their effect. An acute or sharp clyster should be avoided when the

[559]Ibid., 6. 354.
[560]Avicenna, I, cap. 4, f. 57v; cap. 5, f. 64r.
[561]Ibid., cap. 3, f. 69 r5, 70r, 71r.

bowels have been constipated for several days and unnecessary evacuation should be avoided by all means because it cools the body since it destroys the material for the innate heat with a break down of the spirits and obstructions that follow unnecessary evacuations, as Avicenna says.

PURGING BY URINATION

Assiduous provocation of the urine is especially recommended in the regimen of the old men whose health we strive to preserve in this gerontocomia because phlegmatic and serous or watery superfluities congregate in their bodies and increase whose removal through the urinary ducts should be directed through the convenient region of the body. Although there are very many medicinal antidotes which stimulate urination these should be postponed in favor of using celery, honey, and wine as a gentle diuretic, as Galen says,[562] and whatever is grown in gardens that is of good odor such as in addition to celery rue and hyssop but not continual use of these because they excite the senses, as Celsus says.[563] Dill, basil, mint, anise, coriander, nasturtium or cress, rocket, fennel, and in addition asparagus, capers, catmint, thyme, savory, charlock, parsnip especially the wild variety, radish, skirret and onion when diluted in a potion provoke the urine so that you will marvel at their effect.

VOMITING

Vomiting is a movement made laboriously and in a direction opposite to that taken by the food in its passage downward. Asclepiades[564] justly condemned the practice of frequent vomiting beyond measure. For the resumptive regimen, however, he does not flatly forbid it if it is easy and helpful for the old people. It is suitable for the plethoric and all who have become bilious and are broad chested, but it is not helpful for those who are thin and those with a weak stomach. It is useful for old men of phlegmatic com-

[562]Galen, 6. 353.
[563]Celsus, *De Medicina* 2. 31. 32.
[564]Ibid., 1. 3. 17, 19.

plexion in a warm region and is easier for them at the rising of the eastern star called Halobor simultaneously with the sun around June 20, in fact, during almost all the summer, as Hippocrates and Galen[565] have taught. Nevertheless, it is more advantageous in winter than in summer according to Celsus for then more phlegm and severer stuffiness in the head occur. Considering the exuberance of phlegm and the ill of the accidental effects resulting from it as well as the supervacuity of bile in him, the heat, calmness, mobility, and general attitude of the individual, the vomit which is induced in summer should expel his phlegm. They choose the time of midday as preferable for vomiting since thus the exit of the thicker pure phlegm especially contained in the bowels is brought about as well as the expulsion of the bile from which the stomach is cleansed. Thus the abomination resulting from the oily substance is removed, by which appetite is destroyed in the stomach, and the heaviness removed which occurs in the head. This process should not be repeated frequently nor the upsetting of the stomach quickly caused. Nor should the number of days be observed lest it become a force of habit. Along with its assistance vomiting often brings on languor of the body and for many deafness and chilling of the teeth as well as illness to the nose, wherefore Celsus[566] bids that no one who wishes to be well and live to an old age should make it a daily habit. It should not be practiced for the sake of gluttony; on account of health sometimes it can be rightly practiced, according to belief based on experience. Moderation is necessary in the use of vomiting and observation of the season and the time for it should be preceded by bathing and the drinking of a vinegar syrup made with seeds and the eating of salty fish with mustard, melon, and radish, with wines of different kinds, sweet, sour, or acid many times. After two hours water of anise or warm water with honey drunk with olive oil, or with a feather soaked in oil placed in the throat, especially with sesame, vomiting is induced. With[567] the eyes bound with two bandages of silk cloth and a light band over the stomach as it should be when the vomit has been completed the mouth should be rinsed with

[565]Galen, 11. 347; 18 A. 536; 17 B. 619.
[566]Celsus, *De Medicina* 1. 3. 21.
[567]Galen, 7. 235; 16. 142 sq.; 18 A. 484.

wine and rose water, hydromel or vinegar syrup and then a little syrup of apples should be swallowed, or a little mastic *[pistacia lentiscus]* added in water. The vomiter's face should be washed with rodostoma [rose water] or water mixed with vinegar so that the heaviness or ache in the head which sometimes occurs after vomiting may be pacified. He should beware of drinking plain water, going to sleep, anointing or smearing the hypochondrium, going to bathe, and going out soon after washing himself. He should have a meal with food of sweet flavor, good substance, and swift digestion. Theodorus Priscianus [xviii] recommends that certain measures be observed in vomiting for vomiting sometimes brings moisture to the body and relaxes it and sometimés dries it up. If anyone wishes to relax his body and soften his bowels after eating let him wait one or two hours until the entire body is refreshed with sweet and more humid foods. Then vomiting may be undertaken more efficiently. If anyone wishes to dry his body and constrain his bowels, immediately after eating he should shake himself before the juice of those foods descends to the inner part of the intestines so that then they may be forced to accept food more viscid, more biting and pungent to the tongue, of sharp flavor and saltier than was eaten before.

SNEEZING

Sneezing should by no means be excited in the old men of good health concerning whom we are discoursing. Indeed, insofar as it is possible it should be restrained in old age because of its difficulty. For old men are weak and cannot sneeze without hardship, as Aristotle writes.[568] The reason for this is that they cannot elevate the upper parts of the head on account of their weight since the brain is large and heavy and since these parts must be lifted during sneezing. The muscles necessary for this action are weak in old men just as are the muscles of the chest, throat, and face which assist in the process, including those near the diaphragm which support the lower abdomen.

[568]Aristotle, *H. A.* 492b6; *Probl.* 961b9, 962b4.

PICKING THE TEETH AND THE USE OF DENTIFRICE

Those instruments with which at some times one cleans the palate, gums, and teeth should be used by old men. The wooden toothpick should be selected as more comfortable since its nature is astringent and somewhat bitter, such as the bark of roots, nuts, small twigs, cypress sprigs or myrtle. The place where corrosion of the teeth takes place should be cleaned with small twigs or with lentiscus or with a feather, as the poet[569] says:

> Mastick is better; but if pointed wood be not forthcoming, a quill can relieve the teeth.

The teeth can be cleaned with a linen cloth dipped in rose water or wine (not sweet) and rubbed with a powder that restores their powers such as that made from squill, ginger, roses, scrapings of ivory, pumice, and charcoal recently made from wood and with the powder of clay vessels. These should not be used frequently for they discolor the teeth and scratch the gums. Rhazes [335] mentions dentifrice with nut shells; this will keep them straight and hard if used in moderation, for they strengthen the gums and fatten them and prevent cavities from forming in the teeth as well as sweetening the breath although they raise the head and the mouth of the stomach a very little. This is done with the bark of trees which provides astringency and bitterness. But if the teeth are cleaned in this manner very often they lose their gleam, wherefore it is wise not to do so frequently since the result will quickly be a great deal of uncleanliness, the shattering of the teeth and the thinning and weakening of the gums. They say the teeth can be picked all around with staphilinus, that is, wandering pastinaca (or opoponax) to free them from aching.[570]

THE USE OF DENTIFRICE IN PRESERVING THE HEALTH OF THE AGED

Recipe: Burnt deer horn, root of cyperus, spike of roses, one dram; salt crystals, six drams; all these pounded up, sifted, and mixed: use as dentifrice. With this and similar means the usual superfluities of the teeth of old people should be cleaned insofar as

[569]Martial, 14. 22.
[570]Pliny, *N. H.* 19. 88; 20. 30, 32, 264.

is possible. Both regions which betray no feeling as well as those which do should be purged of unnecessary matter, both because of the prime function of the members involved as well as because of the density of the body containing them, such as the brain, which is the seat of the reasoning soul, as Galen[571] calls it, which is contained depressed by bone and thus is purged of its superfluities through the nostrils, palate, ears, and through the sutures of the skull. Then for the sake of its accurate function the eye must be as clean as possible since that which flows to it from the brain is purged through the nostrils and eyelids. Imperceptible evacuations are made elsewhere than through the pores of the skin with the natural heat acting through exercise and the quantity of tempering that is applied to that heat. One of the advantages of exercise as was set forth in its place is to thin out, dissolve, bring together, and then imperceptibly and unobtrusively to evacuate the superfluities gathered in the body which nature is powerless to expel. The beginning of each evacuation of superfluities they say is the completion of the digestion, from which it is cut off, for thus the pure is segregated from the impure. This is done in order that the body may eject the impurities by expulsion lest remaining in the body they should produce a state of discomfort. In fact, none of the impurities should be retained in the body while their expulsion is urgent, certainly not urine or feces. Retention of the urine creates difficulties in urination and illness of the bladder and the parts lying adjacent to it. Such an unusual retention leads to flatulence, a mild form of dysentery, colic, loss of appetite, and nausea of the stomach.

[571]Galen, 3. 700; 5. 288, 521, 606, 649; 6. 73; 8. 159, 174; 10. 636; 15. 293, 360.

Chapter XLI

Retention Opposed to Elimination

Constipation, drunkenness, and obstruction are among those conditions which include retention or a presupposed repletion and are opposed to elimination; these must be observed in the resumptive regimen. Constipation occurs in old people just as it does at any age in men of whatever complexion and in all regions especially in the winter when the retentive power is used to aid the body in conserving its humidity for they say this is nothing more than the victory of the retentive power. However, since constipation is sometimes harmful because it retains the superfluities with foods and medicines controlling the bowels and bladder the harm created by constipation must be resisted. For as Averroes [6.94r] says the things which are more notable in the usage of old age are those in which the astringent power is not found because those things resist in both qualities that which is sought in them, i. e., astringency is lacking in the operations of both bladder and bowels among old people.

DRUNKENNESS

Drunkenness whereby a certain disturbance of the instruments of the senses is brought about in old men of frigid nature in frigid seasons and in a northern region is allowed sometimes by Abulkasim. He does not reject the pleasures of it since it offers relief to severe ills. This does not include that inebriety by which all rational activity is lost, which if frequent is seriously harmful to old men's bodies for it renders the nerves more weak and soft. This subject was discussed in the treatment of wine as part of the diet in chapter XVII.

CONSTIPATION

It remains for me to approach the problem of constipation which is very serious in the resumptive regimen, whether it results from the heaviness of the humors or their viscosity or their amount, for even though the constipation which arises from wine is moderate and light that from food is viscous and heavy, difficult to cure. According to Galen[572] old men are forbidden to eat chondrus, which is a kind of quite nourishing grain but viscous in nature. They should not eat, in addition, cheese and eggs (especially not fresh and quivering), snails, onions, lentils, and pork, much less eels and oysters and everything with hard and indigestible flesh, including hard-fleshed fish, deer, cattle, goat, and gazelle and to abstain from every constipating food and to counteract whatever constipation occurs from thick humors by the use of those things which dissolve and attenuate them so as to accomplish their easy expulsion. Thyme is a quite ideal remedy for this disposition; it relieves the ills of constipation in old people, as Avicenna says.[573] It thins out and dissolves the humor and has the power to comfort the affected viscera by cutting up and diffusing the viscous matter. Such remedies [i.e., thyme] cut through the viscous humors that adhere to the members, make a separation among them, and break them up into small parts. Through the length of the intestines they carry the viscosity like liquid glue. Frequent use of acetic squill *[acetum squillae]* or squill with oxymel for a more pleasing taste is effective especially when there are no other complications. Blood-letting, with flux of the bowels, or other similar methods can also be employed. Because constipation is a closing of the intestinal passages these must be opened by aperient means especially since old men easily run the risk of the affliction called strangury, whereby they urinate drop by drop instead of in a full stream. Diacalamentum, diatrion pipereon, and pepper pounded up with wine, as Avicenna says, aloes and onion if eaten in moderate amounts customarily, and theriac are useful for obstructions as well as athanasia and homorusia. After taking these remedies the

[572]Galen, 11. 495, 736; 12. 157; 15. 480; Pliny, N. H. 26. 49, 55.
[573]Avicenna, II, 714. See also I, fen. iii, doctrina iiii, f. 65 r.

old man's body should be smoothed in a bath with olive oil and food such as water of flesh in spelt and barley. Avicenna also mentions hydromel as very useful for the elderly in case of constipation. Such stoppages should be removed with means appropriate uniquely for the given member, such as the urinary passages, with the seed and root of celery or with stronger means if the obstruction is very hard, as with parsley. If the lung is obstructed then something like hyssop, Venus hair, wood cassia, or such as rob [the juice of any fruit thickened to the consistency of honey by evaporation], which they call *sapa* [thickened grape juice] or dulcor or carenum or more truly defrutum. These are helpful for spewing forth, as Avicenna reports. Therefore it should be constantly borne in mind that for a healthy man who is not cranky a reducing diet is sufficient as long as it is consistent.

Chapter XLII

The Emotions to Be Observed in the Resumptive Regimen

The gerontocomos should not only minister to the body of the old man but to his mind and soul as well, as Cicero says,[574] for these also unless you pour oil on them as onto a lamp are extinguished by old age. Old men's bodies grow heavy with the fatigue of exercise, but their minds are lifted up by it. So much the more should the soul than the body be exercised in the resumptive regimen insofar as the soul is more perfect than the body and dominates it. The exercise of the mind increases its strength to such an extent that many people are cured of their ills through sheer delight. So, just as for the protection of their health and the prolongation of their lives old men willingly obey the doctor's orders, so in respect to what concerns the emotions *(animae passiones)* they should do the same thing even more because the composition and nature of the body all of which the physician strives to preserve and rectify have an effect on the actions of the soul, as Galen says.[575] Thus if those emotions accompany the acquired behavior of the soul it will be difficult for the old man to obey the physician in regard to them. Hence they say that this custom (or habit or behavior) of the soul must be checked by laws, punishment, and by philosophy which will control it, a task which is not easy. Intemperance is one of these emotions of the soul, as the physicians say. Although primarily the emotions are parts of a whole nevertheless they are more principally attributed to the soul than to the body, as Avicenna reports, and especially to that part of the soul called the appetitive, as are the emotions of anger, sadness, joy, fury, fear, envy, and worry. They disturb and change bodies from that consistency which is according to nature, as Galen writes.[576]

[574]Cicero, *De Sen.* 36.
[575]Galen, 4. 779, 787, 788; 8. 191.
[576]Galen, 11. 59; 16. 301; 6. 40; 5. 441, health defined.

Therefore temperance or moderation among these emotions is to be chosen in the resumptive regimen and enjoined upon old men. Since joy and sadness are among the emotions which are associated with or accompanied by the movements of the spirits within and without they declare that joy is useful for old men because it banishes the pain of the body and mind by driving away its torment and leads the individual to happiness. It lends assistance to sluggish and gloomy old people of a cold nature in a cold season and in a chilly region, as Abulkasim reports. By means of such a joy the outflow of the vital spirit and heat is successively regulated by amplifying the first and dilatating the second from the heart to the separate members which when filled with both spirit and heat are extended. The fat and weight of the body increase, especially that of the person grown thin with sadness. The humors of the aged body are equalized and the heat is propelled and spread out to the extremities. Hence Rhazes [97, 111, 112] prescribed that old men should be exercised by or interested in those things which bring them delight, for whatever cogitation of the soul brings pleasure that also gives strength to the body's forces and stimulates its nature; it is of assistance in every action of healthy people. Such thoughts are also listed in the number of those things which humidify the body and accomplish a good digestion. On the contrary, sadness corrupts the digestion and destroys it. Joy also propels the blood to the skin with its dilatation and dissemination; therefore Avicenna counts it among the causes which bring a ruddy color. Hence a moderate and temperate joy is enjoined upon old men. If it exceeds the mean which is set down for them those who are weak in heart and of little heat and spirit die of too much joy suddenly announced to them. Many examples of this well-known phenomenon can be cited. For it happens, according to Galen, that because of its exhalation the spirit is driven swiftly from the heart to the extremities of the entire body. Other emotions similar to joy warn us that the spirits and heat should be enticed or attracted by old men with a light and gradual movement such as hope and love, not exceeding a moderate norm. They say that this approach induces in old men the disposition of youth, than which there is nothing more valuable in the resumptive regimen, for just as the youth in whom there is something of the old man is approved of so the old man in whom there is something of the youth is also approved, as Cicero says.[577] His body may become old but his mind will not. To hope and love should be added security of mind, for it fattens the body, as Celsus says,[578] and a quiet mind is one of the things which make life more blessed, according to Martial.[579] Hope, I say, should be moderate for an immoderate hope will dry up the body. Excessive love also which leads old age beyond its proper nature very quickly is discussed in chapter XLIII. Anger as well from all the emotions (with the exception of joy including its attendant complications) which is listed in the category of sadness Abulkasim says should be adjusted to the frigid nature of old men in winter and in frigid regions in their regimen and must be controlled with natural continence so that both fat and the body heat may be increased and restored. He who becomes excessively angry has abdicated his self-control. All anger, especially after meals, and all contention and agitation of mind as being not only useless but harmful to old men should be avoided. The old man becomes inflamed by such an emotion, his color turns yellow, he is afflicted with trembling, anxiety, and pernicious fever. If anger, however, is moderate it is of benefit to timid souls of frigid complexions for it drives the blood to the extremities and induces blushing, stops the veins, and creates sweating. In the temperament or modification of these emotions which they call the equalization of the habits or individual customs there consists both the protection and restoration of the mind and body since such a temperament is drawn from extrinsic causes which give rise to these emotions. It is in the power of these causes to vary effects in the old man's body and in this manner to cause the emotion to attain equality which in order to restore the health of the old man will not change with another effect that would destroy it.

CERTAIN VOLUNTARY OR NATURAL SENSIBILITIES OR EMOTIONS ATTACHED TO THE SOUL WHOSE EFFECTS ARE TO BE OBSERVED IN THE RESUMPTIVE REGIMEN

Not only do joy, hope, and love, since they are of equal value, wipe away the troubles of old age but they make it gentle and

[577]Cicero, *De Sen.* 38; Seneca, *Ep.* 36. 3.
[578]Celsus, *De Medicina* 1. 3. 15.
[579]Martial, 10. 47.

pleasant because they also carry into operation many other effects of a similar and fitting nature. From among these, the agreeable sensations presented to each of the senses which bring happiness to them are said to be created by the movement of the spirits which serve the powers of sense-perception and place the stamp of joy upon them.

CONCERNING THAT WHICH DELIGHTS THE EARS OF THE ELDERLY

The regimen of old age should not lack the harmony of music which consists in the modulation of song and sound. This entices the spirits of the aged and is accommodated to every old man at whatever season and in whatever region to soothe and delight his ears and his soul, as they say. Music has a great power not only to affect the rational soul but also the part of the soul which feels and which is possessed by brutes as well as humans. According to Abulkasim music was invented in order to induce the spirit toward healthful customs or habits, for the soul is delighted by musical harmonies, as Aristotle says,[580] because everyone rejoices in rhythm and song and in harmonious sounds since we rejoice in movements which are in accordance with nature. They say that the cause of this is a certain natural harmony within us constructed of the similitude of number and sound, according to Plato; Augustine follows him in speaking of the singular example of the nature of religion and adheres to his belief with all his might. He says: No one is harmonically composed who does not delight in harmonies. A sign of this is the fact that man rejoices in harmonies, they say, because infants as soon as they are born rejoice in the songs of their nurses lulling them to sleep, as Galen reports,[581] where he deals with the triple method used by nurses for this purpose: placing the child to her breast, the melody of her voice, and her gentle motion [rocking the cradle]. There is further agreement among the authors that harmony cures the ills of the soul, as may be seen in Plato's *Timaeus*.[582] Music is the most powerful of the arts and possesses a marvellous virtue for soothing the

[580]Aristotle, *Pol.* 8. 3.
[581]Galen, 2. 737; 6. 37 sq.
[582]Plato, *Timaeus* 47 D.

sorrows of the human soul and bringing it happiness. Indeed, in thus acting upon the emotions it may be said that tunes and songs act upon the ills of the spirit as medicines do upon bodily ills. Loaded camels and mules rejoice and are comforted by the singing of their muleteers and drivers, as Abulkasim reports. Thus music changes the soul with its harmony as it does the body. Avicenna [I, 69–70, 73–75] tells us that the same is true of blood-letting operations which drive the blood to the surface of the skin when a song is sung during the process. Asclepiades tells of a certain mad physician who was restored to sanity by a concert, and David snatched Saul away from an unclean spirit with his harp-playing [I Samuel 18. 10–11].

THE ADVANTAGES OF CONVERSATION IN THE RESUMPTIVE REGIMEN

Conversations not only induce the elderly to sleep but increase the blood and spirit in them, helping to complete digestion of the food taken before bed time, cheering the old man's soul and diverting it from sad thoughts. Thus it is assigned in the class of quiet and play which, as Aristotle says,[583] are necessary in life. All this will result if the conversation concerns those subjects which please the mind of the elderly, such as the deeds of a well-spent life. This is true to such an extent that no conversation is more pleasant or suitable than that which praises an old man's past activities, for the habit of old men is to boast about themselves, as Cicero says.[584] A placid and gentle old age is one attached to a lifetime spent quietly and simply. But since there are as many men as there are opinions and judgments and desires *(quot homines tot sententiae)* conversations must be varied in the resumptive regimen according to the desire of the old man concerned. One pursuit delights one old man, other pursuits delight others; there are some who are not hindered from farming by their old age, as they say. Others like history, love stories, accounts of fights and quarrels, the taking of military outposts, and such like, whose reciters or singers they call bards in French, who sing the praises of brave men. In all these old age rejoices more in talking about them than

[583]Aristotle, *Pol.* 8. 3.
[584]Cicero, *De Sen.* 82.

in listening, for old age is by nature loquacious. Hence the poet's words:

> Brave oldsters, brave in babbling alone![585]

This diversity of interest arises from the varied nature of old men themselves so that they are delighted not only in conversation and in riddles but in the pleasures of all kinds of knowledge, sometimes in physical problems in science, sometimes in theological matters and in rhetorical discussions. Certain old people following rather the good in nature and study, as Albertus says, whose complexion of spirit and subtle heat and luminous humor are not constantly freezing with cold nor disturbed with the mingling of heat are delighted with divine and more subtle topics. Those whose organs of imagination are excellently prepared for entertaining images or symbols and are not frozen through temperate and complexional dryness have an intellect bent toward imagination. These rejoice in doctrinal and mathematical studies and such like. Those whose sense organ is quite full of marrow with a lucid spirit not mixed with sluggishness or freezing cold will have an organ of imagination that does not retain figures well and their intellect will be bent toward the senses. These are inclined toward pleasant speculations on natural and mobile subjects insofar as what is mobile is also somewhat divine and marvellous. Those whose spirits are frozen and not very clear because they are thickened with the cold are occupied with rhetorical figures and will be held fast by them nor will they plunge into any speculation on the truth. But conversation will be more pleasant for old men in proportion as the story teller or reciter is of perspicacious talent in matters of rhythm and verse and in every kind of discourse in which the excellently educated old man who is being cared for has been accustomed to take pleasure. Let him be cautious in prolonging, abbreviating, continuing, adorning, and setting in order his opinions according to opportunity so that the course of the conversation should not be turned aside by his long-windedness. Let him be a "little heart" *(corculus),*[586] that is, skillful in introducing jokes, a careful connois-

[585]Maximianus, *Elegies* 1. 204.
[586]A nickname for Scipio Nasica on account of his sagacity: Cicero, *T. D.* 1. 9. 18; *Brut.* 20. 70; Aur. Vict., *Vir. Ill.* 44. 6.

seur of tales and delightful bits of gossip, and good at observing his method of narration without changing his facial expression [i.e., a poker face]. Let him be witty, urbane, *articus,* that is, well educated in the liberal arts, courtly, let him avoid mere blather,[587] that is, stupid and over-eager elocution, let him not atticize or sicilicize [i.e., speak affectedly as an Attic or a Sicilian orator], that is, let him speak consistently in one style. Let him, however, sometimes employ blandishments, ironic scoffing,[588] and let him be sturdy at staying awake nights so that he can carry on amidst all these forms of conversation with complete delight, which he can do beautifully if the old man, although of rather delicate nature, may tolerate more patiently the fellow conversationalist who stays up all night talking with him.

COMFORTS TO THE SIGHT OF THE ELDERLY

The spirits which serve the power of vision rejoice in a moderate light similar to themselves, as the authors agree, because they are either light themselves or bear the image of light. An immoderate or too bright a light is harmful; it dissolves and dissipates the vision of old people in particular since it is already diminished. Lights can blind one so that objects can barely be discerned. Old people need to repair or take care of their eyesight as if with another Euelpides, who was once the greatest of eye doctors. They need to look at some colors in a moderate light which will assist their sight, such as, from among many, the color of things deeply dyed with what they call *coccus, kermes* in Arabic [cochineal kermes] or scarlet, which shines out from roses. Nothing more pleasant is presented to the sight, as Pliny says.[589] Similarly, the color amethyst, which is the color of a precious gem of a violet color, and the color of the mallow flower,[590] which is yellow; it is also the color of the broom flower or of the yolk of an egg. This color was held in the highest honor at weddings among the an-

[587]Auct. Carm. Philomel 56: *blacteram,* bleating of a ram.
[588]Paul. ex Fest. p. 45 Müller: *cavillatio est jocosa calumnatio.* Plautus, *Men.,* prologue; and Apuleius, *Florida,* n. 18, p. 302, 12, mention the affected oratory of the Attic and Sicilian speakers.
[589]Pliny, *N. H.* 9. 140; 16. 32.
[590]Ibid., 37. 121.

cients with their flame-colored garments.[591] Emerald green is also among the colors which assist the sight by concentrating objects of vision which are scattered. Likewise, the color blue, which is between green and black, is agreed among all authors to strengthen the sight of old men.[592] Their sight is harmed, however, by the color white and every light that is too bright. It is good for old people to look frequently at visible objects of great beauty. Avicenna reports that among things which create a good shining color it is pleasant to watch the blood moving toward the skin as it is spread abroad in the body and to sit dressed in fine clothes and to view the sight of those who are suing each other at law concerning pledges in victory and engaging in a divorce proceeding and other affairs.

COMFORTS TO THE SENSE OF SMELL

They say that the very fragrant substances called spices are healthy for old age and that their aid and convenience for human nature are not without value because they contribute to the soundness of the heart, just as with their odor alone they repair the force of the soul by contributing to its spirits and powers. They furnish it with food as well as a proper proportion of air prepared for receiving light and incline the spirit to its aromatization, by which it is restored and refreshed. It is helpful for old men to smear their face and head with the very fragrant rob and with its suffumigations, as Rhazes says [61, 264]. Such fragrances are not to be considered only as a mark of luxury in the resumptive regimen since that would be unnecessary but as a well-known aid to maintaining good health for he who wears a scent does not smell it himself but delights some one else, as Pliny says.[593] The authors are accustomed to call aromatic everything made from the most odorous flowers of all kinds, for their nature is warm, Galen writes,[594] although this is not strictly true, as appears from the rose, violet, myrtle, pond lily, and especially from camphor and sandalwood. Aromas seem to have drawn their name, as one finds in Dios-

[591]Ibid., 21. 46.
[592]Galen, 3. 641; 17 A. 723.
[593]Pliny, *N. H.* 13. 20.
[594]Galen, 17 B. 819.

corides, either from the practice of placing them upon altars accompanied by divine invocations or because they are proven to be inserted into and mingled with the air.[595] For what is odor but a contraction of air, [i.e., a drawing together or concentration of air]? The scent of herbs or simples which bring aid to old age comes from many of them, such as wood aloes. It is of a warm and dry nature to the second degree and very helpful to old men of especially frigid nature in winter in northern regions since it increases and multiplies the vital spirits, Abulkasim reports. It is of thin substance, opens obstructions, dissipates flatulence, and removes humid superfluity especially of the organs of the liver, stomach, brain, and nerves whose strength it repairs. It improves bad breath. The heavy black variety of aloes should be selected. Musk also has its high position as a scent since its odor is most praiseworthy. It is of a warm dry nature to the second degree and increases the strength of the brain and heart. It is very salutary for old people of especially cold nature in winter and in northern regions. Ambra [ambergris] is similarly of warm nature to the second degree and dry to the first degree and is of great assistance with its thinness and heat to the brain and the senses, arouses boldness, multiplies the spirits, and therefore restores old men of especially cold and humid nature in winter in the northern region. According to Abulkasim the lily is to be listed among the scents because it is next to the rose in nobility and to its warmth and dryness is added an especially heavenly aroma. Its root particularly dissolves the supervacuities of the brain and is helpful to old men. Many other flowers abounding with a pleasant odor are prescribed, such as citron peel. Since all aged bodies have diminished blood and spirit they require restoration, as Haly Rodoan writes, with joy and the sight of delightful things such as the sky, the stars, water, and a good color streaked with white, and precious vessels of gold and silver in which the food and drink are served. The vessels should not be made of brass for one must be careful not to serve food in which there is salt or bitterness or fat, such as vegetables and meat, or acidity, or sweetness in brass vessels or to drink from them, for they will beyond doubt cause ziniar [corrosion of

[595]Pliny, *N. H.* 9. 18: *Odorem quidem non aliud quam infectum aera intellegi possit.*

brass filings in acid and salts of ammonia] and ziniar is poisonous.[596] Old men need the pleasure derived from stories which cause laughter and merriment and from suffumigations and pleasant odors. They should not abstain from any kind of hilarity by which the spirit of the old folks can find a relaxation from business affairs and in which it is good to indulge. Care should be taken, however, that giving way to lively emotions old men should not slip into indecent acts and that they should be regarded as decent people. For although we praise a young man who is shamefast we would not ever praise an old man for being so since he ought not to do anything of which he might be ashamed.[597]

[596]Avicenna, II, 750.
[597]Aristotle, *N. E.* 4. 1128b15–20.

Chapter XLIII

Permission and Prohibition of Sex in the Resumptive Regimen

Sex should simply be avoided by old men, as the experts say, and they should live a celibate life worthy of heaven since from the orifices of their veins and small arteries all over the body no superfluity exudes back to the testicles and seminal vessels. This fact must be considered because old men lose much more superfluity than they gain. It happens in general also among old men who are fasting when they engage in sex whatever effusion of semen is made in their testicles is evacuated as superfluity and thus attracts from the entire body whatever superfluity is not like flatulence. Assisting in this process is a friction of the genital parts and a warming of them through frequent coition. When the nourishment is removed, nay rather, snatched away from the old man's members by the first coagulation[598] this then stands more or less in the place of what has been lost. Since the semen itself is a superfluity of the ultimate useful nourishment it happens that the substance of the members is diminished and dried up and the entire body of the aged man becomes weaker than it does from the effusion of any other superfluity, in fact, more than from blood-letting. As was said, the prime part of the food is snatched away by the coagulation. Since in coitus there is also an abundant evacuation of the spirits of motion which is increased by the delight of the act they are ejected with the semen and from all pores of the body just as in a state of enjoyment it happens that the powers which stood in need of the spirits become deficient as lacking their proper instrument. Thus when the warmth and humidity in which the life of the old man consists are evacuated a speedy death results. For

[598]Aristotle, *G. A.* 1. 729a10.

those old men who are in the first stage of old age sex is not entirely forbidden as it is for those more advanced in old age, for the powers of the former are not so weak nor the frigidity and dryness of their bodies so great. A less frequent indulgence in sex is nevertheless advisable for them and great care should be exercised in the act. All this is confirmed by Haly Abbas in the fifty-first opinion *(sententia)* of his *Theorice.* His words are these: Adults should diminish their sexual activity as much as they can; old men should also avoid sex entirely. It is quite clear from his statement that with the exception of youth and adolescence coitus is very harmful to other ages of man, preventing boys from growing and drawing old men into bodily decrease. But if in any way sex may be permitted to old men let the act be carried out at such a great interval of time that the old man may not feel the weakening of strength from it. It is not without its usefulness for those who do not feel languor or pain afterwards. Sometimes it is worse to engage in sex during the daylight; it is safer at night so long as one does not eat food afterwards nor stay awake a long time. Sex is not useful in summer or autumn, although it is more tolerable in autumn. If one can find it possible sex should be completely avoided in summer. Nevertheless, it is difficult for old men as it is for those at other stages of life to curb the use of sex since, as they say, sobriety vanishes when the check rein is removed. So it is with this act because of the great delight it produces. Hence it is possible to commit a great variety of sins due to sex for the power of concupiscence, according to Aristotle, obeys the reason less than do the other powers, as is proven by the fact that the angry man is more obedient to reason than the concupiscent man.[599]

[599]Aristotle, *N. E.*, III, 1111b18–20; VII, 1149b21–23. Celsus, *De Medicina* 1. 1. 4 also discusses the frequency of the sex-act.

Chapter XLIV

The Disposal of Abundant Unnecessary Phlegm in Old Age

Since phlegmatic and extraneous humidities collected in old men adhere externally to their members which by reason of age have already dried up these press upon them and induce the chill of death and the suffocation of the natural heat which makes life short. Therefore the generation of these humidities must be prevented by all means and those which have been generated must be expelled insofar as is possible. Their collection is prevented first of all by the equalization of the resumptive regimen in the six non-naturals, which have been discussed already in their place. Care must be taken in regard to the administration of those things which cause humidities, such as the use of those foods which cause obstructions, including legumes, watery fruits, fresh vegetables, fish, food prepared with milk, boiled wheat, and especially the immoderate use of these, the drinking of cold water particularly of heavy substance, the use of cold things which are touched often, such as rose water, camphor, whose use hastens gray hairs, Avicenna[600] says, opium, mandragora, nenuphar [water lily], and poison hemlock. To these they add excessive sleep after eating and still more between day and night, drunkenness, intoxication, excessive sex, and too frequent use of all these. Extraneous humidity which collects in old men should be counteracted by rectifying or reducing it through the equalizing effect of things which digest it and serve to evacuate it so that its dyscrasy (or distemperance) may be opposed; this is frequently warm. In general use for this purpose are myrobalanus and chebula, both of them highly praised. Their powers are able to consume the supervacuity con-

[600]Avicenna, II, 134.

tained in the stomach, to dry it up with their astringency. They are stimulative to the stomach and purify the blood of its melancholic humor. Thus these herbs are useful for those of melancholic temperament. They brighten up the body and bring a glow to the flesh and skin. For older people of cold and warm nature bezoartic substances have a marvellous power to assist them, as all authors agree. Thus a continual daily mastication of these [calculous concretions] for a year can add youth to the end of life, as Avicenna says. If the mass of these humidities has collected in the old men's chests or lungs, producing a cough and a breathing difficulty and a wracking sound, they say that a good remedy is a syrup of horehound *(prasium)* for old men of frigid nature with asthma, especially frequent among them. This will remove a particularly thick and putrid phlegm, as Mesue [f. 42] says. Hyssop is also good for chest and lung difficulties and for coughs, if there is bad chyme collected in the stomach which has flowed there from elsewhere. The descent of phlegm is from the head to the stomach, as happens with most men and especially at Rome, according to Galen,[601] and in regions which according to their locations are humid. The use of certain warm herbs is also recommended as assisting the digestion, such as cloves, aloes, nutmeg, galanga, cubeb, ginger, cinammon, pepper, three kinds of aromatic reed, and grains of paradise.[602] From among compounds used for the same purpose the more effective are, first, ginger with sugar, citron peel also with sugar, which draws phlegm and black bile contained in the brain. All of these remedies are praised when dissolved in wine, then strained and drunk; this mixture is recommended and penetrates more easily to the separate members. In them it is changed so that the extraneous humid phlegm found in the foramina of the members is disposed of, the power of digestion increased, and the blood restored. The use of these remedies should be estimated to prevent old people of warmer and drier nature from having a more heated liver that almost burns them up. Sometimes they should eat clove in wine or pomegranates mixed with vinegar. Powders which dispose of raw putrid phlegm in old men are those which strengthen the original power and bodily forces especially of

[601]Galen, 1. 630.

[602]See *graine d' aspic* in R. Dunglison, op. cit. 433 *(amomum granum paradisi).*

the stomach without damaging those who are warm in nature. The recipe includes powder of pearls, gold, cubebs, musk, galingale, cypress, spikenard, basil, licorice, and a bit of crocus and sugar in parts of each to make up a pound in all. Nothing finally is thought to be more advantageous for the evacuation of these humidities than agaric, especially when there is need for it, since it draws out phlegm and the black bile contained in the brain and chest. Furthermore, it is suggested that the brain of old men be taken care of lest, becoming rheumatic, it should bring on catarrhs, swellings of the tonsils, and colds. According to Hippocrates these ills do not develop in the very old if a salutary remedy made of substances which have an odor good for the brain has been applied. Placing powdered clove or laudanum or mace upon the coronal commissure of the skull with a smearing of the head with olive oil mixed with spices especially in the winter but rose water in the summer in which mace has been ground up is recommended.

Chapter XLV

The Care of Wrinkles of a Disfiguring Type and Discoloration in Old Age and Their Conversion to Pallor and a Leaden Color

It is impossible to prevent the arrival of wrinkles and gray hairs as described previously no less than of age itself while man passes through all the stages of life until death. It is worth trying to retard them although it is difficult. The difficulty arises from the fact that these changes occur because of the weakness of the third digestive power which it is hard to correct. The reason is that the third power of digestion is situated in the most apparent members in which there is no basis nor strength of nature. These are the vile or inferior members in comparison with the principal members. This is the reason why the error of the second digestion cannot be corrected by the third digestion as the error of the first may be corrected by the second. Hence arises the difficulty of correcting the dispositions and the accidents which occur by reason of the error of the third digestive power. The cures we urge for this situation are of the following sort. For the retardation of accidents beyond the necessary equalization of the six non-naturals (custom being also observed) special efforts must be taken that everything be done in regard to the quantity of the digestion for this is the very root of this intention, as Avicenna reports.[603] For from the corrupted digestion corrupt blood is generated, and hence the humors become impure. Special care must be taken in rectifying the digestive force by certain ingenious means which are nevertheless most rare. The greater difficulties by far are due to the error of the first digestion. Some of these are overcome by the force of the third

[603]Intention implies the subdivision of instructions, as Zerbi uses the term in his treatise on kidney stone (see Introduction).

digestion. First, unguents can be used externally made from black mullein, white bryony, melissa calamintha, celery, and root of lapathum rumex. Another and uniquely special remedy is the assiduous eating of viper flesh prepared in the manner which will be described in its place. This slows the accumulation of wrinkles and in fact removes them. For when the wrinkled skin lacks those elements which renew it by purging with blushing and glowing the skin as far as is possible is restored to its pristine condition so that it may be brought back to its youthful beauty. This is properly brought about by those means which stretch the skin itself and purify the blood. The skin is laid bare and extended when whatever is dead is removed from it and the skin is softened and cleansed by such a gentle extension and soft cleansing and made more subtle. This is most aptly the result of rather frequent eating of viper flesh. By its means the repaired skin is excoriated and renewed with a marvellous power and the superfluities which come up to the skin from the body are expelled. This is proven by experiment by those who eat vipers that from the bodies of those who have vitiated humors in them the superfluities issue forth like scales. All this happens through some strange property of the flesh by which the superfluities adhere to the humors and bring them to the skin, especially that which is thick and earthy among them, and which induce scabies and other ills by which the skin is raised, made swollen, and injured. They say that some Ethiopians[604] who inhabit Mount Athos because they are nourished on viper flesh are free from all poisonous insects both in their hair and their clothing. I shall describe the preferred method of preparing serpent flesh in what follows in its proper place. Nor should I pass over in silence the fact which among authors has great acclaim, that gold is useful in extending human life, as will be discussed a little later (chapter LIII). In addition to these in order to renew wrinkled skin the spirits and blood must be moved toward the cutaneous areas, for this process brings cleansing, red color, and the picture of youthful beauty to the face. Anything which cleanses the skin with a gentle abstersion will do this, removing gently whatever is ugly and dead that exists upon it. There are many ways of bringing the blood to the surface of the skin, such as heat, cold, wind,

[604]Pliny, *N. H.* 7. 27.

which also make the blood thinner. Some other means include pulse *[Lathyrus cicera* Linn.*]*, fresh sucking eggs, water of flesh, fragrant wine, and figs; these generate a thin blood transmitted to the skin and on account of this they create lice, as Avicenna reports.[605] Pliny[606] says figs bring better health to old men and less wrinkles, for they propel nourishment to the skin and are uniquely efficient in opening the passageways of nutrition if they are eaten on an empty stomach and especially with nuts and almonds. A decoction of figs and dates which are not quite ripe often drunk warm at dawn is recommended as helpful. No less effective are four ounces of goat milk with two ounces of fragrant white wine drunk at the same time and continued for days. These two remedies add to the supply of thinner blood and innate heat. Similarly, the eating of bitter almonds whose function is to open obstructions which occur in the extremities of the veins is useful. Almond oil is also quite effective, as Pliny[607] relates, for it removes wrinkles and promotes a healthy facial glow. There are also other remedies devised for the same purpose which move the blood toward the skin with dilatation and diffusion. These are pepper, cypress, clove, and crocus (although it dyes the blood). These should be taken in boiled wine. Iris [flag root] provides a good color to the cheeks. In the entire resumptive regimen the eating of certain praiseworthy foods should not be overlooked for they bring no small aid in promoting a youthful appearance in old people and to the rectification of a leaden color, according to Avicenna:[608] pomegranates, chick peas, fragrant wines, egg yolks, chicken broth, partridge, turtle dove (both well fed), and everything which can conserve the heat of the heart in balance lest it exceed its limits. Thus health is preserved and life and old age extended. Four of these means are praised as more effective than all others; two of them warm up old age with the heat adjusted to that period of life: wine, especially aromatic, whose powers in restoring old age are discussed in their place; and cinnamon, likewise, especially not older than three years, which is very warming in its effect, nourishing and creating happiness,

[605] Avicenna, II, 283.
[606] *N. H.*, 21. 126; 23. 120.
[607] Pliny, *N. H.* 13. 82; 21. 127; 26. 22; 28. 183, 254.
[608] Avicenna, II, 132.

preserving the body from putrefaction and stirring up its natural heat. Two means for humidifying the innate heat of the heart and keeping it in balance are, one, fresh sucking eggs from healthy animals, with sugar; two, chicken broth, or water of flesh, which serve both to heat and humidify equally. To these should be added human female milk, which is very nourishing. Finally, they say that potable gold excels all other means for the same purpose; it will be discussed in chapter LIII.[609] It is prescribed in addition that the old man should be prepared to perspire so that his skin may be cleansed and purged of superfluities. Then he should be fed with nourishing foods so as to acquire a disposition similar to that of youth. Cassius Felix[610] calls local and topical certain other aids applied to the skin by whose power wrinkles are overcome. Experts praise a sap issuing from the tops of trees called dirdar, that is, elm, which cleanses the face of old men, they say.[611] The root of the garden-grown lily also cleanses the face with its juice and brings about a tightening of the skin, says Avicenna.[612] According to Serapio the son sesame oil stretches the wrinkles of the skin and softens it. Pounded bitter almonds will cause the skin to contract when it is smeared around the face and smoothed down, as Avicenna says.[613] Almond oil has similar properties, for Pliny[614] writes that it purges and softens the body, removes wrinkles, increases the glow of the countenance. Pimples, spots, and freckles appearing on the face, especially in women, can be removed with honey, as Celsus[615] says. The flesh of a lion[616] with rose water keeps the face free from blemishes and preserves its fresh appearance. Women use oil of tartar to remove wrinkles. Sesser root made into trochisci is used to clear up the facial skin and the juice of dracontium root [hellebore], water of the root of sea parsley [lovage], barley water, and bean flowers are used for the same purpose. Asses' milk is also good for removing wrinkles and re-

[609]Ibid., II, 444.
[610]See note 512.
[611]Pliny, *N. H.* 24. 48.
[612]Avicenna, II, 447.
[613]Ibid., II, 58.
[614]Pliny, *N. H.* 23. 79, 85; 26. 22; 28. 254; 26. 7, on freckles; 22. 57; 23. 19, 85.
[615]Celsus, *De Medicina* 6. 5. 2.
[616]Pliny, *N. H.* 24. 165.

storing the facial glow, as Pliny[617] writes, for they say that Poppaea, the wife of Domitius Nero, used to take with her five hundred asses with foal and used to bathe her entire body in their milk, thinking that it made her skin softer. The hoof of a white[618] heifer soaked for forty days and nights in liquid until it is dissolved and smeared with a cloth lends a glow to the skin and removes wrinkles. From pharmaceutics, that is, mixed or compounded drugs, is made an antidote of equal parts of water of cheese and wine which are boiled in pomegranate peel until reduced by half; when smeared on the face it removes wrinkles. Dioscorides gives a recipe for removing blemishes and wrinkles made of bitter almond oil and lily root ground up fine and sifted with rose water and wax added to make an unguent [I, 176]. Some people add honey and iris root [blue flag, orris] because they stretch out wrinkles. The root of wild cucumber pounded, sieved, and steeped in water cleanses the face. Fish gluten dissolved in water does the same. Lead oxide whitened in goat oil and used as an unguent is of special use against wrinkles; the lead oxide whitened (which was previously red) with fat of an ass and the juice of caraway seed and pistachio oil or flax seed added is also helpful. Washing the face with a compound of starch and tragacantha [gum dragon] with milk for a day is recommended by Avicenna. For wrinkles already existing in old men especially in the cornea tunic of the eyes a frequently salutary remedy is a fomentation made with boiled barley water, roses, violets, pond lilies, and such like together with an assiduous dropping of female human milk upon the eyes.

[617]Ibid., 11. 238.
[618]Ibid., 28. 184.

Chapter XLVI

The Retardation of Gray Hair

The delaying of gray hair is similarly of great importance in the proper regimen of the six non-naturals. Their primary purpose in reference to hair is attained by the use of those means which evacuate the watery putrid excessive phlegm rather frequently and which destroy and prevent it, properly by vomiting food, as Avicenna reports, and with clysters and rest. This treatment should be varied with the repetition of the same foods of good chyme with temperateness which produce excellent thick blood, that is, foods which are fried in a skillet and such as are cooked in covered containers without water and roasted without juice or gravy. All of this food should be prepared with good digestion in view since they affirm this to be the root of the disposition required for a cure since the corruption of the digestion alters the blood toward corruption also. It is agreed that condiments and spices cut away the material of the phlegm and retard gray hair and conserve youth. Such preparations as theriac and mithridate, which will be discussed in their place, do so also. They must be used for an entire year and taken at mid-day.[619] People say that the frequent chewing of myrobalanus chebula resists gray hair marvellously. Since the old man's nature is quite humid these remedies should be administered while warm, such as mustard, pepper, salt water, and a moderate amount of unmixed wine. A discussion of the causes of gray hair appears in the preceding chapter V, to which copious blood-letting must be added together with the pulling-out of hairs, drunkenness, and excessive sex. Camphor is used to combat gray hairs as well as rose water, elderberry oil and much use of fresh water. Applied externally to the hairs they strengthen them and retard grayness when this method

[619]See R. Dunglison, op. cit., 597, 908 on these terms.

is followed: wash the hair not only in fresh water which is soon dried but with water mixed with herbs such as the pulp of a bitter apple or cucumber *[cucumis colocynthis]*, nutmeg flower, borax *[baurach]*, and the bile of a bull. Liniments adapted for the same purpose are hot oil which restores strength, as Avicenna reports,[620] and similar substances, for they preserve the natural innate heat of the hair and because it is not made moist nourishment penetrates to it. Other helpful substances are pinus silvestris [tar] and humid pitch running thin. Oil of costus is efficacious as well as that of nigella [fennel and nutmeg flower, St. Catherine's flower] and oil of black mustard. The peeling of a leek boiled and smeared on the head inhibits gray hairs, as do oil of unripe or wild olives frequently smeared on and oil of a lily. Elder oil boiled with bitter apple *[cucumis colocynthis]* with seed and flesh first removed and then rolled into a paste boiled three or four times combats gray hairs. The hair should first be soaked in a bath made from a decoction of pistachio, cabbage, and alum. Many people add to this antidote grains of euphorbia lathyris [*cataputia minor,* spurge] ground up and cleaned. Other decoctions include water of oak galls *[quercus infectoria]*, salvia or sage and betonica with which the hair should be frequently washed. When the hair has been frequently washed in water in which much alum and tincture of alum has been dissolved and then dried it should be smeared with the juice of green nuts; this should not be allowed to dry for the hair even if gray will become black. Nor should the suffusion of the hair with good fragrances be omitted for these open the obstructions of the brain and of the sense organs. In this manner the powers of the principal members are repaired and the extraneous humidities which make hair gray are removed together with wrinkles, the face is made radiant and thus both wrinkles and gray hair are retarded. In order to facilitate this process the face should be cleansed of dirt and the pores opened for the expulsion of the excess humors.

[620]Avicenna, II, 533.

Chapter XLVII

The Means of Retarding Baldness

The cure of baldness is difficult, as Avicenna writes, especially since loss of hair comes in the course of nature, as with old men. In fact, there is no remedy to stop the heads of some people from becoming bald through age although it is possible to resist the threat of falling hair before it begins or to slow the process after it has begun. Remedies to conserve hair and to prevent it from falling are made from herbs such as myrtle and grains of ladanum,[621] emblicus, myrobalanus [bennut], chebula, myrrh, aloes, Venus's hair, and nut galls because of their astringency. From the pharmaceutical body of mixtures and compounds those recommended are (as above) myrtle, galls, emblicus boiled twice in rose oil or myrtle oil, one pound of dry wine, a half grain of ladanum, one ounce of pine bark burned to ash, Venus's hair three ounces, one pound of bear fat which is better than goose grease, three ounces of winter cherry, boiled with ladanum in wine until it grows thick; then mix with medicines and lay aside. Dissolve some of it in oil of nard and smear it on the hair. Baldness in old men results from an excess dryness of complexion and lack of blood. Nutritious and delicious foods should be served in the resumptive regimen such as are fat and mildly warm, salty and with vinegar also and astringent foods. The sexual act is to be avoided as well as sarcocolla [tree gum][622] in old wine for frequent drinking of it brings baldness especially to old men, as Avicenna reports.[623] Frequent baths are recommended in fresh water without the use of soap with natron of lichen saxatilis on the head but a mixture of farina, bean, seed of melon, carbonate of lime, and

[621]Pliny, *N. H.* 26. 48.
[622]Ibid., 13. 67; Dioscorides 3. 99.
[623]Avicenna, II, 542, 599.

psyllium is allowed, thickened with ash and the hair of an ass able to reproduce. Grayness may be avoided if the hair is shaved and smeared with the fat of a bear, as Pliny [624] writes. Scanty eyebrows can be repaired with ladanum as well as with lamp-black and soot from a lantern's beak. Drinking and smearing nasturtium can retain falling hair, Avicenna[625] writes.

[624] Pliny, *N. H.* 28. 163. 164.
[625] Avicenna, II, 513.

Chapter XLVIII

The Means of Purifying the Blood

Old men require those substances which cleanse the blood since it has in it no small amount of a mixture of infected serous humidity and fecal matter. The blood can be purified by the use of herbs, pearls, and the juice of fresh fumitory *[fumaria officinalis]* made into a residue, camphor administered in a proper way, myrobalanus, and especially chebula and trifera minor, as Avicenna says, and medicines which wash the blood and soften it such as cassia, fistula, tamarind, violet, plum, infusion of rhubarb, goat serum, borage, lupulus, and medicines which purge the bad humor.

Chapter XLIX

Discussion of the Means for Restoring the Spirit

The gerontocomos ought to strive as earnestly as he can to revive and restore the spirits since they are the principle of life, according to Avicenna. This section will be completed by the use of those things which restore the spirits, such as, among many, thin white fragrant wine which is salutary, as are fresh sucking eggs and especially the yolk. Water of flesh, the brains of acceptable animals, and especially of birds are also used. Very effective are elixir and potable gold, which will be discussed in their place. These things which brighten the spirits with a certain splendor are useful, such as pearls. Ideal also are substances which bring together that which is dispersed and prevent it from breaking up, such as carab and embulicus [emblicus].[626] The best remedies are those which correct the weakened complexion of the spirits and which when chilled must be revived with warm substances such as melissa, arnica, musk, ambra [ambergris], rose water with vinegar, and camphor. There are many other remedies for regeneration and revival with their special quality of effectiveness such as hyacinth [squill], smaragdus, and such like. Some of these operate by separating spirit from substance such as bugloss, which separates the melancholy vapors or fumes from the spirits and the black bile from the blood with its special property. Some clarify the blood and purge it, such as Venus's hair, lupulus, and the juice of fumiterra [fumitory]. There are certain remedies which with a moderate and gentle motion suitable for old age exercise the spirits, such as pleasant thoughts, the sight of desirable things, the hearing of song and harmonies, and so on. There are others which protect the spirits by their venomous quality and by other hidden or manifest properties, such as among many the zedoaria plant

[626]Ibid., II, 228, 374.

[Kaempferia, from Ceylon], the bezoar, and theriac. Other effective restoratives include as the authors agree such things as plasters, liniments, epithemata,[627] poultices of astringents of pleasant odor which combat the diminution of the heart's heat. Among so many salutary aids I must not omit the massage of the spinal column to stimulate its powers, which has been much praised, for nature, the parent of every governing force, properly repairs and protects the duration of human life and is the guardian of the vital spirit. For this purpose we can assign camomile oil and turpentine in equal parts. The Conciliator[628] records the ancient practice of massaging the spinal column praised by the experts in memory of the great benefits hidden in the process of handling that part of the anatomy in this fashion and preserving this area of life with such fine assistance. The beginning of the bones and nerves resides in the nape of the neck *(nuca)* generated from the brain and of the spine, which is the public marketplace of the arteries, nerves, spirits, and powers and is the couch of the spiritual members, containing the marrow of true humidity. Thus very much that is useful is assembled here where the spiritual and protective substance is repaired and manifest assistance rendered to the nerves when they are weak and to the vacillation, tremor, and weariness of the heart. Frequent rubbing of the spine with almond oil is protection against its curvature, which happens to old men, as Judeus [f. cxxii], led by experience, declares.

[627]Of three kinds: liquid, dry, and soft in fomentations, bags filled with dry substances, and cataplasms: R. Dunglison, op. cit. 849.
[628]See note 160.

Chapter L

The Qualities of Snake Flesh and the Method of Preparing It

This flesh has a peculiar virtue in strengthening the third digestive power which is carried out in the members. Eating it extends life, protects the senses, and repairs the youthful state, as Avicenna[629] reports. Finally, it seems to have a very marvellous power often to protect old age. The manner in which it does this has been described in its place earlier. Since some people thus use snakes in the shape of food hence they are called vipers because they give birth by an inner force *(vi)*.[630] When the young vipers in the uterus do not wait for the natural solution of birth they chew out the mother snake's sides and burst out by force. People teach that the vipers should be chosen for eating at the end of spring and the beginning of summer because if it were a wintry spring they would be driven back into the uterus of the mother until the beginning of hot weather from the mountains. Of the vipers those should be chosen which live in dry places, not watery or flooded, and are of a yellow color and especially with white belly and black back, for those with a white back are weak but the black ones are stronger. They say the females are more praiseworthy than the males because the strength of the latter is not excessive. Their sex can be determined by the great number of teeth found in each side of the mouth in the females. In males there is only one. The tame snakes are better than the wild ones. In their appearance they have a flat broad head, a very thin small neck, a straight firm stomach, erect or short tail, a movement with head erect, rapid, with a great noise, and a bold presumptuous aspect. Their feces are expelled from the end of the tail. They should be killed immediately after

[629]Avicenna, IV, Tract. 3, 21; Tract. 2, 12; II, 616.
[630]Isidore of Seville, *Etymologies* 12. 4. 10–12; Pliny, *N. H.* 10. 170.

their capture. The manner of killing is to cut off the head and the tail transversely lengthwise four inches from each end. If after these cuts have been made the snake is still alive and moving with great agitation and much shedding of blood they say you have made the proper choice of a snake. The creature should be eviscerated down its length, completely cleaned with a careful extraction of the bile, then skinned, washed with water and salt or wine, and salt should be placed in its mouth until it becomes a liquid, as Pliny[631] reports. When it has been cut up both lengthwise and across and the entrails removed it should be thoroughly boiled in water or oil with salt and dill and eaten entirely at once or collected piece by piece from slices of bread, as is often done. In addition to what has been said viper broth drives[632] lice away from the entire body. Others say the flesh should be thoroughly boiled in one part water and two parts wine until it comes completely off the bones. Rather weak old men should drink the broth seasoned with spices thrown into the boiling meat. Judeus [f. cxxiv] warns in the cooking of theriac that only burning coals should be placed beneath the pot and at the time the flesh parts from the bones fresh salt should be added and green, not dried, dill. There is another method of preparation of viper flesh in an oven not too hot from which bread has been taken out so as to dry the flesh to such a degree that it can be pulverized for use in electuaries or antidotes helpful in the resumptive regimen. It is even more beneficial if chickens, capons, or pullets are fed on snake flesh thus prepared or at least on wheat and barley or other grains placed in the decoction of snake flesh and drunk by the fowl at the time they begin to moult. It is good for old men to eat now and then the birds thus nourished. Among other salutary advantages of this food Avicenna says finally that it promotes the health of the eye.[633]

[631]Pliny, *N. H.* 30. 117.
[632]Ibid., 29. 121.
[633]Avicenna, II, 146.

Chapter LI

The Qualities of Water of Flesh and the Method of Preparing It

Strength however depleted can soon be restored by the use of water of flesh since it has a marvellous effect upon the principal powers of the body and is the very best remedy for weakness of the heart just as are sucking eggs, as they say. It is one of the more acceptable remedies for restoring a lessened and almost extinct innate heat especially for those who are beating upon the door of death. The method of preparing it is as follows. Take the flesh of an animal acceptable in the resumptive regimen such as an unweaned kid or lamb or a young ram when your purpose is to restore strength of spirits and the old people have failed due to heaviness, disturbance, and general lack of spirits. Cut up pieces of the lighter and more mobile animals, cook them thoroughly until the juice has been removed from the flesh, mix with spices that bring aid to the members, such as cinnamon, cloves, nutmeg [mace], and pearls, gold leaf, and coral melted together by sublimation or whatever method you wish.

Chapter LII

The Qualities of Sublimated Human Blood and the Method of Preparing It

Among very efficient aids for old age is sublimated human blood which they call elixir and praise very highly to such an extent that many have believed it to excel any other remedy for generation of the spirits because of a certain similarity it possesses to human nature itself, so that in the entire realm of nature no one has yet found anything like it especially if the blood is that of a young man of sanguine nature or simply the result of healthy nourishment and the use of good air. The following is the method of sublimating it. Prepare an oven or furnace within which you place a brass pot full of water within whose sides the blood to be sublimated is placed when the water is hot. Then cover the vessel containing the blood with an alembic or cups. Keep the fire continually under the aforesaid pot so that with its brisk heat it may accomplish the sublimation of the water in the first pot when it first becomes white in a wonderful way and adapted for ills produced by bile. Next, collect the second water which is somewhat colored; this is more effective for ills due to phlegm and for phlegmatic bodies, as they say. Keep all these waters completely covered in a glass vessel. They say that if this blood is sublimated according to need and demand its effectiveness will not be reduced especially if its waters are kept apart in several different vessels. Many now use the blood of Spanish pigs which are well fed especially in good air, wishing to reveal this fact to no one as being their own particular secret.

Chapter LIII

The Qualities of Potable Gold and the Method of Preparing It

One cannot sufficiently admire the solicitude and diligence of the ancients who carefully examined everything with the intention that nothing which might promote human health should be overlooked. Gold, which has been discovered to be destructible by nothing else than fire, they found to be a substance whose use in a marvellous way was both a singular and truly unique solace for human nature and a means toward a longer life.[634] For gold has this peculiar property, and after it silver also, to aid the human complexion and to soothe it. By means of gold heart diseases and melancholy which makes a man sad and causes him to talk to himself, which produces ills of the mind in those who are timid and cowardly, when rubbed and scraped furnishes good health and boldness, as is agreed among authors. Hence they say that gold is so called *(aurum)* because it turns the mind *(avertat)* of men, as Festus says.[635] When decoctions containing spices and various dishes are prepared for old people they should be stirred with a wand of gold until they attain a certain reddish color.[636] Gold is thin and temperate; its filings are included among medicines which relieve melancholy and holding it in one's mouth will remove bad breath, they say. Judeus [f. cxxiv] reports that a collyrium or lotion made of gold strengthens the vision and a preserve made in a golden vessel or gold itself mixed into the preserve strengthens the entire body. If what those who write on the subject is true, water of the sun, that is, potable gold, will act very strongly in all these matters for the alchemists ascribe gold to the sun in their desire to dignify

[634]Pliny, *N. H.* 33. 59.
[635]Paulus ex Fest. ed. W. M. Lindsay, p. 8: *quia mentes hominum avertat.*
[636]Pliny, *N. H.* 33. 84.

the metal just as they assign a planet exclusively to each metal and, veiling their knowledge in the manner of the Platonics, they rejoice in the use of metaphor. Gold is used to combat falling hair and tyria *[porrigo decalvans]*. It purges the skin by removing dirt and brings to old men and to the weak person a better health and less wrinkles. They believe that its effectiveness in this respect must be regarded as one of the greatest marvels of nature since indeed the four elements are not corrupted by it or in it, and it is in such harmony with human nature that it does not heat, cool, dry out, or humidify. In fact, in its temperateness it exceeds all else in equality or evenness as it also exceeds everything in weight. There is nothing in nature comparable to gold to such a degree that its powers are regarded in the same terms as those of the human complexion. It is more helpful for all the purposes discussed above because being a product of nature it is more effective than something produced through art can be, as the experts have concluded. But there is a marvellous method of art for preparing gold itself for drinking. It is as follows. Take an ounce of the best gold and two ounces of quicksilver. Place the gold into the quicksilver until it is dissolved. Then place the mixture in an alembic and apply a slow fire to it. Continue until the quicksilver issues forth from the orifice of the alembic. Then collect the denigrated gold at the bottom of the vessel and mix with it four pounds of water of bugloss. Then obturate all together thoroughly in the glass alembic, pour it in such a way that it does not evaporate and keep a steady fire underneath for three days and nights continuously at the end of which time if the process has been followed you will find that the water has not been consumed and the gold itself will be liquefied and made what they call potable. Gold can be dissolved they say in clear water with ammoniac gum and then placed in an instrument to dissolve without salt.

Chapter LIV

Gems Which Are Helpful in the Resumptive Regimen of Old Age

From among gems there are many which are especially helpful in the resumption of old age and by whose properties the old man's nature is tempered and joy and happiness of soul are brought to him. First, there is the carbuncle,[637] which holds the same position among precious stones as gold does among the metals and is agreed to possess more power than any other gem. Jewelers say that chalcedony also strengthens the body's powers as chrysolite does for the spiritual members. Heliotrope, a green stone almost similar to the emerald, sprinkled with a few drops of blood, along with other not inconsiderable virtues can preserve a man and endow him with a long and better life. The pomegranate stone which is of the variety of the carbuncle cheers the heart and puts sadness to flight. The jacinth repairs the body, induces sleep, and lends joy and strength to the heart. Pearls greatly illuminate the spirits and consolidate and restore them. By its special property the stone of the Medes restores the weary, exhausted, and weak. The emerald is good for strengthening the vision. Coral by its property aided by its brightness and clean appearance and solidity with astringence cheers the heart and strengthens it. It is very helpful to place rings with these gems set in gold upon the fingers of the old men.

[637]Pliny, *N. H.* 37. 92, 37, 126, 125, 147, 115, 138, 173, 175, 183, 74, in this order describes these gems.

Chapter LV

Syrups Useful to Old People and Especially Vinegar Syrup

Vinegar syrup is ideal, Abulkasim says, for old men in every season and in every inhabited region. Its nature is equally warm and cold. With its thinness it can open, clean, and thin out and with its excellent power combat humors hot, cold, thin, thick, viscous, or adherent, as Mesue [f. 43] reports. It should be drunk with a julep lest it create cough and dysentery. If it is made with sugar it will benefit all healthy people of whatever age and nature. It can be made with honey temperate in heat and frigidity. When made with roots it becomes warm, opens obstructions, and cuts apart the viscosities of the humors. It reduces thirst less and is less warm than vinegar syrup without roots which they call herbs. It is not recommended in the resumptive regime when it contains very much acidity. Judeus [f. cxxv] writes that with vinegar syrup the powerful acidity dries up humors in a weak body, increases viscosity, and with frequent use often induces dysentery in the intestines, cough in the lungs, and harm to the nervous members.

SYRUP OF CITRON

This syrup because of its power of assisting the stomach's digestion is useful in the resumptive regimen especially for old men of warm and humid nature in summer and other seasons following summer in southern regions. Its frigid nature is listed in the third degree, dry in the second. It allays thirst. In the presentation of syrups the hour should be chosen at which the moon is in conjunction with Venus and Jupiter in the airy and watery signs, as Abulkasim prescribes.

SYRUP OF CITRON PEEL

Among syrups they do not wish to omit the rather frequent use of citron peel as being ideal for a nauseous stomach and for an old man's heart, especially one of cold nature in winter and in cold regions.

GREEN GINGER ROOT AND ROSE HONEY

The same must be observed concerning a syrup made of green ginger root and rose honey, for it is astringent, cleansing, and strengthens the stomach, as Mesue [*Canones Universales,* f. 57r, 66v] says. Syrup of green leek is also ideally unique for old men to remove superfluous thick phlegm; this has been discussed in its place.

VINEGAR OF SQUILL *(ACETUM SCILLAE)*

People have bade a fleshy plump old man to make rather frequent use of vinegar of squill, for it counteracts the heaviness of the humors with its thinness, cutting their thick and viscous materials and preparing them for easy expulsion and sometimes leading forth the black bile, sometimes preserving the body from black cholera and the body from putrefaction. It creates good health, strengthens the stomach which is suffering lassitude and softening, stimulates a more glowing color, and conserves youth in every way while retarding old age.[638] Judeus [f. 57r] reports that he has seen many people whose regime of life was not good; nevertheless, they were saved by the use of vinegar of squill, for it is valuable for a person who lacks very much thinning and breaking up of thick and viscous superfluity.

[638]Galen 14. 567.

Chapter LVI

Electuaries

Special care must be exercised to restore in the resumptive regimen each of the powers which they call those which govern the entire body. Galen[639] named the governing power of the entire body the total collection of its powers. For the removal of the lassitude which affects each of these powers human nature rejoices in the use of suitable aromatics and in other substances which properly promote its welfare. The experts say these substances provide strength and sturdiness to the heart since it is the source and beginning of life, the adornment of the soul, the king of nature, the moderator of the body, and is conceived by divine wisdom. Among the most salutary aids therefore which restore old age are those which unite, restore, and repair the powers of the heart not only with syrups but with electuaries and other means.

ELECTUARY OF GALEN FOR THE MATERIAL SUBSTANCE OF THE BODY

Galen[640] describes one of the most potent electuaries used for the purpose outlined above in his little book *On Secrets* which is useful for the material of the body and for the condition of old age. It opens obstructions, restores innate heat, dissolves corrupt humors, is the best aid to digestion, dispels flatulence and phlegm from the stomach, drives away the ill effects of chill from the joints, provokes the urine, and repairs the strength of the body from every point. The recipe includes up to two drams of Indian leaf [saffron], pepper, long pepper, warm cinnamon, that is, of the

[639]Ibid., 5. 468, 600; 16. 105; 19. 383.
[640]Galen 13: *De compositione medicamentorum locos libri* VIII–X; *De compositione medicamentorum per genera libri* VII.

sharp flower of cynanche, spice of galanga, ammi [bishop's weed], caraway; of mastic, fennel seed, anise, dry ginger, dry river calamint *[melissa calamintha]* up to ten aurei [each two drams fourteen grains, also known as alcobolus]; of cypress, crocus, assar, wood cassia, sweet costum, garden celery seed, three aurei; of cloves, lesser cardamum, cubebs, nutmeg, mace, carpobalsam, wood balsam, foliate pyrethrum imported, acorus [yellow flag iris], two aurei; then pound these all up and sift them. Then with a third part of sugar and three times as much defoamed honey added it is ready for use.

AVICENNA'S CONFECTION OF PHILOSOPHERS

Among these preparations Avicenna's[641] antidote in the *Canon* V is called the philosopher's confection or the material of life. It is ideal for removing phlegmatic superfluities as well as for cheering the soul, restoring the digestion, banishing flatulence of the stomach, and soothing anxiety. In every way it is an accompanying resource for youth and a preservative of it as well as an aid to the memory and the creator of a sound reason; it also counteracts the cold. Avicenna describes it in his book.

THE ELECTUARY OF AMBERGRIS AND OF THE KINGS OF AVICENNA

The electuary of ambergris[642] is considered to be of the same kind and similar to that of the kings and distinguished by not inconsiderable properties which Avicenna calls the medicine of a year, to be taken for an entire year continually. Its use restores the person who is sustaining himself up to the end of his life by the precept of God. Its frequent use ministers to the weakening of the body, checks gray hair, and in every way is the medicine of kings nor should one abstain from it, he writes.

TRIPHERA OF HALY RODOAN

Haly Rodoan wrote this antidote for checking the speed of approaching old age. He calls it triphera, that is, joyous or praised

[641]Avicenna, V, 509v.
[642]Ibid., II, 63.

or victory or juice or that which brings fruit. It assists the digestion, creates a good color, confers youth for a long space of time and counteracts heat and cold and all in all extends a man's life if he observes what is proper. He calls this medicine inda.

THE JOY-CREATING ELECTUARY OF RHAZES AND ALKAPH AND OF MYROBALANUS

The electuary of Rhazes which produces joy is placed among the salutary remedies for old age. Since its property is to dry out excessively it should be administered with something that humidifies or at least it should be rectified with something moist. It produces joy, beauty of complexion, better digestion, and retards gray hair, they say. It is uniquely for this purpose that Alkaph's electuary has served for preserving youth and retarding gray hairs. One may add the electuary of myrobalanus for retarding gray hairs by Rhazes in the third book of *Almansor.*

DIAMUSCUS AND DIAMBRA POWDERS AND MESUE'S ELECTUARY OF GEMS

Mesue's electuary of diamuscus, of gems, and of diambra with its sublimity restores the power of the brain and heart and assists the stomach and the digestion, creates happiness, warms the members of nutrition and assists those of frigid nature. Since these aids increase the powers of the spirits it is urged that old men use them.

MITHRIDATES AND THERIAC

Most noble among other antidotes is that of Mithridates, which that king swallowed daily and is said to have rendered his body safe against the perils of poison. The same is true of theriac, which has no equal among compound medicines, according to Avicenna,[643] especially for equalization of the human complexion and even more that of the heart for which none of the experts doubts that it is a first-rate aid. Indeed, by these means the hilarity of the heart is induced, sadness is removed, and the ills of poison-

[643]Avicenna, V, 508.

ing are healed with a great boon. They preserve health with caution from accidental pestilences and from the evil movements of the humors. They replenish the depleted body and deplete it when it is filled, lending strength in every way to all the powers which conduce to a longer life. The theriac is especially useful. Thus for old men who are not only not temperate but frigid and humid in nature in winter and opportunely in cold regions as the case demands they affirm that these remedies are marvellously effective. Damascenus prescribes that a small quantity of theriac be given to old men whose warm nature brings on wakefulness. This should be done accompanied by cooling and humidifying substances such as barley water, according to Abulkasim, although Judeus and the authority of Galen say weak old men should take theriac with wine, not water, when the digestion of food is completed and after the food has left the stomach. The quantity should be that of an Egyptian bean [forty-two gr.] with two teaspoons of wine but not in the summer. Among the outstanding remaining powers of theriac in addition to what has been mentioned in the category of primary qualities, especially after the composition and fermentation of the mixable herbs, is something divine and unknown in the way of an artificial form coming from the outside rather than from within by whose grace any kind of poison is counteracted, as the authors agree.

THE NOBLE ELECTUARY OF THE CONCILIATOR

When need arises to restore the strength of the old man rather quickly there is prescribed an electuary which more nobly, temperately, and effectively ministers to the suffering of the heart than any other which a subsequent age has discovered. They say a portion of it should be dissolved in excellent muscatel wine or any other unmixed wine and the result should be drunk; in this way those who are rather weak will use it more easily and it will penetrate more quickly. Sometimes it can be mixed with rose water and sugar or infused with borage to the extent of two parts when the power to be restored is only half depleted. For if the old man has broad pores and thin spirit and should make frequent use of it the spirit would be forced to exhale or to issue forth. A sign of this they say is that it makes the body quite fragrant and brings exhilaration to the soul and a more frequent systole and diastole to parts of the face while life is receding. It is the electuary called euporiston, that is, a good invention with a certain divine spirit which was devised by the Conciliator in the difference of opinion cited in chapter 96 of his *Conciliator*.

THE ELECTUARY OF THE MODERNS

In the century a little before our own an antidote ideal for the resumptive regimen has been discovered. The recipe is as follows: selected pearls, one dram; jacinths, emeralds, sapphires, doronics [sardonyx ?], white and red coral up to one scruple; cinnamon, mace, galanga, nutmeg, up to one dram; clove, long pepper, cubeb, wood aloes, storax, calamint up to one scruple; basil seed, one scruple; crocus, one dram; musk, ambergris up to one dram; five grains of citron peel, with spices half a dram; scraped licorice for humidification; one ounce of raisins; of conserve of borage and bugloss, one dram; three drams of purified apple juice, two of rose water; one pound of white sugar. Of these ingredients let a marvellous electuary be made.

MYROBALANUS OR ARABIAN BEN-NUT SPICED WITH CHEBULA AND BELLERIC OR BUCERA BELLERICA

The use of myrobalanus spiced with chebula is greatly praised in the resumptive regimen for it rejuvenates a man with better color, more pleasant breath and perspiration, with a joyful heart and restoration of the liver and stomach, according to Johannes Mesue. There is also Constantinus's use of belleric for strengthening old men.

MUSK

Dioscorides reports that musk drunk or eaten brings an increase of strength to the heart and all the inner organs, with the solace of an increased courage. Therefore they say that four grains of this electuary drunk for several days with two ounces of sublimated water of flowers of crocus relieve old men admirably.

ZEDOARIA [*CURCUMA Z.* OR *KAEMPFERIA ROTUNDA* OR TURMERIC]

Powder of zedoaria in the quantity of one dram with two ounces of aromatic wine added and the same amount of honey furnishes restoration, joy, and strength to the heart, as they say.

A MEDICINE WHICH EXTENDS SOMEWHAT THE LIFE OF THE DECREPIT PERSON WHO IS GRADUALLY DYING

For the extension of the life of a person already as decrepit as possible before the old man exhausts his soul with weeping, especially when the decrepit person is so weak that he stutters out his breath from hardened members as he speaks, so that you may say that he palpitates rather than lives and that he should take the sacraments, this antidote has been devised as the most timely medicine. The Conciliator prescribes equal parts of castor beans, mace, and crocus pounded up and mixed with the best wine, after opening by force the mouth of the dying man to receive the dose. This will be able to protect and extend the life of the decrepit man as it issues forth already from his body at the menacing onset of death. This medicine will serve for a short time. Although this assistance is uncertain the gerontocomos has a duty to try it on his patient. Much that is done in other ways in a sudden peril such as this must be omitted here so long as this remedy is administered as is proper always before the end of life arrives lest, as Theodorus Priscianus says,

> Nature our parent cry out in protest: "The sick man is killed and his fragility is blamed on me."
>
> (*Euporiston,* 3)

Chapter LVII

Death Which Is Natural and Not to Be Lamented, Feared, Nor Wished For

Directed therefore by the gerontocomia the old men will reach the natural end of life beyond which they cannot pass and they will render thus to Nature the debt they owe her, an act through which without sadness and completely without any perceptible violent passion they will experience insensibly the passing away of their souls, for a gentle sleep releases the old man's soul, as Seneca says.[644] Such a death by a reasonable judgment ought not only to occur without lamentation but should not be feared nor longed for although the power of desire may flee from death as the ultimate cause for terror, as it is in Aristotle. Indeed, it is not to be lamented because all things which are according to nature are to be considered as a boon, as Cicero says.[645] Nothing is more in accordance with nature than death for old men. Therefore the old man Ennius said as he was dying:

> Let no one honor me with tears nor wail at my funeral.[646]

It is not proper that death should be feared or longed for since it is among those things which make life more blessed, according to precept, nor should we dread the last day nor long for it, as Martial says,[647] although it is difficult to do this as the mind, presently gazing into heaven, conscious of its rectitude may confess that this greatly desired end is to be in no way dreaded if it leads a man to

[644] Seneca, *Oedipus* 788.
[645] Cicero, *De Sen.* 71.
[646] Ennius, fr. 9, ed. E. Warmington, I, 402.
[647] Martial, 10. 47. 13; cf. Vergil, *Aen.* 1. 604. The reference to Aristotle is *N. E.*, III, 1115 a 26.

the place where he will be eternally happy, which there is no doubt that it does according to orthodox religious belief. For this is the way to eternal glory. By means of better deeds immortality with blessedness follows. This is the life which alone must be called life; I wish that some day, well deserving of it, we may attain it.

Part II

The Elegies of Maximianus On Old Age and Love

Introduction To Maximianus's Elegies

Maximianus the Etruscan as he calls himself, an appellation which must be reduced to Tuscan since the Etruscan race no longer existed in his time, has been called by F. J. E. Raby "in some sort, the last of the Roman poets." This is nonsense; too many poets have been credited with this dubious honor. He is, however, a medieval Latin poet whose work was so popular that he became one of the school authors along with Aesop, Avianus, Theodulus, and Cato. Furthermore, since we are told on the excellent authority of E. R. Curtius that "the Middle Ages was much less prudish than the Modern Period and zealously read Maximianus" we should not wonder that he was much read in schools as "a lesson in prudential morality," as Robinson Ellis says, although children must have been puzzled by some of the racier *Elegies*.

We must dismiss the idea held in some quarters that he was a Christian; many men in his day and after were not professing Christians and survived well enough until the days of the Inquisition and beyond. There is not the slightest evidence of Christian belief in his poems, although Manitius tries to prove it exists. His older friend Boethius on whom he calls in II, 47, was a Neoplatonist and Aristotelian, in other words a thinker who found more consolation in philosophy than in any religion.

Whatever his dates may be he was alive in the age of Justinian, the sixth century. What few biographical facts exist must be gleaned from his six poems, 686 lines in all, probably called *Nugae* by their author. He lived at Rome and had four loves: Lycoris of *Elegy* II, apparently a concubine or live-in partner, who remained the longest with him but finally left him in his and her old age; Aquilina of *Elegy* III, with whom he had a brief but disastrous affair terminated through the cynical greed of her parents; Candida of *Elegy* IV, the cabaret singer and dancer who faded away from him because of her father's interference; and an unnamed Greek performer he met in Constantinople, with whom he survived the most humiliating of all his sexual experiences, a collapse into impotence.

He was sent as he says in *Elegy* V on a mission of state to the East which Lemaire thinks was that of a senator named Festus entrusted with a peace pact by Theodoric perhaps in A. D. 515 (or 498, Wernsdorf). This view is effectively refuted by Fr. Vogel on the grounds that Maximianus would have been too young in 498 or even 515 to suit the context of *Elegy* V in view of the fact that Friedrich Wilhelm has compared the poems in Boethius's *Consolation of Philosophy* and pointed out a number of parallels between them and Maximianus's *Elegies.* Since the *Consolation* was written in 524, the year of Boethius's imprisonment and death, Maximianus must have written after that date; since the *Elegies* are those of an old man they must have been composed perhaps as late as 550, at least during the decline of the Ostrogoth Empire.

Not only Boethius but other Latin poets were used by Maximianus. The fictional elements of elegy he drew from Ovid, Propertius, Tibullus, and Lygdamus; one of his Renaissance editors, Pomponius Gauricus, passed him off in 1501 as Cornelius Gallus, of whose poetry only one line has actually survived; Gauricus (or Gaurico) was also the first to divide the *Elegies* into six poems as we now have them. Lycoris and Candida come from the Palatine Anthology, Martial, and the pseudo-Vergilian *Copa.* Some traits of the old man in the poems may also have been picked up from various sources such as Plautus and Seneca, although most of the sad picture they present looks like Maximianus himself. His Tuscan origin, his stay in Rome, the diplomatic mission to the East seem authentic enough as well as the details of his love affair, reminiscent in *Elegy* V of Goethe's hilarious but also vastly disconcerting experience in *Das Tagebuch* and harking back to Ovid, *Amores* 3. 7, Petronius 132, and *Priapea* 83. 19–45. The address to *mentula* may even have been a source in turn for Bernard Silvestris, *De universitate mundi* (between 1145 and 1153 A. D.), neglected by E. Gilson, according to E. R. Curtius. Merone and other scholars cite numerous borrowings by Maximianus from Propertius, Tibullus,

Ovid, and Vergil particularly; even Martial has contributed his share of echoes to these elegies of the Middle Ages.

Old age as a topic of description and rhetorical analysis and eventually the object of sheer abhorrence appears first among the Greeks in Western literature. The chief trait of Priam and Nestor, the oldest men in the Homeric poems, is beside their loquacity and boastfulness a great pride in their production of offspring, their longevity, and their still indispensable wisdom. These are not particularly revolting features of character and no physical characteristics that might evoke pity are shown by Homer. There are at last a fearful defiance and a pitiful death for Priam which arouse pathos while Nestor is lost sight of at Pylos as Telemachos leaves him. Phoenix, the old tutor of Achilles, is wholly attractive and admirable.

Less dignified and more to be pitied is old age among the lyric poets, Solon, Anacreon, Theognis, and Mimnermos; it is wistful, nostalgic, weak, and self-pitying, although Solon still retains his pride in continuing to learn as he grows old. Aristotle in *Rhetoric* 2. 13 describes old age for the purpose of adapting speeches to the character of different ages as he sees them. Aristotle was often a cynic and his description of old men is sardonic and contemptuous, drawn with broad strokes, sweeping generalities, and a preoccupation with types, not individuals, almost in the vein of Theophrastus, his pupil. All old men are obviously not, despite what he says, cynical, suspicious, small-minded, ungenerous, cowardly, self-conceited, oblivious to the opinions of others, distrustful of the future, living on their memories and the past, loquacious (note Homer, however), loving gain, querulous, and lacking in humor.

Horace may have taken over some of these so-called dominant traits in the description of old age in the *Ars Poetica* 169–75, which is devoted here to practically the same purpose as Aristotle's: the observation of character suited to various ages of man in the writing of drama:

Old age has many troubles; for the wretch
Still seeks, but fears and will not use his hoard;
Or else does everything in fear and cold;
He puts things off and spins his hopes out long,

Slow, greedy of the future, difficult,
Full of complaints, a praiser of the past
When he was young, a censor critical
Of all the modern generation.

Then with a note of hope reminiscent of Cicero's *De Senectute,* the best essay on old age ever written, he continues:

The rising tide of years brings many a joy;
The ebb removes as many.

(John G. Hawthorne, translator)

It is Juvenal who really frightens us with his revolting picture of old age and who sets the tone for most of the descriptions which follow him in medieval literature in *Satires* 10. 187–219:

"Give me long life, Jove, give me many years!"
This only, this, though sick or well, you pray for.
Yet how continuous and how long old age,
How full of ills! Deformed and ugly face
Unlike its former self, a wrinkled hide
Instead of skin, the hanging cheeks, the grooves
Like those an old baboon carves on her jowls
Deep in the shaded jungle of Africa.
Young men differ in so many ways:
This one is handsomer than another; he
Still better than a third, while one man's stronger.
Old men have one appearance only: voices
That tremble like their legs, their heads are bald,
Their noses drip like a baby's; they must chew
Their bread with toothless gums: and so revolting
They are to wife and children and themselves
That even fortune-hunters pass them by.
Their torpid taste finds no more joy in wine
Or food; love fades into a long oblivion,
And if they try, their little tool lies still
And helpless even though they work all night.
Can gray hairs hope for anything from passion?
Should not desire be suspect with reason,
Attempting Venus when it's impotent?
Now see how one more sense is lost. What joy
Can old men take in song, however great
The singer, even the harper Seleucus?
What pleasure to shine with those who wear bright robes?

What difference does it make where he may sit
In the vast theater when he scarcely hears
The blast of horns and trumpets blown together?
The slave who names his caller or tells the hour
Will have to shout to make an old man hear.
Further than this, the little blood that flows
Through his cold body warms with fevers only.
Diseases, forming ranks, leap all around him.

(L. R. Lind, translator)

The Middle Ages present another poet to match Aristotle, Horace, and Juvenal in the description of old age—and to surpass them all: Maximianus. Aristotle had concentrated upon the unpleasant disposition of old men in general and upon their character. Maximianus, like Juvenal, whom he most resembles, dwells upon their physical infirmities and their sufferings. So effective indeed is he in listing the clinical and medical details of old age that he struck a responsive chord in the Renaissance in the *Gerontocomia* by Gabriele Zerbi, who quotes almost one hundred lines from *Elegy* I. Max Neuburger, writing in the *Bulletin of the History of Medicine,* has briefly analyzed the medical aspects of the *Elegies* although he misses what I think may be the onset of enlarged prostate (I, 170) and adds toothlessness which Maximianus curiously does not mention. Cataract or glaucoma also seems to appear at 147–48.

The Middle Ages had already provided Maximianus with a topos or a school theme on the subject of old age called the *vituperatio senectutis.* The topic went back to philosophers such as Theophrastus, Demetrius of Phaleron, Bion, Ariston of Ceos, Musonius, Favorinus, Seneca, and Varro in his *Menippean Satires.* Later writers include Venantius Fortunatus, Corippus, Orientius, Eugenius of Toledo, whose works bear reminiscences of Maximianus, Hrabanus Maurus, and Marbod, who handle the theme and employ some of the same devices, as do Paulinus, Ausonius (who greatly influenced Maximianus), Avitus, and Prudentius. Quotations and echoes of Maximianus occur as Manitius has shown in the works of Hugo of St. Victor, Aimeric, the anonymous *De pravitate mundi,* Giraldus Cambrensis, the *Versus proverbiales,* Geoffrey of Vinsauf, Alexander of Villa Dei, Walter the Englishman, Godfrey of Breteuil, Alan de l'Isle, Nigellus Wireker,

Peter of Riga, Roger of Caen, Baudri of Bourgueil, Walter of Chatillon, Henry of Settimello, and in the so-called *Streitgedichte* entitled *Ganymede and Helen,* in the *De tribus puellis, De nuntio sagaci,* and in *De Paulino et Polla,* a comedy by Ricardo of Venosa (*circa* A. D. 1228–29). E. Baehrens in the *Poetae Latini Minores,* V, 313, has published a fragment of forty lines on old age, probably written in the eighth century, which is practically a cento of lines from Maximianus. Certain other excerpts are called *Proverbia Maximiani.* This is an impressive list of borrowers. As to the widespread use of Maximianus as a schoolbook M. Boas in 1914 could still speak in shocked amazement about it: "*Inest denique in libro tironum institutioni destinato qui minime ad mores pueriles conformandos idoneos complures adeo locos exhibet tenerorum animorum cognitioni alienos pudicaeque indoli erubescendos,* Maximianus."

George R. Coffman has analyzed the idea of old age as it is handled by certain writers from Horace to Chaucer, but he omits Juvenal entirely, who provides some of the most vivid physical details, and ignores the relation between Aristotle and Horace. Useful, however, are his presentation of Seneca, *De Ira* 2. 19. 4: *Senes difficiles et queruli sunt* (from Horace) and of Innocent III (1198–1216 A. D.). This pope wrote an important item in the list of passages on old age in "*De incommodis senectutis*" from his treatise *De Contemptu Mundi sive de Miseria Humanae Conditionis,* utilizing Horace. Coffman also refers to Vincent of Beauvais, *Speculum Doctrinale,* chaps. 101–103, who quotes both Horace and Maximianus. In the fourteenth century Coffman reaches England and Rollo of Hampole, John Bromyard, and finally Chaucer, who knew Maximianus well, and to whom G. L. Kittredge had come already in 1888 in an article entitled "Chaucer and Maximian": *The Pardoner's Tale,* 727–38, translated and adapted from Maximianus 1. 221–36, and *The Reeve's Prologue,* 3855–98. These poems are "among the most amazing in all of Chaucer's work," as Coffman says, and are based on Horace and Maximianus, *Elegy* V, but chiefly on the latter. The emphasis on sexual impotency which Coffman regards as so important in Maximianus, whom he calls "the only successor of Horace," is also found if he had looked for it in Juvenal. The latest medieval use of Maximianus seems to be the pseudo-Chaucerian *Court of Love* 792–98 = Maximianus, 1.

97–98. Coffman sums up the *Elegies* thus: "In essence these elegies are a blending of lascivious eroticism, in degenerate Ovidian or Ausonian vein, and of universal cynicism and pessimism, with a final touch of Stoicism." This somewhat exaggerated and distorted estimate shows that prudery dies hard especially among scholars.

The eighteenth-century edition of Maximianus by J. C. Wernsdorf assembles much useful material in its testimonia and commentary. It is an honor to American scholarship, however, to say that Richard Webster's edition with full *apparatus criticus* and commentary (Princeton University Press, 1900) is the most complete and useful for our time, despite the fact that Webster refuses to believe in the reality of Maximianus as an actual living person but only as a character in his own dramatic monologues. This view reminds me of nothing so much as the stubborn refusal of some German critics to believe in the reality of Goethe's Roman love-affair in the *Roman Elegies*. If Webster is right, then all the Roman elegists must be charged as he charged Maximianus with a similar lack of real feeling, with mere formalism, rhetoric, and artificiality, and any historical allusions in their elegies must be similarly interpreted as not referring to their real authors. Although Webster thus throws out the baby with the bath his commentary is valuable as well as his text based on eighteen manuscripts including Etonensis (A) usually considered the best, although as he says no one of them is good enough to be followed in all cases.

Maximianus is much influenced by Catullus, Vergil, Ovid, and Ausonius as well as by dozens of other writers. Almost every line in his poems parallels, echoes, or imitates some word, phrase, or line in another author; he also uses proverbs effectively. Classical Greek and Latin and medieval Latin literature is pillaged right and left but the effect on the reader who may not perceive his borrowings is still vivid and fresh and gives the impression of a lively talent working from personal as well as literary experience and materials. The technical elements of his versification include repetition of sound in word-endings, leonine and ophite or serpentine verses (I, 77–78; III, 5–6; V, 99–100) where the first half of the first line is identical (or practically so) with the second half of the second line. Chiasmus, assonance, alliteration, oxymoron, hiatus, rare elisions, paradox, rhyme, ellipsis, synizesis, comparison, litotes, the mixture of sepulchral and erotic language, false quantities, etymological play on words (e.g., III, 48, Boēti, a false quantity but a play on the Greek βοηθεῖν = *fer opem*), amphiboly (IV, 7: *candida* . . . Candida), parody, antithesis, *cumulatio verborum* are all in his bag of tricks.

Croce has made a useful distinction between the poetic and the practical personality of a poet. Whatever may be the exact delimitation of each of these in Maximianus the practical elements point to his birth around 490 or 495; his association with Boethius, perhaps even as his pupil, which may have taken place around 510; the publication of his elegies in the first decade of the second half of the sixth century; and his embassy to the East around 550, with his death perhaps around A. D. 570.

The psychological and poetic personality is also fairly perceptible from his poems. They are clearly those of an old man who looks back over a career which was not wholly undistinguished either in public or private accomplishments. He was an orator much acclaimed for his skill in the law courts; a man-about-town much admired in Rome; a hunter and an athlete of great prowess who excelled at wrestling, racing, and swimming; a poet from youth onwards who won in competition at dramatic composition; a lusty and competent drinker; a long-time bachelor who finally succumbed and took a concubine—a not unusual way of life in his time—and then in the relentless course of time, an old man afflicted with many ills but one who knew how to make poetry out of his sufferings. All in all, he lived a full and exciting life and one worthy of a better end.

His love affairs seem to have begun with Lycoris, who was also the most enduring of his companions. These experiences hold first place in his memories and constitute the story line of the last five poems, somewhat more than half of their entire bulk, although each has its own quality of bitterness, frustration, and disappointment mingled with its delights as well. If, as Szöverffy believes, Maximianus was a satirist his elegies do not reveal that objectivity which characterizes Juvenal, for example, in the Sixth Satire. Maximianus's loves are real; he suffered personal defeats, and he does not stand apart as a detached observer; he feels guilt, despair, and humiliation without any attempt to conceal or deceive. His love life is accompanied by laments for his old age; they appear even in *Elegy* II, which records the galling loss of Aquilina because of her parents' greed, where one might suppose that he could have reached some accommodation with them and continued his affair instead of losing heart so suddenly. I suspect that his pride was wounded too severely for him to continue the association.

Only a deep sense of personal tragedy can account for the frank and unflattering description he gives us in *Elegy* IV of his affair with Candida, in which he was again thwarted, this time by a ridiculous revelation in a dream, while his reputation as a man of some social standing was ruined by his incoherent babble. The most ambiguous of the six elegies, it is at once the most painful and the most heart-felt of his experiences. *Elegy* V, a brief and tumultuous encounter with an unnamed Greek cabaret performer, is of course extremely embarrassing in its outcome but no more so than it was for the much younger Goethe as he tells it in *Das Tagebuch* in a similar situation. For Goethe it was, when over, a rather hilarious adventure, one more in a series of frolics in the company of the Duke Karl August of Weimar; for Maximianus, however, his fiasco was damaging to his pride to say the least, even though it could have been forgiven considering his age. The address to *mentula,* his elaborate *apologia pro sua calamitate,* carries Maximianus to a height of impassioned rhetoric well in keeping with his reputation as an orator which dissolves in laughter as he perceives the girl's genuine disappointment at his failure to function adequately and from which, in a perverse sort of way, he wins a rueful victory. She too is moved to utter her own hymn of praise to the member in question and to achieve an even more effective level of eloquence than Maximianus's own. Its combination of passion and pathos makes this elegy perhaps the finest of all six and was clearly intended to crown the series of poems with a striking climax. Indeed, Maximianus's deft changes of mood and sentiment, from simple affection to harsh irony, from acute self-condemnation to philosophic calm, from idyllic reflection to bitter despair, from youth to manhood to old age, his alternate theme, together with an often rapid and abrupt change of tense which reflects these shifts of feeling and mood, are the characteristics of a complex nature perhaps abnormally sensitive to some of the most difficult and challenging aspects of his life. Not the last of the Roman poets nor the first of medieval poets, Maximianus is like every original and gifted mind unique in the history of elegy, a product of his own troubled age, one in transition between the classical and post-classical periods but nonetheless amazingly modern as well in some of its social phenomena. His emphasis upon the free expression of his individual nature and erotic instincts looks back to the *Pervigilium Veneris* and forward across the centuries to the revival of Latin love poetry among the Italian humanists. Maximianus is thus like every truly classical poet not only in harmony with his own times but a part of a long line of succession in a tradition which extends from ancient Greece and Rome to our day. Certain of his genius but unable to discover certainty in human relations, he is assailed by pride and desire, doubt, guilt, and failure, to find at last a partial resolution and sublimation for his anxieties, his discontent, and his physical and mental stress in his poetry.

The Elegies of Maximianus

I

Jealous old age, reluctant to hasten my end,
Why come a laggard in this my worn-out body?
Set free my wretched life from such a prison:
Death is my peace and life a punishment.
What I was once, I am not: the best has perished;
Illness and fear possess what's left of me.
Life is a bore in my grief, though once it was happy,
And what is worse than dying is my wish to die.
While young and handsome, while mind and sense remained,
I was a speaker renowned throughout the world.
Often I fashioned the lying songs of a poet,
And often my fictions brought real glory to me.
Often I won the decision in cases at law,
Deserving the tribute awarded my nimble tongue.
What can be deathless now when my body's failing,
Alas, what portion of life remains to the old!
Not less than these talents was the grace of my sublime beauty;
When it is absent there's nothing else can please,
Not even virtue, more precious than tawny gold,
Through which a noble soul shines even more.
If I was minded to fit my bow with swift arrows,
The creatures I hunted fell to my missile's aim.
If I was pleased to circle deep glens with my dogs
I killed many beasts, and everyone cried "Hurrah!"
Good sport I had when I went to the sweaty gymnasium
To twist slippery legs and arms on the wrestling pad.
Now I would beat every runner who ran with me,
Now I would top competition at tragic song.
This charming mixture increased the worth of my talents

As always a varied work of art shines more,
For whatever is wont to please when considered alone
Pleases the more when joined with an alternate grace.
My patience, unconquered amid these resources of virtue,
Scorned all the menacing crises of daily life.
Bareheaded I bore the assaults of wind and rain.
Neither the heat nor the cold was oppressive to me.
I swam in the chilly waters of Tiber at flood
Nor feared to entrust my limbs to its treacherous bed.
I was able to rest with a slumber however little
And nourish my body with only a little food.
But if some drunken friend should happen to find me
And made it a night and day carousing with me
Father Bacchus himself stopped drinking in sheer amazement
And he who could beat all others went off in defeat.
It's not easy to bend the will in such challenging matters,
To make one mind bear two ways of living that clash.
In this struggle of choice also they tell that the great
Socrates once was deserving of victory's palm.
Here too they remind us stern Cato prevailed in his strength.
Not circumstances but evil deeds bring us to vice.
Unshaken, whatever the choice, I was borne to both sides.
Every sadness and sorrow yielded before my mind.
Always content with little, I loved poverty,
And, desirous of nothing, was master of my affairs.
You only subdue me, you grim old age, to your will,
To whom everything yields which was able to overcome all.
We sink down in you, you possess everything that grows weak;
At the end even you consume yourself with your ill.
Thus adorned with my merits the entire province had hoped
I would live among them as one who had married a wife.
But it was more sweet to dwell with a head held high
And to suffer no bondage of wedlock, however pleasant.
I walked through the center of Rome with my boyish appearance,
Admired wherever I went by the girls, every one.
And whichever girl could be courted, or perhaps had been courted,
Blushed to the ears when she looked on my youthful face
And soon with a smile sought to hide her fugitive self,
Yet not in her flight with a wish to conceal herself wholly
But rather to give me a glimpse of some part of her,
Rejoicing the more in the fact she was scarcely concealed.

Thus handsome I was to all and I pleased everyone,
I was engaged to all of the girls in general,
But only engaged; since nature created me bashful
And chaste in my heart I was resolute unto the end.
For while I desired to marry a beautiful woman
I remained a cold bachelor upon a wifeless bed.
Every girl seemed to me ugly, a country jake too,
And none of the girls seemed worthy to be my wife.
I was horrified at both the skinny as well as the fat ones,
None of the short ones pleased me, not one of the tall,
Since I delighted to play with the middle-sized only
For a greater pleasure is found in the golden mean.
Soft lustfulness dwells in the middle parts of our body,
This is the seat where the mother of love resides.
I looked for the slender girls, not the ones who were skinny;
The fleshy members are suited to service of flesh.
Let her have a body which pleases when squeezed in embrace
Just so the bones do not hurt when you press her side.
I despised pale girls except the ones who had faces
Which blossomed to pink of the rose with a quiet blush.
Venus herself prefers this tint before others,
The Cyprian loves her flower wherever it grows.
Bright golden hair and a lowered milk-white neck
Seem to be found rather more with an innocent face.
Eyebrows coal-black, bold features, languorous eyes
Would set my heart on fire whenever I saw them.
I have loved bright-red, slightly pouting lips,
Which when I tasted them gave me a full round kiss.
On slender necks gold seemed to shine more precious
And in my view to glow more brightly than gems.
To mention these features once sought for is shameful for old men,
And that which once was quite proper is now a sin.
Different things please different men; not everything
Is fit for all ages; what suited once now harms.
The boy delights in games, old age in sternness:
Between them both there stands the young man's charm.
Silence and sadness befit this one, but that one
Becomes more brilliant with joy and chattering tongue.
He carries all with him, turns rolling time about,
Nor lets it run its course in whichever way.
Yet now since age is useless, heavy, long,

Since live I cannot, give me power to die.
O what a harsh condition of life oppresses
The wretched: but death's not subject to human will.
Death's sweet to the old but, hoped-for, it recedes.
Yet when it's bitter it comes at break-neck pace.
Defunct in so many parts of me some day
I'll go still alive into the roads of hell.
Now hearing is less, taste less, my very eyes
Grow dim; I barely know the things I touch,
No smell is sweet, no pleasure now is grateful:
Devoid of feeling, who's sure that he survives?
Lethean oblivion comes upon my mind
Nor can it now, confused, remember itself;
It rises to meet no demand, with the body weakens,
Is stupefied, concentrating on its ills.
I sing no songs; the greatest joy of song
Has fled; true grace of voice has perished quite.
I arouse no public, write no alluring poems,
Seek favorable judgments with suits by no means savage.
The handsome looks I loved have now departed,
And now I seem to be as dead as they.
Instead of my healthy red and white complexion
A pallor stains my face, bloodless as death.
My parched skin dries, stiff tendons stand out on it,
And claw-like hands now scratch my itching limbs.
Once smiling eyes now weep with endless tears,
Both night and day deplore their punishment,
And where neat eyebrows brought together lashes
Now a rough forest overhangs and covers
As though the eyes were stowed in some dark cavern:
What fierce and frightful thing they see I know not.
To gaze at an old man now brings fear, nor can you
Believe that he's a man, who lacks man's reason.
If I read books, the letters split in two,
The page I knew seems larger than it was.
I seem to see a bright light through the clouds;
The clouds themselves are bright within my eyes.
Daylight is gone though I still live; who will
Deny that hell is fenced with opaque darkness?
What madman has convinced him to believe
Such things, to wish it worse than he had prayed for?

Now come his ills, a thousand perils come,
And now sweet banquets and delights grow harmful.
We must abandon everything that pleases;
That we may live, we are deprived of living.
I whom no raw or adverse foods had troubled,
See how a regimented diet burdens!
I liked big meals; soon I'll regret I ate them.
It's better to abstain; abstention grieves me.
That which was good for me now is forbidden.
My pampered taste is gone that once delighted.
The gifts of love and wine are now unpleasant,
Whatever once beguiled life's humdrum course.
Dejected nature abides, which hour by hour
Dwindles and dribbles away with its own weakness.
No medicines avail though I often take them,
Nor anything which once could soothe my cares.
Thus with my food I lose whatever's served:
The bladder grows tighter with each loss of urine.
Just as one wishes to prop the tottering ruin
And tries to throw up some supporting timbers
Right then long time destroys our careful efforts,
Brings down the building with the props we fashioned.
Why do not public spectacles relieve me
Nor can disguise so many ills of life?
Shameful to the old are shining faces and garments,
To live without them now is shameful to the old.
It's a sin to love jests, dinner parties, and song.
O wretches, for whom joys are held a sin!
What's wealth to me if you remove its uses?
However rich, shall I be always poor?
No, it's a sin to depend upon my riches,
Which once you have it's wrong to dissipate.
Not otherwise did Tantalus thirst after
The nearby waves, restrained from offered foods.
I am become the guardian of my wealth
To keep for others what is lost to me
Just as the dragon in the gold-leaved garden
Watchfully guards the apples not his own.
Thus cares concerned with everything torment me,
Thus no repose is given to my soul.
I who can't pile up wealth strive to retain it,
Yet feel that while I keep it I've kept none.

Trembling, doubtful, the old man is expectant
Of ill, dreads foolishly his every act.
He praises the past, despises the present years,
Thinks only that is right wherein he's wise,
That only he is learned, he is skilled,
And, because he's wise, he grows more foolish still.
He talks much, though you hate it, and repeats it,
Then trembles and abandons what he said.
His listener's gone but he keeps right on talking:
Brave oldsters, brave in babbling alone!
He fills the air with clamoring in vain:
Nothing's enough; he shrinks from what once pleased him.
He laughs with those who mock him and, applauding
Himself, grows happier in his very shame.
First fruits of death, age flows down in his limbs,
Seeks his extremities by these degrees:
His carriage, color, walk as he goes by,
His shape are not the same as they once were.
His cloak falls down from shoulders hunching over
And what was short now seems to him quite long.
We shrink together, grow wonderfully smaller;
You'd think our very bones have been diminished.
We can't look upward; old age now looks downward
At earth from which it came, soon to return,
Becomes three-footed, four, like little babies,
And creeps in sorrow on the filthy ground.
All things seek whence they rose, seek out their mother,
Go back to nothing, which nothing was before.
Thus leaning on his cane old age decaying
Strikes sluggish earth with his repeated blows
In rhythmic steps that bring a sure applause.
His wrinkled mouth sends forth such words as these:
"Take me, my mother, pity your child that suffers:
Nourish my tired limbs upon your breast.
Children abhor me, my appearance has so changed.
Why keep your offspring looking horrible?
I've nothing to do with life, I've fulfilled its chores:
Restore dead limbs, I pray, to their native soil.
Why torture miserable men with added pain?
No mother's heart can bear such punishment."
This said, he props with cane his tottering legs
And seeks the rough straw of his neglected bed.

When he lies down he looks like death itself.
You see the bones alone of his shrunken body.
The more that I lie down the more I live
By lying down: who'll think my bed life-giving?
The torture's being alive: we burn with sunshine,
The clouds are harmful, cold and air annoy us,
The dewdrops injure, we melt in a little shower,
The gentle days of Spring and Fall afflict us.
Thus itches trouble, thus wracking cough fatigues us.
Sick old age has nothing but complaints.
Do those survive to whom the air itself
And light, by which we're guided, are rendered heavy?
Rest also, which for all is very pleasant,
Sleep flies away, scarce comes back late at night,
Or if it ever honors our tired limbs
Disturbs and horrifies with what strange dreams!
Soft couches are like hard and jagged rocks;
Though thin, the bed clothes press with heavy weight.
I'm forced to rise at midnight in distress
And suffer much lest I should suffer worse.
I'm conquered by an infirm body; whither
I do not wish I'm dragged unhappily.
All inner parts of nature now are loosened,
Need nods its head, both well and ill, no matter.
Bowed age comes forward burdened with its evils
To teach itself to bend beneath their weight.
Thus who would wish to bear these pains much longer,
To die by slow degrees with fading spirit?
Better to die with death than death in life
And bury sense together with one's members.
I don't regret the long year's ruin of all:
It's wrong to say that nature's laws are bad.
Strong bulls grow weak within the course of time,
The handsome horse grows ugly presently.
The lion's anger is checked when its day is done,
The tiger's pace is slowed with harsh old age.
The rock itself is worn with long duration.
There is no work which does not yield to time.
It's better I should thwart events to come
And thus anticipate unhappy days.
Less is the pain to bear sure, sudden ruin
Than fear that which the longer borne is worse.
But who can say what other ills may come?

These too are hard for old men to remember:
Insults, contempt, sharp losses come in turn,
No friends to help in their adversity.
The very boys and girls now think it shameful
To call me master, putting up objections.
They mock my gait, they mock my countenance
And shaking head, which once they feared. Although
I may see nothing, yet I shall look on this.
This pain is heavier for wretched me.
Happy the man who's worthy of calm days
To close a tranquil life with joyful end:
Full harsh it is for the wretched to remember
Good times, but worse their lofty plunge to ruin.

II

Lo, lovely Lycoris too much loved by me,
Our minds, our very lives one and the same,
Though we had lived for many years united,
In loathing has rejected my embrace
And now seeks other younger men and loves.
She calls me ugly and decrepit, old,
Nor wishes to recall joys shared with me
Nor that it's she who made me an old man.
No, rather, she, ungrateful, faithless, feigns
The fault is mine that she despises me.
A while ago when she saw me passing by
She spat these words, then covered up her face:
"I loved this man? This man loved my embrace?
I often kissed him softly? What a horror!"
She gags, spews out our former love like vomit,
Calls down abundant curses on my head.
Look what long age now brings, that some one once
Beloved can be foully treacherous.
Was it not better for me to spend that time
Where no one could despise me, undeserving,
Than, after that which was delight has perished,
To live destroyed by insults I deserve?
There's nothing left of the life we lived; time with it
Has taken all, the final hour drags by.
And yet, though snowy locks surround her brow
And now time stains her with its darkish age-spots,

She still looks stunning, thinks well of herself,
And now disdains the years she spent with me.
I will admit she keeps her youthful figure
And hidden flames remain beneath the ash.
Even you, the years, I see, spare something lovely,
All grace of former beauty does not die.
Young men feed on remains of bygone loves;
Whatever the present, the past does not displease.
They set before their eyes their earlier actions
And nourish imagination on vanished deeds.
And since all use of limbs deserts me now
I have no one's embrace which I can cherish;
But grief alone remains for wretched folk.
As many joys I had, their loss I weep for.
No one suffers all things, not all are able
To do all: conquered, the woman wins, man loses.
As with the herds, the present alone abides;
Will nothing remain of the past which we'll remember?
When brute beasts shun the fields new to them
And swift-paced flocks seek pastures they have known,
The bull lies down beneath the shade he loves,
And the lost sheep go back into their fold,
The nightingale sings best in her familiar thicket,
And their own lair is sweet to wild animals,
Do you desert what is well known and proven
For lodgings with which you are not acquainted?
Is it not better to trust what's sure and certain?
Novelty always brings some strange results.
I'm aged, but your hair's as white as mine:
Our equal age brings harmony of soul.
If now I cannot, remember, once I could:
Suffice it to please you that I pleased before.
Old reverence still remains for worn-out farmers,
The soldier loves what he saw in the veteran,
The rustic weeps for the bullock which has served him,
The rider honors the horse with whom he aged.
Time has not spoiled me so of my earlier blooming:
Look, I make verses and sing sweet ditties for you.
Let gravity and age be reverenced by you,
Wish me long life because you knew me once.
Who damns his own life in reproaching others

And strives to close their path when they keep going?
If you disdain to call me friend or brother,
Then call me father: the word bears the love of both.
Let pride yield to honor, let mercy yield to love.
Reason and not blind force will ever prevail.
We have bemoaned long years as much as is proper:
It's hard to keep on remembering our sorrow.

III

Now it is worth our while to mention youth
And speak but little of my own old age,
To clear the reader's mind of unnerving thoughts
And make him care to learn my woeful tale.
Madly in love with you, Aquilina, I fell,
Pale and sad but madly in love with you.
What love could be, or Venus's fire, I knew not:
I suffered rather in shy rusticity.
No less smitten by the same desire
She wandered; her whole house could not contain her.
Songs, tasks she loved so much all lay abandoned,
Nothing but love was her heart's constant care.
She found no way to feed her hidden passion,
No studied words to let me know her plight.
Her bootless zeal brought her only the sight of me,
Fostered her anxious heart with that sole light.
My tutor held me, the sternest of all mothers
Kept guard on her, one evil piled on evil.
They watched our eyes, our nods, our very blushes
Designed to reveal the secrets of our hearts.
While we could we suppressed our love in silence
And wove with varied art sweet stratagems.
But after our shyness burst its tender cover
Nor could conceal the flame that burned within,
We soon began to seize both time and place,
To speak with lifted eyebrows, with our eyes,
Outwit our guards, to place our footsteps softly
And prowl all night without a single sound.
It was not long before her mother sensed
Our secret love and fought our fire with fire.
She scolds and beats: flames flourish with her blows

As fire usually grows when fuel is added.
Our blazing hearts spring up with redoubled ardor,
And thus heartache is mingled with raging love.
Panting with passion, she seeks me; she believes
That she has bought me through her sufferings,
Proud to say so, to strip back her torn gown.
No, even rejoicing, she credits me with this:
"For you," she cries, "I'm happy to bear my beatings:
You're the sweet price I pay for so much blood.
Let only your faith be sure and your will unshaken:
Suffering which brings no loss deserves not the name."
I writhed to feel these goads and still in love
I languished, no salvation's hope I had.
Not daring to speak, I nursed my wound in silence,
But, numb and weak, distress had need of voice.
"Bring me your merciful aid, Boethius, lone
Investigator of the universe.
For though you see me often absorbed with cares
You cannot know the causes of my grief.
At last perceiving the plague from which I suffer,
Bid the closed doors to open with gentle words."
"Tell me: whence comes this sudden wasting fever?
Tell me: you'll be relieved if I know its name.
There is no cure for an ill undiagnosed,
The hollow furnace roars when its fire's enclosed."
While shyness is loth to speak, to admit its guilt,
He recognizes the signs of my hidden ill,
Then says: "An ill revealed shows its hidden cause.
Be brave: so great a suffering will earn you pardon."
Prostrate at his feet, I broke shamefast silence
And told him all in order while I wept.
"Tell me," he said, "can you win the girl with presents?"
"My sense of duty shuns this," I replied.
Dissolved in laughter, he shouted: "What stiff resistance!
Tell me when Venus's love was ever chaste?
Cease to have pity on her the boys all love.
Here you will sin if you wish to be so sinless.
Loves are nourished by tender bites and scratches,
Something adapted to blows does not flee from wounds."
Meanwhile he softens with gifts the hearts of her parents
And draws them to me quite easily, for a price.

Blind love of gold now conquers their love for her:
Her parents began to favor their daughter's sin,
To permit clandestine trysts, to join our right hands,
To celebrate all day with us in sport.
What they allowed grew dull, love's ardor died:
Cool hearts survived the sickness they had suffered.
She, seeing that I had ceased to press my cause,
Turned love to hate and, still a virgin, left me.
I cast off empty cares, my heart was cured;
I suddenly learned how wretched I had been:
"Hail, holy virginity, always abide intact;
Because of me you'll be completely chaste."
After the news was brought to that great man
He saw I had escaped from passion's waves,
"Flourish," he said, "young man, you've mastered your love;
Take up the trophies of war from those you've defeated.
Let the weapons of Venus, the bow of Cupid, yield,
And let Minerva, mighty in warfare, yield."
The power to sin thus permitted removed my desire
To sin, and the very wish to do so was gone.
Sullen, displeased, we parted from one another;
The reason for parting: a chaste and virtuous life.

IV

It remains to tell you of other embarrassing ventures
And to nourish the heart with a story to make you laugh.
For a listless chagrin accompanies silly old age
While an idle song is what I have need of now.
Thus we're beguiled by the varying seasons of years
And changing the time (and the place) is pleasant to me.
There was a girl whose candid appearance had given
The name of Candida, comely in various ways.
I saw her playing the cymbals that hung from her body,
Giving out manifold sounds when she clanged the brass.
Now with her snowy fingers, now with the pick
She struck up the chords and uttered a dulcet tune.
Thus pulled in different directions by a beautiful girl
She plucked me for her enjoyment in various ways.
Suddenly charmed by her dancing I fell in love
And began to suffer in silence my pleasing wounds.

Her separate features once seen it was joy to remember,
They clung to my fevered spirit both night and day.
Often as though I had seen her my mind rejoiced
Although I was far away from her voice and hand.
Often, as if she were present, I talked to myself,
I sang the sweet songs which she was accustomed to sing.
How often insane, how often they thought me mad.
Nor were they mistaken, I think; I was not quite sane.
Some one would say, who well knew my blinding passion:
"He's singing, he is; Maximian loves a singer."
It's certainly hard to conceal the fever of love:
Often the fury's revealed though one's lips are sealed.
For suddenly pallor and blush stain a countenance
And require that one keep a close check upon his voice.
No less did my sleep betray my innermost cares;
The dreams were faithless to which I entrusted my secret,
For when sleep's forgetfulness pressed down on drowsy sense
My tongue, all unknowing, confessed its sinful deeds.
"Candida," I cried out, "hurry: why do you linger?
Candida, night goes by; dawn, hostile to lovers,
Returns." As the father of my beloved was lying
By chance nearby on the grassy ground with his friends,
Troubled, he shook his frame as he heard her name,
Jumped up, believing his daughter was present there.
Looking all round he spies me breathing the deep
Sleep of exhaustion, forgetting to close my lips.
"Are the light illusions of sleep true dreams or false?
It seems to me that he's stirred by true love," he said.
"At least I believe that familiar forms can return
To the mind; a deceitful image tricks his desire."
He stands there astonished and tries to seize my strange murmurs
And asks in his silent prayers that I utter more words.
Thus I who was held by all in respect before
Am betrayed, and made miserable because of my fault:
And now I'm unhappy because my whole life's without loving,
And I am ashamed as an old man unable to sin.
My vices desert me, indignant pleasure flees,
Now that which I cannot do I wish I had done.
This also I may recall, that a later age
Gives me the same sorrows it brought me in happier times.
But who can explain such a quirk of nature which causes
A noble and wise man to wish what is harmful to him?

Sometimes we are seized by our vices and willingly dragged,
And stupid souls wish for that which they cannot retain.

V

Sent to the East, with my mission as legate accomplished,
To fashion a pact of peace that brings quiet to all,
While I tried to prepare a treaty between two kingdoms
I fell upon battles abominable to my heart.
Here, taking me up as an offspring of Tuscan race,
A Greek girl ensnared me with all of her native wiles.
For although she pretended that *she* had fallen in love,
She made me rather to fall in love with her.
Awake through the night she stood at my windowsill
Singing so sweetly some kind of a song in Greek.
Now there were tears and groans and sighs and a pallor
And anything you might suppose that she could not feign.
Thus as I pitied too much the afflicted lover
I became rather the one to be pitied instead.
She was an outstanding beauty with modest face,
With sparkling eyes, and pleasing no less with her skill;
She was trained to speak with her fingers, to improvise songs,
Playing the lyre meanwhile with its answering sounds.
In my stupor I likened her tunes to the Siren songs
And in my madness became another Ulysses.
And I who could not avoid great rocks in the ocean
Was borne in my ignorance onto the cliffs and shoals.
Who can describe her steps as they moved in rhythm,
Lifting her feet to dance with renewed applause?
A thrill it was counting her curls as they shook with her motion,
And it was a thrill to see her dark hair on white skin.
Her nipples stood firmly forth, bewildering our eyes,
While her breasts you could squeeze in the hollow of your hand.
Ah, how her writhing loins stirred the spectator's lust
And the round plump thighs that joined her stomach beneath!
I was afraid to press hard on her tender limbs:
Her bones seemed to crack as I clasped her in my embrace.
"Your arms are big," she cried, "they hurt me extremely:
My legs under yours do not bear the weight of your body."
My erection subsided, my passion for her grew cold
And this is the mishap that makes me ashamed of my member.
No mingled coagulants give forth a milk so hardened

Nor will any watery spume become love's sweet liquid.
I fell for her, I admit, ignorant of Greek guile,
I fell like the simpleton Tuscan old man I was.
When Troy was defeated though Hector himself was defending,
Could not her tricks overcome a single old fool?
I abandoned my zeal for the task with which I was entrusted
Now wholly subject to your commands, fierce Cupid.
Nor am I ashamed to describe the wound which I suffered;
Great Jove himself was subject to flames like these.
The first night with her was at hand, I discharged my function;
My performance was almost too strenuous for an old man.
The next night my powers forsook me, my unfulfilled ardor
Departed, and I was as sluggish for love as before.
Angered, she kept on demanding the tribute I owed her,
Urging and scolding: "Pay up your debt!" she cried.
But neither her clamor nor gentle coaxing availed:
What nature denies that nobody else can supply.
I blushed in embarrassment. Shame robbed me of my will
And terror itself left me paralyzed for the sweet task.
Then she began to stroke with her hand my limp member
And to tickle me with her fingers seductively.
Her touching did nothing to rouse up my torpid fire:
Coldness persisted in the midst of the flame as before.
"What cruel female has snatched you away from me?
Exhausted from whose embrace do you come to my arms?"
She cried. But I swore my mind was consumed with worries
Which kept me from turning my harassed heart toward sex.
Suspecting a trick, she said: "You don't fool this lover:
A love that is sure of itself has a thousand eyes.
Come, get it up, don't abandon our jolly game;
Cast off your cares and return to the joy we were sharing.
Of course the weight of your worries is dulling your senses:
Shifting the load now and then makes the burden less."
Then completely naked and sprawled all over the bed
I shed hot tears and spoke as follows to her:
"Alas, we old men must admit our shame and our fault
Lest you should think the fires of love have died.
Poor wretch that I am! My will power isn't to blame!
I'm cleared of that charge by the witness of infirmity.
Look, I surrender my worn out weapons to you;
Dull with their rust, I commit them to your kind care.
Do what you will, I'm defeated. The enemy's stronger

Just because my ardor has cooled, my forces are weak.''
At once the wanton began to exercise her lively arts
And desired me then to revive myself at her flames.
But when she perceived my beloved member had perished
Nor saw it perk up as though its load had been lifted
She raised a lament, scratched and torn on her widowed bed,
Soothing my grief and its damages with these words:
''Pecker, the busy provider of festive days,
Once the delight of my heart and a treasure to me,
What dirge can I moan for you, drowned in your tears,
What songs shall I sing you worthy of such great merits?
You were accustomed to please me when I was horny
And to divert my passion with fun and games.
You were my fondest guardian throughout the night,
The dear companion of sadness as well as joy.
You were the most faithful confidant of my secrets,
Standing at guard with indulgent intimacy;
Where has your fervor gone, which would strike and please me?
Where is its crested and wound-producing head?
You're certainly limp, no longer suffused with a blush,
Pale, with your head held low, you're certainly limp.
My blandishments, charming songs do nothing for you
Nor anything which could coax your passion avails.
Here I shall weep for you just as if you were dead:
Yes, it is dead because it lacked careful attention.''
As she was tearfully singing with subdued voice
I burst into laughter and uttered the following words:
''While you deplore, dear woman, my languorous member,
You reveal that you're troubled with malady worse than mine.''
She, in a fury: ''You're wrong, you traitor, dead wrong!
I'm not lamenting a private, but general chaos.
This member creates the race of humans, the herds,
The birds, the beasts, whatever breathes in this world.
Without it there is no coming-together of sexes,
Without it, the consummate joy of marriage is gone.
This it is draws two minds to a single agreement
In order to transform into one body two souls.
With its loss a beautiful woman loses her beauty
And if he has lost it a man turns ugly as well.
If this sparkling seed is not sown in a shining soil
It becomes but another deceptive and deadly weed.
Pure trustfulness, well-kept secrets whisper to you,

O truly our bountiful, beautiful, fruit-bearing blessing!
You are very happy, I say, suited for the happy,
Lo, take and use the delights that are kindred to us!
All things yield to you, whatever's more lofty, at will,
The mightiest scepters yield to your sweet commands,
They do not lament their subjection, they rejoice at your sway:
The wounds of your anger are rather propitious wounds.
Wisdom herself who guides the entire world
Stretches out at your bidding her hands once invincible.
The virgin lies stricken in bed with your wished-for wound
And joyfully lies in a pool of freshly shed blood.
Lacerated, she bears it in silence and smiles at her pain,
And, a friend to him who has served her, she even applauds.
It is not fitting to be always limp, soft for action;
Bold deeds are mingled among the games that you play.
Now you use cunning, now an exceptional force,
And thus you are able to bear both your toil and its pains.
For wakeful hardships are often destined for you,
Storms, ambuscades, harsh scoldings, losses, and shipwreck.
You frequently soften the hearts of terrible tyrants,
And bloody Mars becomes meek as well for your sake.
And after he conquered the Giants and thoroughly smashed them
You shake off the trident from the grasp of angry Jove.
You force the raging tigers to a mutual affection,
By you the lion is rendered both gentle and tame.
Your virtue is marvellous, so is your patience: the conquered
You love, and you often love to be conquered yourself.
When overcome you lie low you resume strength and vigor,
And once again you defeat and then are defeated.
Your anger is brief, your pity is great, joy recurring,
And whenever your power is lost your purpose remains.''
She fell silent at last, surfeited with her long sorrow:
She left me as though the last rites of death were accomplished.

VI

Cut off, I pray, your wretched complaints, wordy age.
Will you not cease to reveal this failing of yours?
Let it suffice to have touched upon shamefulness lightly:
Reproaches too long drawn out bring their own reproach.
The road to death is the same for all, but the manner

Of exit from life is not the same one for all.
This road is trodden by boys, young men, and the aged,
This way will be equal for rich men as well as poor.
Therefore on the trodden path no one can avoid
It's better to travel with footstep that hurries along.
Unhappy as though from a funeral I arise:
Although my member is dead I shall live in my art.

A Bibliography on Gabriele Zerbi

Bacon, Roger, *Libellus Rogerii Baconi . . . de retardandis senectutis accidentibus et de sensibus conservandis . . . ;* London: Joseph Barnes, 1590; Short title catalogue no. 1181.

Bacon, Francis, *Instaurationis Magnae Pars Tertia: Historia Vitae et Mortis;* London, 1623.

Baffoni, A., "Un precursore dei moderni geriatri: G. Z."; *Studia Humana,* Ser. 2, Vol. 2 (1950):119–25.

Bandtlow, F. W. O., *Die Schrift des Gabriel de Zerbis: de cautela medicorum;* Leipzig: Inaugural Dissertation, Zeulenrode i. Thür., 1925.

Cornaro, Luigi, *Discourses on a sober and temperate life . . . wherein is demonstrated, by his own example, the method of preserving health to extreme old age.* By Lewis Cornaro. Translated from the Italian original. A new edition, corrected, London, Printed for Benjamin White, 1779.

———, *The immortal mentor; or Man's Unerring guide to a healthy, wealthy and happy life.* By Lewis Cornaro. In three parts by L. C., Dr. Franklin, and Dr. Scott; Mill-Hill, near Trenton, published by Daniel Fenton, Philadelphia. Printed by Brown and Merritt, 1810.

———, *The art of living long; a new and improved English version of the treatise by the celebrated Venetian centenarian Louis Cornaro,* with essays by Joseph Addison, Lord Bacon, and Sir William Temple; Milwaukee, Wis.: W. P. Butler, 1905.

———, *How to Live One Hundred Years;* Girard, Kansas: Haldeman-Julius Publishing Co. (Little Blue Book No. 93).

Crummer, L., translation of Zerbi's *Anatomia Infantis; American Journal of Obstetrics and Gynecology,* 13 (1927).

Dall' Osso, E., "Gabriele Zerbi visto attraverso le pungenti postille di Berengario da Carpi"; *Pagine Stor. Med.* 1, 4 (1957):12–23.

Dunglison, Robley, *A Dictionary of Medical Science;* second ed., Philadelphia: Blanchard and Lea, 1860; 21st ed., 1893.

Flenker, Hellmut, "Die 'Gerentocomia' des Gabriele Zerbi"; Dissertation in Medical History, Kiel, 1965.

Freeman, Joseph T., *Aging, Its History and Literature;* New York: Human Sciences Press, 1979.

Galen, *Opera Omnia,* ed. C. G. Kühn; Vols. 1–20; Leipzig: C. Cnobloch, 1821–33 (reprinted).

Lind, L. R., *Studies in Pre-Vesalian Anatomy: Biography, Translations, Documents;* Philadelphia: The American Philosophical Society, *Memoirs* No. 104, 1975.

Mancini, Clodomiro, "Un codice deontologico del secolo XV (Il 'De cautelis medicorum' di Gabriel de Zerbi)"; *Scientia Veterum: Collana di Studi di Storia dellu Medicina diretta e curata da G. Del Guerra,* No. 44; Pisa: Casa Editrice Giardini, 1963.

Marini, Gaetano, *Degli archiatri pontifici,* 2 vols.; Rome: Pagliarini, 1784.

Münster, Ladislao, "Studi e ricerche su Gabriele Zerbi: Nota I. Nuovi contributi biografici: la sua figura"; *Rivista di storia delle scienze mediche e naturali* 41 (1930):64–83.

———, "Il primo trattato pratico compiuto sui problemi della vecchiaia: la 'Gerontocomia' di Gabriele Zerbi"; *Rivista di Gerontologia e Geriatria,* 1 (1951):38–54.

———, "Il tema di deontologia medica: Il 'De cautelis medicorum' di Gabriele Zerbi"; *Rivista di storia delle scienze mediche e naturali,* 47 (1956):60–83.

Nascher, I. L., *Geriatrics: the Diseases of Old Age and Their Treatment, Including Physiologic Old Age, Home and Institutional Care and Medico-legal Relations,* with an introduction by A. Jacobi; Philadelphia: Blakiston, 1914; second ed., 1916.

Putti, Vittorio, Berengario da Carpi: *Saggio biografico e bibliografico seguito dalla traduzione del "De fractura calvae sive cranei";* Bologna: L. Cappelli, 1937.

Richardson, Bessie Ellen, *Old Age Among the Ancient Greeks; the Greek Portrayal of Old Age in Literature, Art, and Inscriptions, With a Study of the Duration of Life Among the Ancient Greeks on the Basis of Inscriptional Evidence;* New York: AMS Press, 1969 (a reprint of the 1933 edition, The Johns Hopkins University Press); bibliography, pp. 363–72.

Riesco, José, "Gabriel de Zerbis, Medico y filosofo Humanista"; *Giornale di Metafisica,* 19 (1964):90–97.

Sanuto, Marino, *I diarii;* Venezia: a spese degli editori, pubblicato per cura di G. Berchet, 1879.

Sarton, George, *Introduction to the History of Science;* 3 vols. in 5; Baltimore: Williams and Wilkins, 1927–48.

———, *Appreciation of Ancient and Medieval Science During the Renaissance* (1450–1600); New York: A. S. Barnes, 1961.

Shock, Nathan W., *A Classified Bibliography of Gerontology and Geriatrics;* Stanford University Press, 1951.

Tacuinum Sanitatis, *The Medieval Health Handbook,* ed. Luisa Cogliati Arano; New York: George Braziller, 1976.

Thewlis, Malford W., *Geriatrics: A Treatise on Senile Conditions, Diseases of Advanced Life, and Care of the Aged;* with introductions by A. Jacobi, M. D., LL. D., and I. L. Nascher, M. D.; St. Louis: C. V. Mosby, 1919.

Tiraboschi, Girolamo, *Storia della letteratura italiana,* etc., VI (Milano, 1824):685–90.

Valerianus, Joannes Pierius, *De litteratorum infelicitate libri duo;* Venice: Jacob Sarzina, 1620; new edition by Egerton Brydges, Geneva: Typis Gal. Fick, 1821.

Villanova, Arnaldo da, *The Conservation of Youth and Defense of Age;* Woodstock, Vermont: The Elm Tree Press, 1912.

Zeman, F. D., " 'Gerontocomia' of Gabriele Zerbi: Fifteenth Century Manual of Hygiene for the Aged"; *Journal of Mt. Sinai Hospital,* 10 (1944):710–15.

———, "Life's Later Years: Studies in the Medical History of Old Age." Pt. 8. "Revival of Learning"; *Journal of Mt. Sinai Hospital,* 12 (1945):833–46.

On the six non-naturals, see L. J. Rather, "The Six Things Non-natural: A Note on the Origin and Fate of a Doctrine and a Phrase," *Clio Medica,* 3 (1968):337–47; Saul Jarcho, "Galen's Six Non-Naturals: A Bibliographic Note and Translation," *Bulletin of the History of Medicine,* 44 (1970):370–77; Peter Niebyl, "The Non-Naturals," ibid., 45 (1971):486–92; Jerome J. Bylebyl, "Galen on the Non-Natural Causes of Variation in the Pulse," ibid.: 482–85. See also the opening lines of the *Tacuinum Sanitatis,* ed. Luisa Cogliati Arano; New York: George Braziller, 1976.

A Bibliography on Maximianus

EDITIONS

Maximiani philosophi atque oratoris clarissimi ethica suavia et periocunda; Utrecht, 1473.

Maximiani Libellus Nugarum; Paris, 1500.

Corneli Galli Fragmenta, ed. Pomponio Gaurico; Venice, 1501.

Wernsdorf, Jo. Christianus, *Poetae Latini Maiores,* VI, pars 1; Altenburg, 1780–84.

Baehrens, Emil, *Poetae Latini Minores,* V: 313–48; Leipzig: Teubner, 1879–86.

Petschenig, M., ed., *Maximiani Elegiae;* Berliner Studien für Classische Philologie und Archaeologie, XI: 2; Berlin: S. Calvary und Co., 1890.

Webster, Richard, ed., *The Elegies of Maximianus;* Princeton: Princeton University Press, 1900.

Prada, G., ed., *Maximiani Elegiae;* Abbiategrasso: De Angeli, 1919.

Agozzino, T. di, ed., *Elegie;* Bologna: Silva, 1970.

BOOKS AND ARTICLES

Alfonsi, L., "Sulle elegie di Massimiano"; *Atti dell' Reale Istituto Veneto di Scienze, Lettere,* ed. Arti 101 (1941/42):333–49; 102 (1943):723; see Aevum, 1942, 86–92.

Anastasi, Rosario, "Boezio e Massimiano"; *Miscellanea di Studi di Letteratura Antica* 2 (1948):1–20.

———, "La IIe elegia di Massimiano"; *Miscellanea di Studi di Letteratura Christiana;* Catania, 1951.

Ashton-Gwatkin, Frank, Max: *Poet of the Final Hour being the Elegies of Maximianus the Etruscan;* London: Paul Norbury Publications, 1975.

Boano, G., "Massimiano e le sue elegie"; *Rivista di Filologia Classica* 27 (1949):198–216.

Boas, M., "De librorum Catonianarum historia atque compositione"; *Mnemosyne* 42 (1914):17 ff.

Bröring, Julius, *Quaestiones Maximianeae;* Münster, 1893.

Coffman, George R., "Old Age from Horace to Chaucer. Some Literary Affinities and Adventures of an Idea"; *Speculum* 9 (1934):249–77.

Curtius, E. R., *European Literature and the Latin Middle Ages,* translated by Willard Trask; London: Routledge and Kegan Paul, 1953, pp. 50, 58, 113, 290.

Dapunt, A., *Der Elegiker Maximianus;* Diss. Innsbruck, 1949.

Ellis, Robinson, "On the Elegies of Maximianus"; *American Journal of Philology* 5, 1 (1884):1–15 (I); 5, 2 (1884):145–63 (II).

Hartung, A. E., "The Non-comic Merchant's Tale, Maximianus and the Sources"; *Mediaeval Studies* 39 (1967):1–25 (Toronto).

Hunt, J., "Adnotatiuncula in Maximianum"; *La Parola del Passato* 33(1978):59–60 (on *Elegy* IV, 39).

Kittredge, G. L., "Chaucer and Maximian"; *American Journal of Philology* 9 (1888):85–86 (The Pardoner's Tale).

Lekusch, V., "Zur Verstechnik des Elegikers Maximian"; *Serta Harteliana,* Wien. 1896, 257–62.

Lemaire, M., *Poetae Latini Minores,* VII; Paris: Didot, 1826.

Lind, L. R., *Latin Poetry in Verse Translation from the Beginnings to the Renaissance;* Boston: Houghton Mifflin Co., 1957.

Lindsay, Jack, *Songs of a Falling World,* etc.; London: A. Dakers, 1948.

Lutz, Cora E., "A Medieval Textbook"; *Yale University Library Gazette* 49 (1974):212–16; a discussion of MS 513 in the Beinecke Library, containing Maximianus, Theodulus, and Avianus, commonly read in twelfth- and thirteenth-century curricula.

Manitius, M., "Über den Dichter Maximian"; *Rheinisches Museum* 44 (1889):540–543.

———, *Geschichte der lateinischen Literatur des Mittelalters,* III; München: C. M. Beck, 1931.

Merone, E., "Per la biografia di Massimiano"; *Giornale Italiano di Filologia* 1 (1948):337–52.

———, "Maximeana"; ibid., 3 (1950):322–36.

Moricca, U., "Di un nuovo codice delle Elegie di Massimiano"; *Athenaeum,* 1918, 135–42.

Neuburger, Max, "The Latin Poet Maximianus on the Miseries of Old Age"; *Bulletin of the History of Medicine* 21 (1947):113–19.

Nizard, P., *Collection des Auteurs Latins;* Paris: Garnier frères, 1850 (prose translation).

Prada, G., *Quae inter metri dactyli disciplinam et sermonem latinum in Maximiano poeta exsistunt quaestiones;* Ticini: Mattei, 1914.

———, *Sul valore e la parentela dei codici di Massimiano;* ibid., 1918.

———, *Lamenti e Guai d'un Vecchio;* Abbiategrasso, 1919.

Puget, L., *Collection des Auteurs Latins—Oeuvres complètes d'Horace . . .* publiées sous la direction de Nizard; Paris: Didot, 1903, p. 610.

Raby, F. J. E., *A History of Secular Latin Poetry in the Middle Ages* I, sec. ed.; Oxford at the Clarendon Press, 1957.

Riché, Pierre, *Éducation et Culture dans l'Occident Barbare 6e–8e Siècles;* Paris: Editions du Seuil, 1967; pp. 68, 128.

Schanz, M., *Geschichte der röm. Lit.*, IV, 2 (1920):76–78.

Schuetter, W., "Neues zur Appendix des Elegien des Maximianus"; *Philologus* 104 (1960):116–26.

———, *Studien zur Überlieferung und Kritik des Elegikers Maximian;* Wiesbaden: Herter und Schmid, 1970.

Spaltenstein, F., "Structure et intentions du recueil poetique de Maximien"; *Études de Lettres, Bulletin de la Faculté des Lettres de l'Univ. de Lausanne et de la Société des Études de Lettres* 10, 2 (1977):81–101.

Strazzulla, V., *Massimiano etrusco elegiografo;* Catania, 1893.

Szöverffy, J., "Maximianus a Satirist?"; *Harvard Studies in Classical Philology* 72 (1967/68):351–67.

Traube, L., "Zur Überlieferung der Elegien des Maximianus"; *Rheinisches Museum* 48 (1893):284–89.

Vogel, Fr., "Maximianus der Lyriker"; *Rheinisches Museum* 41 (1886):158–59.

Waddell, Helen, *The Wandering Scholars;* London: Constable; New York: Barnes and Noble, 1966.

Walker, Hoveden, *The Impotent Lover accurately described in six elegies upon Old Age, with the old doting lecher's resentments on the past pleasures and vigorous performances of youth;* London: Peacock and Bible, B. Croyle, 1688, 1689 (two editions).

Wilhelm, Friedrich, "Maximianus und Boethius"; *Rheinisches Museum* 62 (1907):601–14.

I have followed the edition by Petschenig in making my translation.

Index